"Our diets have a significant impact on our brain health and overall well-being. But in today's world, there is so much confusion about what we should actually be eating. *Food* by Mark Hyman, MD, helps consumers cut through all of the nutrition confusion and provides a road map for leading a healthier life."

—Maria Shriver, journalist and founder of the Women's Alzheimer's Movement

"Dr. Mark Hyman's new book is the perfect antidote to misconceptions about diet and nutrition. In clear, concise terms, he tells us exactly what foods we should be eating or avoiding in order to win and maintain lifelong wellness. If everyone followed this advice, we could reduce the incidences of preventable disease and lower the cost of health care for everyone."

— Toby Cosgrove, MD, CEO of Cleveland Clinic

"Just about every time someone leaves the doctor's office, they are told to exercise and eat well. Sadly, at this point in our collective human history, there is still not wide consensus on how to do either properly. With nutrition in particular, it feels like near daily whiplash. Yesterday coconut oil seemed a panacea, by tomorrow you may hear it causes heart disease. Dr. Mark Hyman, who has diligently dedicated his life to wellness, has a new book that may offer some much-needed relief. *Food* goes between the lines of nutrition research, providing a clear road map for the confused eater." *—Sanjay Gupta, MD*

"Mark Hyman knows as much about food and our health as any human being alive. His new book, *Food*, is an invaluable guide to what we should eat and, perhaps more importantly, what we shouldn't to get healthy and stay healthy."
— *Gary Taubes, author of* The Case Against Sugar

"Finally, a book that puts common sense and integrity back into the discussion about what to eat — despite decades of being fed a steady diet of nonsense by so-called 'trusted authorities.' Bravo, Dr. Hyman. This book is good medicine." — *Christiane Northrup, MD*

"Food has turned out to be a much more powerful medicine than we were all taught, yet for so many of us, the many different diets available paint a confusing picture. In his new book, Dr. Mark Hyman has provided exactly what we need: an expert analysis, clear-headed description, and effective solution to what the heck we should all be eating to optimize our health and longevity. This may be the most important book you read on this critical topic, and Dr. Hyman is one of the precious few with both the expertise and writing skill to make this information available and digestible."
— *Dale Bredesen, MD, author of* The End of Alzheimer's

"In the diet wars, no battle is more contentious than low-fat vegan versus high-fat paleo. Mark Hyman finds common ground with paleo-vegan ('Pegan'), a plant-based diet supplemented moderately with animal foods (as 'condi-meats'). *Food* offers a delicious recipe for restoring our health, as we care for the planet."
— *David Ludwig, MD, PhD, author of* Always Hungry?

"Food and the way we produce and consume it is at the center of most of our world's health, environmental, climate, economic, and even political crises. With his new book, Mark Hyman, MD, shows us that food is powerful medicine, and it contains information that speaks to our environment and our genes, programming our body with messages of health or illness."   —*Deepak Chopra*

"It has never been easier to harm ourselves with food, and at the same time, it's never been easier to heal ourselves. By the end of *Food,* you feel more empowered than ever and more at ease than ever to create the latter."
     —*Steven R. Gundry, MD, author of* The Plant Paradox

"Most people know that a good diet is the cornerstone of health but are confused about what to eat. Low-carb, low-fat, Paleo, plant-based, raw-food, vegan, or vegetarian diets? In *Food,* Dr. Hyman cuts through this confusion and empowers readers with confidence and clarity about what to eat."
     —*Chris Kresser, MS, LAc, author of* The Paleo Cure

"Nutritional science can be confusing. Dr. Hyman makes it easy to understand and to implement in an effort to empower you to simplify your life."
     —*Dr. Joseph Mercola, founder of Mercola.com,*
     the most-visited natural health site

"Dr. Hyman sets the record straight. Your food decisions will become effortless, and you'll be happier and healthier than ever."
     —*Vani Hari, author of* The Food Babe Way
     and founder of FoodBabe.com

"Good health starts at the end of your fork. With straightforward, thoughtful advice, Dr. Mark Hyman clears up the food confusion and shows you how to eat to heal and nourish your body, while also delighting your taste buds."

—*JJ Virgin, celebrity nutrition and fitness expert and author of* The Virgin Diet

"We have more knowledge about food and more options than ever, and yet people are getting sicker and sicker because of lifestyle diseases. Where did we go wrong? How did we stray so far from real food and get to the point where most people are accustomed to boxed meals loaded with twenty unidentifiable ingredients and others are finding themselves lost in grocery stores, perplexed and bewildered to the point of panic, wondering what the heck they can and should eat? *Food* is the definitive guide for achieving food peace. It will show you that what we eat matters, but it doesn't have to be that complicated. Mark Hyman is a masterful clinician and teacher. Let him show you the healing power of foods and make eating easy, fun, and delicious."

—*Daniel G. Amen, MD, founder of Amen Clinics and author of* Change Your Brain, Change Your Life *and* Memory Rescue

"Dr. Mark Hyman's *Food* offers a masterpiece of truth-telling, a subversive reproach to the industrial systems that threaten our very health—and it explains how each of us can flourish by making better food choices. This could be the most useful book you will read."

—*Daniel Goleman*

"Dr. Hyman has eloquently addressed the most important nutrition question in *Food*. This book is essential for anyone who is looking for answers on how to use food to improve their functional health."

— *Jeffrey Bland, PhD, founder, Institute for Functional Medicine, author of* The Disease Delusion

"What exactly has industrial agriculture done to your food supply and how does it affect your health and your environment? How can you be a conscious consumer when you hit the grocery stores? What is the difference between grass-fed and organic? Does organic matter? And seriously, what the heck should you eat? Mark Hyman, MD, answers all of these important questions in his new book, *Food*. Read it!"

— *Dave Asprey, creator of Bulletproof Coffee and author of* Head Strong

"Food is at the center of our well-being, and how we get our food is directly connected to the health of our planet. But we're drowning in bewildering information and advice about what to eat. In his new book, *Food,* Mark Hyman, MD, breaks down all the science into practical advice about what to eat and what to avoid. This is a manual for how the food we eat can help us thrive."

— *Arianna Huffington, author of* Thrive

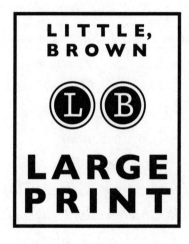

LITTLE,
BROWN

LB

LARGE
PRINT

Books by Mark Hyman, MD

The Eat Fat, Get Thin Cookbook
Eat Fat, Get Thin
The Blood Sugar Solution 10-Day Detox Diet Cookbook
The Blood Sugar Solution 10-Day Detox Diet
The Blood Sugar Solution Cookbook
The Blood Sugar Solution
The Daniel Plan
The Daniel Plan Cookbook
UltraPrevention
UltraMetabolism
The Five Forces of Wellness (CD)
The UltraMetabolism Cookbook
The UltraThyroid Solution
The UltraSimple Diet
The UltraMind Solution
Six Weeks to an UltraMind (CD)
UltraCalm (CD)

FOOD

WHAT THE HECK SHOULD I EAT?

Mark Hyman, MD

LITTLE, BROWN AND COMPANY

LARGE PRINT EDITION

This book is intended to supplement, not replace, the advice of a trained health professional. If you know or suspect that you have a health problem, you should consult a health professional. The author and publisher specifically disclaim any liability, loss, or risk, personal or otherwise, that is incurred as a consequence, directly or indirectly, of the use and application of any of the contents of this book.

Little, Brown and Company
Hachette Book Group
1290 Avenue of the Americas, New York, NY 10104
littlebrown.com

First Edition: February 2018

Little, Brown and Company is a division of Hachette Book Group, Inc. The Little, Brown name and logo are trademarks of Hachette Book Group, Inc.

The publisher is not responsible for websites (or their content) that are not owned by the publisher.

The Hachette Speakers Bureau provides a wide range of authors for speaking events. To find out more, go to hachettespeakersbureau.com or call (866) 376-6591.

ISBN 978-0-316-33886-8 (hardcover) / 978-0-316-43997-8 (large print)
LCCN 2017958899

10 9 8 7 6 5 4 3 2 1

LSC-C

Printed in the United States of America

For all those who have ever wondered,
"What the heck should I eat?"
this book is for you.

Contents

PART III

WHAT ELSE YOU NEED TO KNOW ABOUT FOOD

PART IV

THE PEGAN DIET AND HOW TO EAT FOR LIFE

FOOD

Introduction

My guess is that you picked up this book because food confuses you. Why do I say that? Because I have been studying nutrition for 35 years, and even the experts are confused by the science. If the people we look to for nutritional guidance keep changing their views, it's no wonder that the rest of us are befuddled and mystified.

When you wake up in the morning, do you wonder what you should eat that day? Are you sick of being mixed-up and confounded by conflicting media reports about the latest research on which foods are good or bad for us? One day eggs are unhealthy, and the next day they are a miracle food. One year the government tells us to eat six to eleven servings of carbohydrates (bread, rice, cereal, and pasta) as the foundation of our diet, and the next it tells us to cut carbs. The US Dietary Guidelines told us 35 years ago that all our health problems were derived from eating fat and recommended we eat fat "only sparingly." Then, more than three decades later, they suddenly learned fat wasn't so bad for us. We were just recently told, in the 2015 US Dietary Guidelines, "Uh, don't worry about fat; there is no restriction on how much you can eat because the research shows no connection between obesity or heart disease and dietary fat. And that cholesterol we told you to avoid for fear of dropping dead of a heart attack? Well, we were wrong about that, too, so skip your egg whites and enjoy your whole eggs."

Of course, the $1 trillion food industry provides us with all sorts of "healthy" options: low-fat, high-fiber, whole-grain, gluten-free—most of which are the opposite of healthy. My food rule is if there are health claims on the label, what's inside is probably unhealthy. Multigrain Frosted Flakes, anyone?

All of this is enough to make you give up and just eat whatever you want, whenever you want, and in whatever quantities you want. It feels like nutrition whiplash.

This is the reason I have written this book. I want to help you undo all the beliefs about food that are making you fat and sick and replace them with a new understanding that will lead to health and longevity.

In the landscape of eating, there are many beliefs and dogmas, from vegan, Paleo, vegetarian, Mediterranean, and raw food, to ketogenic, high-fat, low-fat, omnivore. How can they all be right? There are benefits to each of these diets, but an all-in approach to one or another may not be the all-in answer.

Humans are adaptable. For generations we have consumed varied diets native to all sorts of environments from all over the planet, from arid desert landscapes to frozen Arctic tundra. So, should you be eating 80 percent carbs from mesquite, acorns, and wild plants, as the indigenous Pima of Arizona did for thousands of years, or 70 percent fat from whale blubber and seal, as the Inuit of the Arctic have traditionally eaten?

The good news is that science continues to refine and illuminate fundamental principles of good nutrition, and we know now more than ever what a good and healthy diet really looks like. I refer to these basic nutritional principles as the Pegan Diet, mostly as a spoof on the fanaticism of my Paleo and vegan friends, who often get hotheaded and emotional when defending their points of view. It's sort of like the Hatfields and the McCoys.

The sad truth is that much of what we eat is not really food. At least, it has been so adulterated and processed we may as well not call it food. It is more of a food-like substance. And as a result, most of us are confused, baffled, and frustrated, not knowing whom to believe or what to eat.

I've also written *Food* because I believe that cultivating and consuming real, whole food is the answer to many of our world's problems. How we grow it, produce it, and eat it affects almost every aspect of our lives and our society. *Food* is an honest how-to guide designed to answer the question, "What the heck should I eat?"

Now, you might be thinking, *I know what food is.*

It's the stuff you eat to provide fuel for your body so you can live. But it is so much more. It is medicine. It is information. Food literally controls almost every function of your body and mind. And it connects almost everything that matters in our lives. Food connects us to one another and to our bodies; it can reinvigorate our health, bring families together, restore vibrant communities, improve the economy and the environment, reduce pollution, and even help our kids get better grades and avoid eating disorders, obesity, and drug abuse; food can even reduce poverty, violence, homicide, and suicide. Our industrial food system drives many of these problems by enabling a national diet of sugary, starchy, overly processed, nutrient-depleted foods laden with pesticides, herbicides, hormones, antibiotics, and other harmful chemicals.

This book is meant to be a road map, based on the best and latest science of what to eat. What you put on your fork is the most important thing you do every day. It influences your capacity to live a rich, energetic, connected, soulful life — a life in which you have the energy to care for yourself, to love your friends and family, to help your neighbor, to fully show up for your work in the world, and to live your dreams. If you enjoy real, whole, fresh foods that you cook using real ingredients, you are positively affecting everything around you.

Simply put: Food is the doorway to living well and loving well — and to fixing much of what's wrong with our world.

HOW THIS BOOK WORKS

Each chapter in Part II of this book examines a different food group (meat, dairy, grains, vegetables, fruits, etc.) and aims to provide a full view of it, starting from the science and shifting to the experts—what they got right and what they got wrong. Each of these chapters contains a guide for how to integrate environmental and ethical guidelines into your shopping practices, as well as lists of what to eat and what not to eat—because, after all, isn't that what we all really want to know? No part of this book involves deprivation and suffering. I want you to wake up every morning feeling good, enjoying life, and ready to eat great food. I think you'll find that this book is not so much about what you can't eat as it is about what you can—delicious, whole foods full of flavor, texture, and culinary surprises.

In Parts III and IV, I will show you how to use food as medicine to reset your body and to eat in a way that promotes health, and I'll introduce you to simple guidelines and nutritional principles that synthesize the research on food, health, and disease and the environment. These guidelines are flexible and allow for a varied diet that is inclusive, not exclusive.

You will also learn which nutritional supplements are essential for health and healing. According to government data, 90 percent of Americans are deficient in one or more nutrients. In a perfect world, none of us would need supplements; however, given modern-day stressors, the depleted nature of our soil, the fact that our food is transported over long distances and stored for periods of time, and our exposure to an increasing load of environmental toxins, we all need a basic daily supply of vitamins and minerals to tune up our biochemistry.

You may notice that some information appears in more than one chapter. I've repeated certain important facts because they apply to more than one food group, and I know that some readers will skip around the book rather than read from start to finish. Better to say something twice than have you miss it altogether.

Even though this book contains a great deal of scientific information about food, my hope is that it actually empowers you to simplify your life. Cooking and eating become infinitely easier when you leave all the artificial stuff behind and focus on real, whole foods. It's easier to remember what's what. Ask yourself, Did a human being make this or did nature? Nature made an avocado, but not a Twinkie. Any five-year-old would understand that. Now let's bust all those harmful nutritional myths and learn to embrace delicious, yummy foods that you love and that love you back.

PART I

ENDING FOOD CONFUSION, FEAR, AND INSECURITY

The science of nutrition is confusing. But it shouldn't be. There's nothing more natural, or fundamental, in our lives. The miracle we humans have always known is this: Food exists specifically to energize, heal, repair, and uplift us. Every bite you take is a powerful opportunity to create health or promote disease. When I say it's miraculous, I'm talking about *real* food, the kind that comes from the earth and fuels and sustains us, *not* the industrialized, hyperprocessed, hyperpalatable junk that degrades us and makes us sick. Which kind will you allow into your body? The choice is yours to make. Now let's dig into the real story about food, get clear about what the science shows and what it doesn't, and learn how to eat well for life.

Before we dig in, let's start off with a little pop quiz. Answer the following questions based on your current beliefs about food. The answers appear at the end of Part I. Don't cheat!

NUTRITION IQ QUIZ

True or False?

1. Oatmeal is a healthy breakfast.
2. You should avoid egg yolks because they raise your cholesterol and cause heart attacks.
3. Orange juice is a great way to start the day.
4. Red meat is unhealthy and causes cancer and heart disease.
5. The best way to lose weight is to eat a low-fat diet.
6. Gluten-free food is healthy.
7. If you want to lose weight, you should eat less and exercise more.
8. Dairy is nature's perfect food; it is essential for kids to grow and build bones and can prevent fractures.
9. You should avoid butter because it has too much saturated fat and causes heart disease.
10. Vegetable oil is better for you than butter.

My guess is that most of you got most of the answers wrong. I certainly was taught that all these statements were true—and I believed it! But they are not true. Tragically, those myths contribute to our growing burden of obesity and chronic disease. The purpose of this book is to separate fact from fiction, to bust myths and tell the truth about what we know, what we don't, and what we need to eat to thrive.

Starting at a young age, we are all taught that we should "love thy neighbor as thyself." Yet many of us neglect ourselves by eating low-quality industrial food that robs our health, makes us heavy and sluggish, clouds our minds, and dampens our spirits. If we fed our neighbors like most of us feed ourselves, we would all be in big trouble.

Many of us focus primarily on work, hobbies, and friends and tend to ignore our basic needs for good food and regular fitness and deep relaxation and quality sleep. We don't connect the dots between what's on our plate and our mental, physical, emotional, and spiritual well-being. Food is not just calories; it's medicine. And most of us don't realize how quickly our health would bounce back if only we thought of it that way. The question, then, is, How do we eat to create abundance, health, joy, happiness, and energy every day? How do we eat to prevent and even reverse most illnesses?

Chronic disease affects half of all Americans— among the culprits are dementia, autoimmune diseases, heart disease, diabetes, cancer, neurological problems, depression, attention deficit disorder, auto-immune disease, allergies, reflux, irritable bowel, thyroid disorders, hormonal and menstrual problems, and skin problems, including eczema, psoriasis, and acne. The costs are staggering. Medicaid and Medicare are the single biggest drain on our federal budget. Annual spending on health care in 2016 was $3.35 trillion, or $10,345 per person (nearly $1 in $5 of our entire economy). And 80 percent of that goes toward the ongoing treatment of chronic lifestyle diseases that are preventable and reversible.

We all know food can harm — that drinking soda and eating junk food is bad for us. But how many of us believe food can heal? How many of us believe that food can cure depression, diabetes, arthritis, autoimmune disease, headaches, fatigue, and insomnia? That it can prevent and reverse dementia and heart disease or a hundred other common diseases and symptoms?

This is the biggest scientific discovery since the germ theory of disease in the mid-1800s and the development of antibiotics in the 1920s: *Food is medicine.*

Food is the most powerful drug on the planet. It can improve the expression of thousands of genes, balance dozens of hormones, optimize tens of thousands of protein networks, reduce inflammation, and optimize your microbiome (gut flora) with every single bite. It can cure most chronic diseases; it works faster, better, and cheaper than any drug ever discovered; and the only side effects are good ones — prevention, reversal, and even treatment of disease, not to mention vibrant optimal health.

Yet, sadly, doctors learn almost nothing about nutrition in medical school. That is changing, as more and more physicians face the limitations of drugs and surgery when it comes to healing the lifestyle-related diseases that cause so much suffering today. As director of the Cleveland Clinic Center for Functional Medicine and The UltraWellness Center, and chairman of the board of the Institute for Functional Medicine, I am a strong advocate for practitioner education and clinical research to prove that the use of food as medicine is effective at treating chronic disease. I have treated more than 10,000 patients using food as my main "drug," and its benefits far exceed those of any prescription I have written. These cutting-edge centers have created programs that rely on functional medicine. Instead of labeling and treating diseases based on their symptoms, functional medicine addresses the root causes of disease. And when it comes to chronic illnesses, the culprit is nearly always food. Don't get me wrong: We still treat patients holistically using advanced testing, carefully selected combinations of supplements and medications, and other lifestyle tweaks to create balance and healing. But our main "drug" is food. It's that powerful when applied correctly. Functional medicine is the best model we have for addressing our chronic illness epidemic. It is the medicine of *why*, not the medicine of *what*. It is about why you have the disease, not just naming what disease you have. It strives to treat the underlying cause of the disease, rather than merely suppressing its symptoms.

SO, WHAT EXACTLY ARE WE EATING?

Most Americans don't eat food anymore. They eat factory-made, industrially produced food-like substances, or Frankenfoods, that contain trans fats, high-fructose corn syrup, monosodium glutamate (MSG), artificial sweeteners and colors, additives, preservatives, pesticides, antibiotics, new-to-nature proteins, and heightened allergens caused by genetic breeding and engineering. We call these anti-nutrients. If someone were to hand you a plain box of food with only a nutrition label and ingredients list on the outside, you would have a hard time guessing what it is—you couldn't tell if it was a Pop-Tart or a Pizza Stuffer. This should make us all stop and think.

For example—this "food" item has thirty-seven ingredients. Read them and then see if you can guess what it is:

Ingredients: Enriched Bleached Wheat Flour [Flour, Reduced Iron, B Vitamins (Niacin, Thiamine Mononitrate (B1), Riboflavin (B2), Folic Acid)], Corn Syrup, Sugar, High Fructose Corn Syrup, Water, Partially Hydrogenated Vegetable and/or Animal Shortening (Soybean, Cottonseed and/or

Canola Oil, Beef Fat), Whole Eggs, Dextrose. Contains 2% or Less of: Modified Corn Starch, Glucose, Leavenings (Sodium Acid Pyrophosphate, Baking Soda, Monocalcium Phosphate), Sweet Dairy Whey, Soy Protein Isolate, Calcium and Sodium Caseinate, Salt, Mono and Diglycerides, Polysorbate 60, Soy Lecithin, Soy Flour, Cornstarch, Cellulose Gum, Sodium Stearoyl Lactylate, Natural and Artificial Flavors, Sorbic Acid (to Retain Freshness), Yellow 5, Red 40.

Of course you can't tell, because it is not real food. It is a food-like substance. In fact, it is Twinkies.

Should we really be putting this in our bodies?

Now let's look at another example—see if you can guess what this is:

Ingredients: Organic Hearts of Romaine Lettuce

Pretty obvious, right? An avocado doesn't have an ingredients list or a nutrition facts label. Neither does a steak. They are just food.

The food industry has invited itself into our homes and encouraged us to "outsource" our food and cooking. They got us out of the kitchen altogether. We have raised at least two generations of children who don't know how to cook a meal from scratch using real ingredients and who spend more time watching cooking on television than actually cooking. Today's industrial food-like substances have hijacked our taste buds and brain chemistry. Sugar is highly biologically addictive. And not by accident. Food giants have taste institutes, where they hire "craving experts" to identify the "bliss points" of foods to create "heavy users." (These are terms companies use internally to describe what they do.) A top executive at Pepsi told me how excited he was that they had learned how to grow and harvest human taste buds in the lab. It would allow them to easily road test their new products and create even more addictive drinks or junk food. Our industrial food system, sponsored and supported by our government policies, has taken over our bodies, minds, and souls. It's like the invasion of the body snatchers. Most of us have no clue. And worse, most of us blame ourselves for our bad habits, cravings, and weight gain.

Health is the most basic human right and it has been taken from us.

COOKING OUR WAY OUT OF OBESITY AND DISEASE

I have been writing about, lecturing on, and using food as medicine for a long time, and I've seen the health benefits in thousands of my patients. But it wasn't until I participated in the movie *Fed Up* that I took a step back and realized just how bad the epidemic of industrialized food has gotten in our country. The film exposes how the sugar industry drives our obesity epidemic, and I was asked to go to South Carolina to talk to a low-income family about their health. I looked at this family's health crisis, tried to understand the root causes, and worked to help them pull out of their scary downward spiral. Three of the five were morbidly obese, two had pre-diabetes, and the father had type 2 diabetes and kidney failure and was on dialysis. The family survived on disability and food stamps (or SNAP — the Supplemental Nutrition Assistance Program). They were under financial stress and felt hopeless. This vicious cycle of poverty and poor health affects more than 150 million Americans (including tens of millions of children) who are in some way struggling with the physical, social, and financial burden of obesity, chronic disease, and their complications.

And so it was with this family. The mother, father, and sixteen-year-old son were all morbidly obese. The teenager had 47 percent overall body fat, and his belly was 58 percent fat. To provide some perspective, the normal range for total body fat for a man is 10 to 20 percent. He said he was worried he would soon be 100 percent body fat. His insulin levels were sky-high, which drove a relentless cycle of sugar cravings and food addiction, leading to the storage of more and more belly fat. Obese at sixteen, he had a life expectancy thirteen years *shorter* than those of kids with healthy body fat, and he was twice as likely to die by the age of fifty-five as were his healthier friends. His father, at age forty-two, had renal failure from complications of obesity. The whole family was at risk.

They desperately wanted to find a way out but didn't have the knowledge or the skills to escape the hold industrialized food had on them. They blamed themselves, but it was clear they were not at fault. They were victims.

When I asked them what motivated them to want to change, the tears began to flow. The father said he didn't want to die and leave his wife and four sons. His youngest boy was only seven years old. The father needed a kidney transplant to save his life but wouldn't be eligible until he lost forty pounds, and he had no clue how to lose the weight. None of the family members knew how to cook. They didn't know how to navigate a grocery store, shop for real food, or read a label. They had no idea that the frozen chicken nuggets they were buying had 25 different ingredients and only one of them was "chicken." They had been hoodwinked by the "health claims" on the packaged foods that were making them fat and sick—including "low-fat," "diet," "zero trans fats," and "whole-grain." Whole-grain Pop-Tarts? Cool Whip with *zero* trans fats?

Here's a fun little fact about food labels, serving sizes, and marketing: In 2003, the food lobby coerced the Food and Drug Administration (FDA) into allowing food companies to label their products as trans-fat-free *if* the product had less than ½ gram of trans fats *per serving.* So, the makers of Cool Whip can state that it is a trans-fat-free "food" because there is less than ½ gram of trans fats in a 2 tablespoon serving, despite the fact that Cool Whip is *mostly* made up of trans fats. *They can legally lie.* Finally, in 2015, the FDA ruled that trans fats are not safe to eat, or non-GRAS (GRAS is an acronym for generally recognized as safe). But they've given the food industry a long time to get trans fats out of products. So beware. Read ingredients lists and don't eat anything with the word "hydrogenated" on the label.

The parents in this South Carolina family grew up in homes where practically everything they ate was either fried or came from a box or can. They made only two vegetables—boiled cabbage and canned green beans. They didn't have basic cooking tools, such as proper cutting boards to chop vegetables or trim meat. They had some old, dull knives that were hidden in the back of the cupboard and never used. Everything they ate was premade in a factory. They lived on food stamps and disability payments, spending about $1,000 a month on food, half of which went toward dining out at fast-food restaurants—that was their main family activity! They were trapped in a food desert and a cycle of food addiction. The conversation has changed now that science has proven that processed foods—and especially sugar—are addictive. When your brain is hooked on drugs, willpower and personal responsibility don't stand a chance.

But there is a way to break the cycle with real whole food.

THE CURE IS IN THE KITCHEN

I realized that the worst thing I could do to this family was to shame or judge them, prescribe them more medication, or tell them to eat less and exercise more (a subtle way of blaming them). Instead, I wanted to teach them to cook real food from scratch and show them they could eat well on a tight budget and feel satisfied.

When I looked through their fridge that first day, I was surprised to see a bunch of fresh asparagus. The mother explained that she used to hate them. "Once I had asparagus out of a can; it was nasty," she said. "But then a friend told me to try one off the grill, and even though I didn't want to, I tried it and it was good." My theory about vegetables is this: If you hate them, then you most likely never had them prepared properly. They were canned, overcooked, boiled, deep-fried, or otherwise highly processed and tasteless mush. Just think of overcooked Brussels sprouts or tasteless canned peas. The worst!

So we got the whole family washing, peeling, chopping, cutting, touching, and cooking real food—whole foods like carrots, onions, sweet potatoes, cucumbers, tomatoes, salad greens, and even asparagus. I showed them how to peel the garlic, cut the onions, and snap the asparagus to get rid of the chewy ends. I taught them how to sauté the asparagus with garlic in olive oil, how to roast sweet potatoes with fennel and olive oil, and how to make turkey chili from scratch. We all cooked together. The family even made fresh salad dressing from olive oil, vinegar, mustard, salt, and pepper, instead of dousing their greens in the bottled dressings laden with high-fructose corn syrup, refined oils, and MSG that they once favored.

The youngest boys came running into the kitchen, lured away from their gaming consoles by the sweet, warm smells of chili and roasting sweet potatoes, fragrances that had never wafted out of their kitchen before. We all sat down at their table to eat the freshly prepared food, and they were surprised at how delicious and filling it was.

After a happy, healing meal of real food, cooked in less time and for less money than it would have taken them to drive to Denny's and order deep-fried chicken nuggets, biscuits, gravy, and canned green beans, the nearly "superobese" son turned to me in disbelief and asked, "Dr. Hyman, do you eat real food like this with your family *every night*?" I said, "Yes, we do." This child had been struggling with getting healthy, hoped to go to medical school, and wanted to help his family. I think it became clear that if this family were to simply choose real food, cooked at home—even on a budget—they would be on the right path to achieving these dreams and so much more.

When it came time to head home, I left amid tears of relief and of hope for a different future for this family. I gave them my *Blood Sugar Solution Cookbook* and a pocket guide called *Good Food on a Tight Budget* from an organization I work with called the Environmental Working Group. Five days after I left, the mother texted me to say that the family had already lost eighteen pounds collectively, and they were making turkey chili again. When I checked in nine months later, the family had lost 200 pounds collectively. The mother had lost one hundred pounds. The father had lost forty-five and was able to get a new kidney. The son had lost fifty pounds but had gone to work at a fast-food place and gained it back. However, he is back on track — and he went from a high of 338 pounds to 210 pounds — a 128-pound weight loss. And now he is applying to medical school!

If a family living in one of the worst food deserts in America and surviving on food stamps and disability income can do this, then any family can.

COOKING OUR WAY OUT OF THIS MESS ONE MEAL AT A TIME

Time and money are the biggest perceived obstacles to eating well. In most cases, neither is a true obstacle. Americans spend eight hours a day in front of a screen. On average, we each spend two hours a day on the Internet — something that didn't even exist 20 years ago! But we can't find the time to plan, shop, and cook for our families? True, it might cost a little more to buy fresh meat, fish, and produce than to eat processed junk and fast food. But it also doesn't have to. In fact, studies have shown that eating real food is not more expensive than eating processed food. You don't have to buy grass-fed steak (although that's ideal). You can eat well for less. To put it in perspective, Europeans spend about 20 percent of their income on food, Americans only 9 percent. We have to value our food and health. What we don't spend on the front end we pay for on the back end at the drugstore and the doctor's office.

What's missing is the education—the basic skills, knowledge, and confidence—to purchase and cook real foods. When you don't know how to cook a vegetable, how can you feed yourself or your family? My experience in South Carolina taught me that it is not a lack of desire to get well that holds people hostage to the food industry and the marketers. Without the confidence that comes from knowing how to prepare quality foods, people are left vulnerable to the aggressive marketing tactics of the food industry, which is all too eager to sell us highly addictive, poor-quality, man-made food-like products that fatten us up, along with their bottom line. Major packaged food companies are like drug dealers pushing their addictive products.

We have to cook our way out of our addiction to bad food. Shopping, cooking, and eating are political acts with far-reaching benefits to our health, the earth, the economy, and beyond. Michael Pollan, in his book *Cooked,* says, "The decline of everyday home cooking doesn't only damage the health of our bodies and our land but also our families, our communities and our sense of how our eating connects us to the world."

Cooking is fun, freeing, and essential to achieving health and happiness. Unfortunately, we have handed over the act of cooking, this unique task that makes us human, to the food industry. We have become food consumers, not food producers or preparers, and in doing so, we have lost our connection to our world and to ourselves.

I aim to help rebuild that connection for you.

UNTANGLING THE RESEARCH ON FOOD

Part of the reason we're so confused about what we should eat is that nutrition research is hard to conduct. Ideally, scientists would take two groups of people, feed them different diets (making certain they don't eat anything else), and follow them for 30 years. That will never happen. Humans, unlike lab rats, can't be contained in controlled environments for any sustained amount of time, so the results of nutritional studies are never as definitive as we might like them to be. The key to drawing accurate conclusions is to weigh all the evidence from basic science, population studies, and controlled experiments and combine it with a pinch of evolutionary common sense. The science of nutrition is often squishy, and this accounts for the kind of contradiction and misinformation we've seen from scientists and experts over the decades. For example, the American Heart Association, or AHA (which receives much of its funding from the food and pharmaceutical industries), recently declared coconut oil harmful because it contains saturated fat, despite the fact that there has not been a single controlled trial or study showing that organic virgin coconut oil causes heart attacks. The AHA study on fats was funded in part by canola oil processors. The sponsors of the AHA include many of the big food companies, such as Kellogg's, PepsiCo, General Mills, Nestlé, Mars, Domino's Pizza, Kraft, Subway, and Quaker—almost all of which have swapped out saturated fats for omega-6 vegetable oils, which the AHA tells us to eat more of to prevent heart disease. The AHA also receives hundreds of dollars every time its heart-healthy checkmark of approval is used on foods like Lucky Charms—high-sugar junk known to cause heart disease. Increasingly, many scientists point out the potential harm from swapping out saturated with refined vegetable oils or PUFAs (polyunsaturated fatty acids).[1]

The demonization of coconut oil is based on an outdated theory that saturated fat causes heart disease. More than seventeen meta-analyses have found no such link. If we accepted the recommendation of the American Heart Association that we eat less than 5 percent of our calories as saturated fat, we would have to ban breast milk. (It contains a whopping 25 percent of its calories as saturated fat.)

Most nutritional research relies on large studies of populations and their eating patterns, and data is obtained mostly through dietary questionnaires or food-recall surveys, in which participants are given a food-frequency questionnaire every year. Do you remember every single thing you ate this month? How about this week, or even in the last twenty-four hours? And how closely does that represent what you have been eating over the past five years or five decades? It is a fact of life that people often under- or overreport their consumption, depending on what they think sounds healthiest. For example, if you believe that dessert is bad for your health, you will likely underreport how much ice cream you ate last week.

Another factor we need to consider is who is funding the study. Is there any conflict of interest? If a study is paid for by a food company, it is eight times more likely to turn up positive findings for that company's product.[2] If the National Dairy Council funds studies on milk, then milk is likely to be found beneficial. If Coca-Cola underwrites studies on soft drinks, soda is likely to be found blameless for obesity and disease.

Furthermore, even scientists are sometimes guilty of supporting their preferred theories with a near-religious fervor. As a result, they believe only the studies that confirm their points of view. We call this cherry-picking the research. After reading scores of papers on human nutrition over 35 years, even I get confused. But I find my way beyond the headlines because I understand the methods and can analyze the actual data to learn what the studies demonstrate—or, equally important, what they *don't* demonstrate. I have spent hours and hours wading through data and deciphering all the geeky science so you don't have to.

As a doctor, I have also seen how my patients respond to different dietary and nutritional interventions. I have developed a way of eating that frees you from a dangerous fear of food and creates a sane, sustainable, flexible diet. I don't take money from any vested interests, nor have I spent my life proving any particular nutritional school of thought. I have been both a vegan and an omnivore. I have eaten low-fat, high-carb diets and low-carb, high-fat diets, and I have recommended and overseen all sorts of regimens for tens of thousands of patients over 30 years of medical practice and advocacy.

Once, I advocated and prescribed low-fat vegetarian diets, but as new research convinced me that fat was good, I changed my recommendations. I am not married to a particular point of view. I am curious about what lies beneath the money and the egos behind the research. I am interested in one simple thing: What should we eat to stay fit and healthy? I want to live long, feel great, and avoid disease, and I don't want to eat anything that will threaten that goal. And I want the same thing for you.

THE NEED FOR A NATIONAL FOOD, HEALTH, AND WELL-BEING POLICY

A final reason for dietary uncertainty is that our food system has become so political. Government policies heavily influence our dietary guidelines and dictate which foods are grown, how they're grown and processed, and how they are marketed. Our food policy also determines which foods are at the foundation of all our government food programs, such as food stamps, or SNAP, which feeds more than 40 million people; school lunches; and WIC (Women, Infants, and Children Food and Nutrition Service). The outsize influence that industrial food and agriculture lobbyists have on our policies encourages a food system that engenders disease. For example, in the 2016 election, the American Beverage Association and the soda companies spent more than $30 million fighting taxes on sugar-sweetened beverages. It was only because a deep-pockets organization and a billionaire (the Arnold Foundation and Michael Bloomberg) spent $20 million opposing them that soda taxes passed in four cities. Also, why do the 2015 US Dietary Guidelines recommend we cut our consumption of added sugars to less than 10 percent of our calories,[3] while the same USDA's SNAP program (food stamps) spends about $7 billion a year for the poor to consume soda and sugar-sweetened beverages (about 20 billion servings a year)? (Soda is the number one "food item" purchased by those on SNAP.) No wonder the costs of chronic disease overwhelm our federal budget. We need to transform our food system and address one of the biggest threats to our well-being: our lack of a coordinated and comprehensive food policy. Our nation's and the world's health crises are not driven by medical issues, but rather by social, economic, and political issues that conspire to drive disease—or, as the physician and global health activist Paul Farmer calls it, "structural violence." And our food system is at the nexus of where our current crises come together. The effects of the way we grow, produce, distribute, and consume food undermine the public good and subvert what's left of the public's trust in government. Here are just some of the consequences of our food policies:

- A health care crisis that results from lifestyle- and food-driven chronic disease affecting half of all Americans[4]
- Escalating federal debt due mostly to the fiscal burden of chronic disease on Medicare and Medicaid[5]
- An "achievement gap" due to childhood obesity and food-related illness that drives poor school performance, resulting in diminished global economic competitiveness[6]
- National security threat due to the lack of fitness of military recruits[7]
- Environmental degradation[8] and climate change[9] from petrochemical-based agriculture and concen-

trated animal feeding operations (CAFOs)—how most of our meat is raised in the United States

- Poverty, violence, and social injustice due to effects of a poor diet on behavior[10]

Our current food policies promote the consumption of sugar and unhealthy processed foods by allowing:

- Unregulated food marketing that targets children, the underserved, and minorities and pushes the sugar-sweetened beverages and industrial foods responsible for our epidemic of childhood obesity and racial disparities in health, predominantly in the African American and Latin American communities.[11]
- Lack of clear food labeling to help consumers make informed choices.[12]
- Subsidization of commodities[13] used in processed food (high-fructose corn syrup and soybean oil) that have been linked to poor health. Only about 1 percent of the farm bill supports healthy food. The price of soda has decreased almost 40 percent since the 1970s, while the price of fruits and vegetables has increased almost 40 percent.[14]
- A food stamp program (SNAP)[15] that supports consumption of sugar-sweetened beverages. (The single biggest line item, as noted previously, in SNAP is $7 billion a year for soda. That's almost

20 billion servings of soda for the underserved each year.) It is the number one "food" bought with food stamps.

- US Dietary Guidelines[16] that reflect not science but rather food lobby influence, forming the basis for all government programs, including school lunches, which allow sugary sweetened low-fat milk but not whole milk. In fact, in 2016 Congress directed the National Academy of Sciences (NAS) to review how the US Dietary Guidelines were developed. The NAS report was released in late 2017. They found significant problems with the process, including food-industry influence and conflicts of interest of scientists on the Dietary Guidelines Advisory Committee. Is there any evidence that we should be drinking three glasses of milk a day? Not at all. The report also found the committee ignored significant portions of the scientific literature. For example, they ignored many large studies that showed no link between saturated fat and heart disease, or studies showing the harm of cereal grains.
- Lack of taxation on sugar-sweetened beverages despite clear evidence that taxation results in reduced consumption and provides a funding source for public health measures to fight obesity and chronic disease and improve the health of communities.[17]
- Lack of regulation of irresponsible relationships[18] between food industry and nonprofit organizations

entrusted with public health. This is compounded by community and philanthropic activities or "corporate social responsibility" programs by the food industry designed to control or subvert efforts at reform (examples: food-industry donations to the NAACP led that organization to oppose a soda tax; more than 40 percent of the annual budget of the Academy of Nutrition and Dietetics comes from the food industry).

- Lack of adequate funding for nutritional science or community-health-based interventions for chronic disease (like the Daniel Plan, which Rick Warren and I created with Drs. Mehmet Oz and Daniel Amen, or community health workers from Partners in Health, the group founded and run by the aforementioned Paul Farmer).[19]
- Use of antibiotics for prevention of disease in animal feed, which puts our health at risk by creating drug-resistant superbugs.[20]
- Persistent opposition to change by the food industry through lobbying and active opposition to any initiatives for soda or sugar taxes. Soda companies spent $30 million to oppose soda taxes in just four states in 2016. They also regularly take legal action[21] to oppose warning labels, taxes, and more.

There are many ways to address these issues. However, food injustice and its far-reaching effects on the health of our population, economy, and environment warrant a comprehensive review and reform of our food policy. We have more than eight federal agencies governing the largest sector of our economy: the food industry. The agencies and their policies are often at odds with one another and produce results that do not promote our well-being. For example, the US Dietary Guidelines advise us to dramatically reduce sugar-sweetened beverage consumption, yet the government "crop insurance," or farm subsidies, supports the production of corn, which is turned into high-fructose corn syrup, making it so cheap that it is ubiquitous in our food supply. That is why the vice-chair of Pepsi, when I asked why they use high-fructose corn syrup, replied that the government makes it so cheap he can't afford not to use it. The lack of a coherent policy benefits special interests and undermines the public good. Reforming our food system, creating a national food, health, and well-being policy, and ending food injustice are key parts of creating a healthier nation.

SHIFTING OUR FOCUS BACK TO REAL FOOD

Part of the confusion around what we should and shouldn't eat is due to something called *nutritionism*. Nutritionism is the science of breaking down dietary components into their individual parts, such as one vitamin or one type of fat, and studying these in isolation. This approach is helpful for evaluating medication, where there might be a single molecule designed to target one specific pathway and one particular disease. But it's not helpful for understanding food. The things we eat contain many different components, which interact with one another and with the biochemical complexity of our bodies. In the real world, no nutrient acts in isolation. But pretending that they do plays into the food industry's hands, allowing claims of benefits from this nutrient or that one, depending on what's in fashion today: If suddenly everyone's talking about the benefits of fiber or vegetable oils, or the dangers of saturated fat, manufacturers can tailor their ingredients (and their ads) to take advantage. Multigrain Froot Loops?

I want to emphasize this: People don't eat ingredients; they eat food. And they often eat foods that contain dozens of different ingredients, many different types of fats, proteins, carbohydrates, vitamins, minerals, phytonutrients, and more. For example, olive oil, which people think of as a monounsaturated, or "good," fat, also contains about 20 percent saturated fat, 20 percent polyunsaturated omega-6 fat, and even a little bit of omega-3 fat, as well as a host of disease-busting antioxidant polyphenols. Beef also contains all different types of fat and many vitamins, minerals, and antioxidants. The nutrition world is shifting away from focusing on individual nutrients and toward focusing on dietary patterns, whole foods, and complex assortments of foods...in other words, the way we *actually* eat.

GETTING CLEAR ON WHAT THE HECK WE SHOULD EAT

I truly believe that the health experts of the world could all agree on what constitutes good nutrition, even though there seems to be so much conflicting information and debate. If we all tapped into our common sense, we would agree that we should be eating real, whole, local (when possible), fresh, unadulterated, unprocessed, chemical-free food. This book gets into the nitty-gritty of what it really means to eat this way.

Together, we can reframe the narrative around food choices. We can take back our health from those who gain by keeping us confused. I don't want to label all big food companies and the media as evil profiteers; however, it is clear that they stand to benefit from keeping us consumers and eaters disoriented. Our government allows corporations to privatize profits and socialize costs.

In the headlines, blanket statements and confusion sell. Just think of articles that have taken the Internet by storm: "Lettuce Is Worse for the Planet than Bacon." "My Vegan Diet Almost Killed Me." "Coconut Oil Isn't Healthy." These headlines aim to trick us, and once we are good and frustrated, the big food companies can make a lot of money by providing convenient, easy, hassle-free products that claim to take away the guesswork. In the 1950s, General Mills invited all the major food companies to gather in Minnesota to address the backlash at the time against processed food. They collectively decided to make convenience their core value. Convenience was the strategy. They actively subverted a home-economics movement that taught families to cook and garden. They invented Betty Crocker and created a cookbook that integrated pro-cessed food—Ritz crackers, Velveeta cheese, Camp-bell's soup, and more—into the recipes. My mother used these recipes all the time. Big food companies told us that they were actually lifting a load off our backs by making the preparation of our meals easy and cheap, but all they really did was make us sick and fat.

Your confusion around food is not just a personal dilemma. It can impact your family and your commu-nity. Collectively, our confusion sends the message that we're not responsible for what we put into our bodies; we can let big food companies and the so-called experts shoulder the responsibility for us. In essence, when we feel defeated, they win, but when we feel clear and unaffected by trends, conflicting news reports, and unethical marketing, we win.

This is an exciting and complex time. With every purchase, we have an opportunity to vote for a health-ier planet and create a healthier society, and with every bite we have the opportunity to nourish and heal our bodies. Part II of this book is designed to help you understand each aspect of your food—from its effect on your biology and health to its effect on our environment, our animals, and the people who make our food. It has been estimated, by the Consultative Group on International Agricultural Research (CGIAR), a partnership of fifteen research centers around the world, that when all agricultural activities are taken into account—from fertilizers to packing and transportation—agriculture accounts for up to a third of greenhouse gases.[22] What you put on your fork is more important than the car you drive, for both your health and the environment.

And where does my authority on this subject come from? It comes from this: I have seen thousands of incredibly ill patients become thriving, healthy humans by taking a comprehensive approach to wellness in which they eat real food, reduce stress, incorporate movement, build better relationships, and find joy in their own personal way. What connects their experiences, however, is and will always be food. I have never seen anyone evolve to be the best version of him- or herself by eating a really crappy diet.

One hundred years ago we didn't need a label to tell us that our food was local, organic, and grass-fed; all food was whole, real, unadulterated, traditional food. Fortunately, there is a strong desire among conscious consumers to get back to that way of life and to heal our conflicted relationships with what we eat.

So, let's take back our health, starting with our food.

ANSWERS TO THE NUTRITION IQ QUIZ

You didn't think I'd forgotten about the Nutrition IQ Quiz that started Part I, did you? As you'll see in the following answers, the statements are all false. Read the rest of the book to learn which of your food beliefs and conventional wisdoms are true, and which are potentially harmful myths. And, perhaps most important, to finally answer the question, "What the heck should I eat?"

1. Oatmeal has been touted as heart-healthy because the bran it contains reduces cholesterol. However, there is often a ton of sugar in instant or microwavable oatmeal. Don't believe health claims on the label or endorsements from the American Heart Association. The AHA gets $300,000 when a product's company puts the AHA's seal of approval on the label. And oatmeal spikes insulin and blood sugar, which makes you even hungrier.[23] It's definitely not heart-healthy and it promotes weight gain. Oat bran itself is fine, but not instant oatmeal. And steel-cut oats are not that much better.
2. After decades of avoiding eggs because we were told that cholesterol caused heart attacks, the 2015 US Dietary Guidelines officially exonerated them, finding no link between dietary cholesterol and heart disease. Now eggs are a health food.[24]

3. Orange juice is essentially soda with some vitamins. One 12-ounce glass contains about the
   same amount of sugar as a 12-ounce Coke. Definitely not a health food. Eat the orange instead.

4. Red meat has been vilified for decades as a source
   of saturated fat and a cause of heart disease. It
   turns out neither meat nor fat is the enemy;
   indeed, meat is a great source of protein and key
   nutrients. We go into great detail about meat and
   the science behind it in Part II.

5. We now know the main cause of weight gain. It is
   insulin, our fat-storage hormone. When you eat a
   low-fat diet you almost automatically eat a high-
   carb diet. In a review of fifty-three studies comparing low-fat and high-fat diets for weight loss, the
   high-fat diets won every time. The higher the fat,
   the lower the carbs, the greater the weight loss.[25]
   It's not about the calories themselves, but how
   those calories affect your metabolism. Fat speeds
   up your metabolism and burns body fat. Carbs
   slow it down and promote weight gain.[26]

6. Gluten-free processed foods are definitely not
   healthy. They contain sugar, other types of high-
   glycemic flour, thickeners, and more. Gluten-free
   cakes and cookies are still cakes and cookies.
   Other gluten-free foods are great—avocados,
   chicken, broccoli, apples.

7. The lie we have all been told is that weight loss is
   only about calories. Eat less, exercise more. A

thousand calories of Pepsi are the same as a thousand calories of almonds. Nonsense. This makes no intuitive sense, and science has proven that calories that spike your blood sugar and insulin (sugar and starch) promote weight gain, while calories that don't spike blood sugar and insulin—especially fat and vegetables and some protein—actually speed up your metabolism.

8. Dairy is nature's perfect food, but only if you are a calf. It does not promote healthy bones or prevent fractures. It has more than sixty naturally occurring hormones that can cause cancer and weight gain. And low-fat milk is even worse. Is a glass of milk better than a Coke? Yes. Is it better than water? No.[27] You will learn much more about the risks and problems of consuming dairy in Part II.

9. Butter has been on the "don't eat" list for decades. But now we have found out that margarine and butter substitutes kill tens of thousands of people a year. It turns out saturated fat is not the enemy we all thought it was, and it's been shown to have no effect on heart disease.[28]

10. Other than extra virgin olive oil, vegetable oils (polyunsaturated fats) are a relatively new food. They were invented in the early 1900s, and our consumption has increased a thousandfold since then. Seed, bean, and grain oils (sunflower, soy, corn) are unstable, oxidize easily, and create

inflammation. Most of the studies showing that these oils are beneficial include healthy anti-inflammatory omega-3 fats (from fish oil, flax-seeds, and walnuts). When you look at just the omega-6s (from refined vegetable oil), these oils increase the risk of inflammation as well as heart attacks.[29]

If the answers to the quiz surprised you, visit www.foodthebook.com to sign up for my newsletter and receive a weekly food fact and recipe directly from my kitchen.

So, what are the big questions of our time surrounding food? Well, first, where has all the real food gone? What exactly has industrial agriculture done to our food supply and how does it affect our health and our environment? How can we be conscious consumers when we hit the grocery stores? What is the difference between grass-fed and organic? Does organic really matter? How can we use food as medicine? And seriously, *what the heck should we eat?*

Read on.

PART II

WHAT THE HECK SHOULD I EAT?

In this part of the book, I will address the title question, item by item, choice by choice. What the heck *should* we eat? Nowadays, nutrition experts usually warn us to avoid certain foods and embrace certain others if we want to be healthy. But often, they can't agree on which is which. And their wisdom always seems to be changing. I'll cut through the confusion by tackling key food categories and reviewing the best science to give you the basics.

Here's my promise to you: If you take the time to read through each section that follows, not only will you walk away with new information, but you'll also let go of the anxiety and worry that most people have around the basic question, "What the heck should I eat?"

Let's get started!

MEAT

NUTRITION IQ QUIZ

True or False?

1. Red meat contains high levels of saturated fat, which causes heart disease.
2. If you avoid meat you can easily get all the protein you need from plants.
3. Cattle evolved to eat grass in the wild, not grains and beans like corn and soy.
4. Liver is one of the most nutritious foods you can eat.
5. Eating bacon is as strongly linked to cancer as smoking cigarettes.
6. The government strictly regulates what cattle are fed.
7. Grilling meat helps reduce contaminants and chemicals.

Answers

1. False: Red meat contains various types of fat—not only saturated fat, but also omega-6 fats (more

in corn-fed feedlot cows) and omega-3 fats (in grass-fed meat). Furthermore, the link between saturated fat and heart disease has been disproven. Studies of more than 600,000 people in nineteen countries found no link between saturated fat and heart disease.[1] Another study of 135,000 people from eighteen countries and five continents over ten years showed a lower risk of heart disease and death from eating saturated fat.

2. False: You'd have to eat a lot of vegetables, beans, and grains to meet your daily protein requirements. You would have to eat 3 cups of lentils to get the amount of the right amino acids and protein you get from one 4- to 6-ounce serving of meat, chicken, or fish. And as you age, you need more and higher-quality protein to maintain muscle mass and health. Plant proteins contains low levels of leucine, the rate-limiting amino acid for maintaining and building muscle, whereas animal protein contains high levels of leucine.[2]

3. True: Cows, sheep, and goats should eat grass and forage. But factory-farmed animals are fed cheap grains and candy and ground-up animal parts, not to mention hormones and antibiotics to fatten them up fast.

4. True: Liver contains high levels of vitamins, proteins, and nutrients. But eat liver only from organic, grass-fed, or pasture-raised animals.

5. False: There is evidence linking processed meats to colorectal cancer. But the association has been overblown. I wouldn't binge on processed meat, but it's not the bogeyman we may think from reading the headlines. Eating one piece of bacon every day raises your risk by one half of 1 percent.

6. False: The junk, toxins, hormones, and antibiotics that are legally added to livestock feed would make you shudder.

7. False: Cooking meat at high temperatures can produce toxic compounds. It's best not to overcook it or grill it at high temperatures.

> Get a new food fact and weekly recipe directly from my kitchen. Sign up for free at www.food thebook.com.

Eating meat will clog your arteries, cause cancer and type 2 diabetes, and take years off your life, right?

Absolutely not.[3] But you could be excused for believing that. A lot of people do, meat lovers and abstainers alike. This food that we've eaten all our lives has become the most controversial thing on our plates. It's where many of today's raging food fights—warring nutritional theories, the abysmal state of our nation's health, the environmental impact of agriculture, the unethical treatment of animals (cows, pigs, chickens)—all come together in one big, messy collision. Is meat really bad for us, or really good for us? If we want to live long, healthy lives, should we eat a lot of it, a little, or none at all?

Let's start by acknowledging that humans first domesticated sheep, cows, and pigs as far back as 10,000 BC.[4] Humans have been eating meat for about as long as our species has existed. In fact, scientists who study modern-day hunter-gatherers, who live and eat very much like our Paleolithic ancestors did—with a meat-heavy, low-sugar diet—find that they typically have no signs of heart disease, diabetes, or other chronic diseases.[5] Animals have always held a central place in the human diet. So, from an evolutionary perspective, it's hard to imagine that this food

that has been such an integral part of our existence —
a food that helped sustain civilizations across the globe
for millennia — has been slowly killing us all along.

In recent decades, the anti-meat advocates and scientists have tried to scare Americans by linking meat to
everything from cancer to heart disease, diabetes, and
even obesity. But time and time again the research has
shown that the opposite is true. As our ancestors knew,
meat is a nutrient-dense food that can help *prevent* disease and nutritional deficiencies when consumed in
combination with plenty of plants and vegetables — or
as part of what I like to call a Paleo-vegan, or "Pegan,"
diet. Of course, that's not to say that there isn't a dark
side to meat consumption. Most of the meat consumed
in America and other developed countries, sadly, comes
from factory farms, where animals are subjected to cruel,
unsanitary, and often unimaginable conditions. These
industrial behemoths contribute to climate change, pollute the environment, and, in some cases, abuse their
workers. We should do all we can to avoid propping up
this industry. But that does not negate the fact that the
right meat can — and should — be an essential part of
the average American's diet. There are valid personal,
spiritual, religious, ethical, and environmental reasons
for not eating meat. There are not, however, good scientific or health reasons to avoid good-quality, organic,
grass-fed, sustainably raised meat in the context of an
overall healthy diet, what I call a Pegan diet.

THE SCIENCE OF MEAT

When you think of meat, you probably think of protein. But protein exists in virtually every food. Even vegetables contain it in small amounts. As meat became demonized over the last half century, many Americans began seeking out alternatives, in some cases quitting meat altogether. An estimated 5 percent of Americans now identifies as vegetarian.[6] But that's a difficult path to maintain for long. While plant alternatives to meat are increasing in popularity, there is no getting around the fact that meat is the single best source of protein (and also many vitamins and minerals). You may have heard that legumes have a lot of protein, for example. And they do—for plants. But they lack a number of critical amino acids. Eggs are another source of protein, containing 6 grams each. But the average adult needs between 60 and 90 grams of protein each day, and even more if you're active. You need about 30 grams, three times a day, to maintain and build muscle. If you rely on eggs, then you'd have to eat a whole lot of omelets. Fulfilling your protein requirements with non-meat foods requires enormous planning and effort, more than most people can manage. You also need to make sure to get all the essential amino acids—the ones that we need but our bodies can't make—from the protein you eat. Only quinoa, buckwheat, and soy are plant sources that contain all nine of them, but they can be found in complete form in all animal foods. To give you an idea of how plant protein ranks next to animal protein, here's a side-by-side comparison of the two.[7]

Grams of animal protein per 100 grams of:

- Veal: 36.71
- Beef: 36.12
- Lamb: 32.08
- Pork: 28.86
- Chicken: 28.74
- Tuna: 25.51
- Sardines: 24.62
- Cheese: 23.63
- Salmon: 22.10
- Crickets: 20.50 (yes, they're protein-packed)
- Eggs: 12.58

Grams of plant protein per 100 grams of:

- Peanut butter: 22.21
- Almonds: 20.96 (but almond milk: 0.42)
- Oats: 16.89
- Tofu: 9.04
- Lentils: 9.02
- Black beans: 8.86

As you can see, you'd have to eat a whole lot of black beans, oats, or tofu to deliver the protein in just a small serving of meat. That doesn't mean meat should be your only source of protein. You can get a portion of your daily protein from plants. But for most people, especially as we age and need more protein to maintain our muscle mass, animal protein is important.

WHAT THE EXPERTS GOT RIGHT

For all of human history, with the exception of a period beginning midway through the second half of the twentieth century, meat was considered by experts and ordinary people alike to be a vital part of the human diet. Indeed, there has never been a voluntarily vegan indigenous society anywhere on the planet.[8] In fact, the word "vegan" wasn't coined until 1944. Yes, some studies show that eating meat harms our health, but the devil is in the details, and in this case that means the design and type of study. As you're about to see, the scaremongering crumbles under the weight of scientific scrutiny. Did the nutrition authorities get anything right? They did. There is some relevance to warnings about eating too much red meat—conventionally raised beef comes from animals that are fed improper diets, which in turn can harm us. Even the way we cook meat can damage our health. For the most part, however, meat has gotten a bum rap. The science doesn't support meat as the disease-creating thing we thought it was for decades.

WHAT THEY GOT WRONG

Anyone who has lived in America over the past 50 years has heard the dire warnings about red meat. It causes cancer. It causes heart disease. It's practically deadly. How did we end up with all this hysteria and misinformation?

Two words: saturated fat.

The discovery a half century ago that saturated fat raises cholesterol levels led to the widespread demonization of meat. We cut back on meat, we chose "lean" meat, and we trimmed and skimmed all the fat off our meat. Back then, scientists were convinced that high cholesterol was the number one culprit behind the nation's epidemic of heart disease, which contributed to more than a million deaths per year. Their theory was simple — too simple. It was introduced by scientist Ancel Keys at the World Health Organization in Geneva in 1955 and was known as the lipid, or "diet-heart," hypothesis. The theory went like this: When you raise cholesterol, you increase heart disease. And when you lower it, you reduce heart disease. Initially, Keys and his colleagues targeted all dietary fat as the primary cause of high cholesterol. But over time they zeroed in on saturated fat, which typically raises cholesterol more than unsaturated fats does. And since saturated fat is found primarily in animal foods, Keys argued, then meat must be bad for you. This line of thinking was endorsed and promoted by the American Heart Association, which told Americans to put down their plates of bacon, eggs, and sausage and back away from the breakfast table. In fact, all foods that contained saturated fat became "bad" almost overnight—even fatty plant foods such as coconuts, nuts, and avocados.

Today, we know that thinking was horribly oversimplified and entirely wrong: Heart disease is a complex condition that involves not only cholesterol but inflammation, blood sugar, triglycerides, and a host of other factors. And the impact of saturated fat on cholesterol is not so simple either. Some forms of saturated fat raise LDL cholesterol, the so-called bad kind. But at the same time, saturated fat raises HDL cholesterol, the kind that *protects* you from heart disease.[9] Saturated fat also has a beneficial impact on the size and density of the lipoprotein particles that carry cholesterol in your bloodstream. It creates LDL particles that are large and fluffy (like cotton balls),[10] which are less *atherogenic* (heart-disease-causing) than the small, dense LDL particles created by sugar and refined carbohydrates (starchy foods), which increase inflammation and promote plaque formation in your arteries.[11]

This new data on saturated fat has been uncovered in numerous studies and embraced by many cardiologists and nutrition experts. But the outdated idea that saturated fat causes heart disease has not gone away so easily. After introducing the lipid hypothesis in the 1950s, Keys followed up with the Seven Countries Study in 1970, which pushed the idea that nations that consume relatively low amounts of saturated fat have low rates of heart disease. Unfortunately, Keys cherrypicked the data—he reported on the small number of countries (7) that fit his hypothesis and ignored those that did not (15), such as Brie-and-butter-loving France.[12] Newer studies that involved forty-two countries found that fifteen countries had no link between saturated fat and heart disease. Despite its flaws, the Seven Country Study took hold and became enshrined in our food policies, which continue to this day to call for drastic reductions in America's meat and saturated fat intake.

Reducing saturated fat intake has remained one of the most persistent recommendations in the government's Dietary Guidelines for Americans, which are updated every five years. The most recent guidelines, released in 2015, called for Americans to limit their intake of saturated fat to no more than 10 percent of their daily calories.[13] The American Heart Association's equally outdated recommendations are even more drastic. They advise Americans to limit their saturated fat intake to no more than 5 to 6 percent of daily calories, which for the average person is slightly less than a 3-ounce serving of ground beef or 1-ounce serving of cheddar cheese.[14] On its website, the Heart Association tells people to "limit red meat" and to avoid other foods with saturated fat such as lamb, pork, and skin-on poultry. The heart association advises, "Eating foods that contain saturated fats raises the level of cholesterol in your blood. High levels of LDL cholesterol in your blood increase your risk of heart disease and stroke."[15]

Meanwhile, research shows that fixating on LDL

cholesterol can obscure other causes of heart disease. A nationwide study that looked at almost a quarter million adults admitted to hospitals with heart attacks found that almost 75 percent of these patients had LDL levels that were categorized as either "low" or "optimal" under the current cholesterol guidelines.[16] Long-term studies like the famous Framingham Heart Study show that while LDL cholesterol is associated with heart disease, HDL cholesterol, which increases when we eat saturated fat, actually *lowers* our risk of heart attack.[17]

At the same time, the largest and most comprehensive studies of dietary fat intake have found no link between saturated fat consumption and heart disease.[18] One tightly controlled clinical trial published in the journal *BMJ* in 2016 compared people who were fed diets rich in saturated fats from milk, cheese, and beef to people who were assigned to eat foods in which most of the saturated fat was removed and replaced with corn oil, an unsaturated vegetable oil. The study found that the vegetable oil group had lower cholesterol levels but higher mortality rates.[19] Another large review of the most rigorous research on saturated fat, published in the *Annals of Internal Medicine*, found no link between saturated fat and heart disease and concluded that the current dietary guidelines that tell us to avoid saturated fat and increase PUFAs, or refined vegetable oils, are not supported by scientific evidence.[20]

One of the most striking rebukes to the saturated

fat mythology that grew out of Keys' Seven Countries Study came in 2016. In a study published in the journal *Food & Nutrition Research*, scientists analyzed data that was gathered over 16 years from forty-two different countries and looked at the relationship between various foods and heart disease.[21] Their study was far more comprehensive than the Seven Countries Study—and their results were completely antithetical to what Keys found. In fact, they found no link between red meat and heart disease. If anything, their results indicate that a higher intake of animal fat and animal protein is *protective* against cardiovascular disease. The foods found to be the biggest drivers of disease were high-glycemic carbohydrates like potatoes, bread, and cereal. The lead author of the study, Dr. Pavel Grasgruber, said the findings made it clear that the conventional dietary advice should be flipped on its head.

"This study flies in the face of accepted wisdom on diet," he told one news outlet.[22] "It is quite clear consumption of dairy products and meat is not linked with heart disease risk, as was traditionally believed. The biggest problems are cereals, wheat and potatoes, which increase the risk of heart disease."

Outdated ideas often take a long time to die, which is why many in the medical and nutrition establishment refuse to change their thinking on saturated fat. But some are beginning to come around. In 2016, one of the nation's most respected cardiologists, Steven Nissen, who is the chairman of cardiovascular medicine at the Cleveland Clinic, the number one heart hospital in the world, and a colleague of mine, published a major editorial in the *Annals of Internal Medicine* that took the dietary guidelines and their saturated fat recommendations to task. "The best available evidence does not clearly support the widely held belief that Americans should limit saturated fat and cholesterol in the diet," he wrote.[23]

And in 2017, at a major cardiovascular medicine conference in Switzerland, the president of the World Heart Federation, Salim Yusuf, a world-renowned cardiologist, was even more blunt about the myth surrounding saturated fat and heart disease: "Contrary to common beliefs, the current recommendations to reduce saturated fat have no scientific basis."[24] So, he asked, what does cause heart disease? "Carbohydrates are probably your biggest culprit. So, when you eat a hamburger, throw away the bun, and eat the meat!"

I couldn't agree more. And if I could choose between a bagel or butter, I would choose the butter.

WHAT WE STILL DON'T KNOW FOR SURE

Even though saturated fat has been exonerated as the cause of heart disease it once seemed to be, that does not mean you should go crazy with it. I don't believe you should be eating limitless amounts. We're still working out precisely how much saturated fat is "healthy," though the latest wisdom suggests that it's fairly neutral. It's not harmful, but it's not necessarily a health food. One big caveat: When combined with sugar or refined carbs (what I call "sweet fat"), it is deadly. You hear a lot of advice these days to eat meat and butter "in moderation." But what exactly does "moderation" mean? For that we need more research. In the meantime, don't be afraid to toss a little grass-fed butter into your pasture-raised organic eggs. And don't feel guilty about ordering the grass-fed steak instead of the halibut the next time you dine out.

EIGHT THINGS YOU SHOULD KNOW ABOUT MEAT

1. It's More Than Protein and Muscle

Animal foods are our only source of vitamin B_{12}, which is essential for life itself. Meat also provides vitamin E, vitamin D, and the other B vitamins. It contains enzymes that we need to access nutrients, essential amino acids, and cancer-fighting antioxidants like beta-carotene (which our bodies convert into vitamin A), lutein, and zeaxanthin. Meat contains minerals such as zinc, selenium, magnesium, sodium, and potassium. And it also contains iron, which is particularly important for women, a great many of whom are anemic due to menstruation. It's true, as vegans point out, that all these minerals (and even protein) are available in vegetables and legumes and other foods. But our bodies' internal systems have to work to convert them into a form we can use, whereas nutrients in meat are much more bioavailable. A clinical study in the *American Journal of Clinical Nutrition* found, for example, that people assigned to follow diets that include beef, poultry, pork, and fish gain more muscle and lean body mass than people who are put on vegetarian diets consisting of plants, dairy, eggs, and grains.[25] Diets that contain animal protein have also been shown to help preserve muscle mass and reduce "protein breakdown" in the body to a much greater extent than vegetarian diets.[26] Protein is required to maintain and build muscle. With the loss of muscle (sarcopenia) comes age-related hormonal changes including pre-diabetes (which causes heart disease, cancer, and dementia), higher levels of stress hormones like cortisol, and lower levels of anti-aging hormones like growth hormone and testosterone. That's why studies show that as you age you need more protein to prevent disease and death. It's no wonder we evolved to eat meat.

2. Stop Worrying About Bacon Causing Cancer

If you're like most people, you probably saw the terrifying news in late 2015. "Processed Meats Rank Alongside Smoking as Cancer Causes," blared a headline in the *Guardian*. "Bacon, Hot Dogs as Bad as Cigarettes," read another. These headlines were referring to a World Health Organization (WHO) report that concluded that eating processed meats like bacon, ham, deli meat, and sausages raised the risk of colon cancer by 20 percent.[27] Many people who saw the news were understandably worried. Some, perhaps, even swore off bacon altogether. But the report's findings were widely exaggerated.

Here's why. The report found that the effects of red meat per se on our health were not conclusive. And while it did link processed meats to cancer, the effect was relatively small. The 20 percent increase referred to the *relative* risk of cancer, not the *absolute* risk. The average person has a fairly low likelihood of developing colon cancer in his or her lifetime: roughly a 5 percent risk. When the WHO says that eating bacon every day increases the risk by 20 percent, what it means is that your lifetime risk would climb from 5 percent to 6 percent if you ate four pieces of bacon every day for your whole life. That's only a 1 percent real increase in the risk. For a piece of bacon once in a while, that's probably a risk I am willing to take, especially in the context of an overall healthy diet. If you consider the absolute risk rather than the relative risk, the increase is not as frightening as the headlines would lead you to believe.

As I mentioned, the risks associated with eating meat are often distorted. In fact, it's debatable whether the WHO's warnings about meat being linked to cancer are even accurate. One paper published in the journal *Obesity Reviews* looked at thirty-five large studies of cancer and meat consumption and concluded that there was little risk at all.[28] In fact, an analysis of the Women's Health Study of 37,547 women over almost nine years found that the women who consumed the most meat actually had the lowest rates of colon cancer.[29] So why do some studies find that meat consumption is linked to cancer and others find the opposite? One reason is the healthy-user bias. In most studies, people who report higher levels of meat consumption also tend to engage in other "unhealthy" behaviors like smoking, heavy drinking, neglecting fresh fruits and vegetables, and eating more processed foods and sugar—all of which are linked to higher cancer rates. On the other hand, people who do the "healthy" thing and avoid red meat are also more likely to exercise several times a week, eat lots of veggies, and avoid cigarettes. We make the mistake of thinking it's meat that causes disease, when it's everything else those people are eating and doing. This explains some of the misleading cancer findings in nutrition studies.

Of course, not all processed meat is the same. Much modern processed meat is full of sugar, fillers, and additives such as gluten and preservatives. Stick to whole-food processed meat—such as sliced turkey and roast beef, or traditionally prepared salami or bacon from organic producers such as Niman Ranch. My neurosurgeon friend, as a practical joke, once sent a hot dog instead of a brain biopsy to the pathologist. The pathologist called back alarmed because he found bone, hair, nails, and teeth in the specimen. Know where your meat is coming from.

3. We Are What Our Meat Eats

You've probably heard the old saying that you are what you eat, right? Well, that's false. You are what your food eats! That's scary because all of our worst fears about how modern, industrialized animals are fed and treated are essentially true — in fact, the truth might be even worse than you imagine. Factory-farmed animals are fed cheap, mass-produced grains because it fattens them quickly at low cost. That means they're eating GMOs and pesticides. They're pumped full of hormones and antibiotics because these make them bigger and fatter, too.[30] And it gets scarier: Under federal regulations, it's perfectly legal to feed livestock and poultry things you would never eat or want any animal to eat. Yet "additives" that are allowed under the law include "feather meal" (ground-up feathers); both dried and unprocessed "recycled" animal waste (that's poop to you and me); food adulterated with waste from rodents, insects, or birds (more poop, but only after it has been heat-treated to kill the germs); "polyethylene roughage replacement" (that's plastic filler); bacteria, including some that are resistant to antibiotics; toxic chemicals such as PCBs and dioxin; and a long list of other substances that don't sound like anything you would want to feed an animal.[31]

Sadly, many factory farms are willing to feed their animals whatever it takes to fatten them up as quickly and cheaply as possible, with no regard for proper nutrition or the quality of the meat they produce. In January 2017, a flatbed pickup truck accidentally spilled its cargo on a Wisconsin highway, creating a remarkable scene. The truck, destined for a factory farm, was carrying hundreds of thousands of red Skittles to be used as feed for cattle.[32] The spill left a blanket of red candies scattered across the road, but what was most disturbing about the accident was that it revealed a little-known fact about factory farming: that it's not only legal but common for producers to feed their cattle all sorts of sugar, candy, Kool-Aid powder, potato chips, and molasses.[33] Some producers even boast about it. In 2012, the owner of United Livestock Commodities in Kentucky told a local television station that in response to rising corn prices he started feeding his cattle cheap, defective candy that would have been destined for landfills.[34] A video even showed that the cattle were being fed candy that was still in its wrappers. Agriculture experts say this has been going on for years and is perfectly legal. In fact, many beef producers throw all sorts of food waste into their animal feed—things that are considered unfit for human consumption, but somehow perfectly fine for the animals we eat.

4. Why Grass-Fed Meat Is Best

It's hard to deny all the problems with factory farming. It damages the environment with the widespread use of fossil fuels for fertilizers and agricultural chemicals. It drains and pollutes local water supplies, releases toxic chemicals into the atmosphere, and contributes to climate change. It relies on the rampant use of antibiotics in animal feed to promote bigger and fatter animals that are more resistant to the diseases that spread easily in crowded, clustered pens and holding cages. And it involves the unimaginably cruel and horrendous treatment of animals. But there is yet another reason to frown upon factory farming: It results in less nutritious meat. The alternative to factory-farmed meat — grass-fed meat — is not just better for the environment and better for the animals, but better for you, too. Grass-fed meat is so nutritionally superior to factory-farmed meat that it is practically a different food.

Cows, sheep, and goats are ruminants, meaning they have four-chambered stomachs designed to extract the nutrients they need from grass, hay, and other forage. Pigs are omnivorous — they earn their reputation — but are healthiest when allowed to roam and eat whatever plants or natural foods they find on the ground, like acorns, fruit, and grubs. These are the foods they evolved to eat. But that is not what they are fed on factory farms. Instead they're forced to eat corn, soy, wheat, and other crops that are extremely cheap because they're subsidized by the federal government. Roughly half of all the soy and 60 percent of the corn produced in the United States are used as feed for livestock.[35]

How does all that affect their health and the health of their flesh? Terribly. Cattle raised on grain can develop bloating, liver abscesses, and other fatal conditions. One study in the *Journal of Animal Science* reported that up to a third of feedlot cattle develop liver abscesses as a result of "aggressive grain-feeding programs."[36] But studies show that the incidence of these diseases decreases when cattle are fed their natural diet of grass and hay.[37] Conventionally raised livestock are also more susceptible to infections that can linger in their meat. In a 2015 investigation, Consumer Reports tested 300 samples of beef purchased at stores across the country and compared the conventionally raised beef samples to "sustainably" raised beef that was grass-fed, organic, or raised without antibiotics. The investigation found that 18 percent of the conventional beef samples were contaminated with superbugs—the hazardous bacteria that are resistant to three or more classes of antibiotics—compared to just 6 percent of grass-fed beef samples, and 9 percent of samples that were organic or raised without antibiotics.[38] The investigation also found that three of the conventional beef samples contained a type of antibiotic-resistant bacteria called MRSA (methicillin-resistant *Staphylococcus aureus*), which kills more than 10,000 people in the United States every year. The grass-fed, organic, and non-antibiotic samples contained none of these potentially lethal bugs. The conventional beef was also more likely to harbor *E. coli*.

"We know that sustainable methods are better for the environment and more humane to animals," said Dr. Urvashi Rangan, the executive director of the Center for Food Safety and Sustainability at Consumer Reports.[39] "But our tests also show that these methods can produce ground beef that poses fewer public health risks."

Three decades of research have shown that grass-fed beef and pasture-raised meat are significantly healthier than grain-fed, factory-farmed meat. Grass-fed meat has much better types of fat than grain-fed (more omega-3s, fewer omega-6s, and more CLA, or conjugated linoleic acid). When livestock are fed grains and other foods that are not part of their natural diet, the levels of inflammatory omega-6 fatty acids in their meat rise, while the levels of beneficial omega-3 fats plummet. If they're fed a natural diet, the reverse happens. Grass-fed meat contains up to five times the omega-3 fats as conventionally raised meat, and much lower levels of omega-6 fats.[40] In grass-fed beef, the ratio of omega-3 to omega-6 is a healthful 1:1. In grain-fed beef, the ratio is more like 1:7. Grass-fed meat has higher levels of critical nutrients including the B vitamins, vitamin E, and the antioxidants lutein, zeaxanthin, beta-carotene, superoxide dismutase, and glutathione, a powerful cancer-fighting compound that's also found in fresh vegetables.[41] Grass-fed beef also contains much higher levels of beneficial minerals[42] like potassium, phosphorus, zinc, and iron.[43]

5. Grass-Fed Meat Contains a Remarkable Fatty Acid

It's true that meat contains saturated fat, but that's only part of the story, and, as it turns out, it's not a problem. Forty percent of the fat in beef is monounsaturated and polyunsaturated fat—the same kinds that are found in olive oil, seafood, and nuts. The type of saturated fat in steak is also noteworthy: Much of it is stearic acid, the kind that doesn't increase your total cholesterol level. Meat also contains an unusual healthy, naturally occurring trans fat that's actually great for you. It's called CLA, or conjugated linoleic acid.[44] It exists in only a few foods, and the richest known source is the fat of ruminants (cows, sheep, and—top of the list, in case you're an adventurous eater—kangaroos) that eat grass. CLA is a powerful antioxidant that slows the growth of cancerous tumors. It also prevents plaque from forming in your arteries and causing atherosclerosis. It reduces the risk of heart disease and type 2 diabetes,[45] lowers triglycerides, and helps with weight control and metabolism.[46] All animal foods contain CLA, but grass-fed meat and dairy are far and away the best source of it: They contain up to 500 percent more CLA than grain-fed meat and dairy products.[47]

6. Organic or Grass-Fed Meat Is Worth the Extra Cost

In its 2015 investigation, Consumer Reports performed a cost analysis of ground beef from different sources, and here's what was found:[48]

Conventionally raised meat, per pound: $4.95

Organic: $5.62

Raised without antibiotics: $6.55

Grass-fed: $7.38

Grass-fed and organic: $7.83

There was roughly a 50 percent price difference between the lowest- and highest-quality beef, which is a considerable amount of money if you're feeding a family. This is because grass-fed animals are much slower to reach market weight since they're not plied with cheap grains, corn, candy, or antibiotics to fatten them up, and they are generally leaner, with less meat on their bones than factory-farmed animals. Grass-fed cattle require additional land and high-quality pastures as well. Keep in mind that you're paying for meat that's not only humanely raised and sustainably produced, but more nutritious, less likely to be contaminated, and ultimately better for your body.[49] Americans devote about 10 percent of their salary to food, while Europeans spend 20 percent, and some countries even more. Think about all the ways we waste money ($5 specialty coffees, for one). Reorganizing your budget to focus on your health and quality of food will make you feel better now and save much more in health care costs later. But best of all, you don't necessarily have to pay a high price for grass-fed meat if you know where to shop and which resources to use. I'll provide a list of those a little later in this chapter. The big takeaway: We need less meat than we are eating. We don't need a 12-ounce steak, only a 4- to 6-ounce one. I urge you to focus on high-quality meats rather than high quantity.

7. We Should Return to Organ Meats

Have you ever watched one of those *National Geographic* specials where a pack of lions takes down an antelope or a zebra? There's a reason they always go straight for the liver when they devour their kill: It's one of the most nutrient-dense organs in the body. The liver contains a wide range of vitamins (especially A and B_{12}, but also folate and C, which we usually associate with plant foods), minerals (especially copper, phosphorus, iron, zinc, and magnesium), and other substances, like CoQ10, that we need for good health, as well as ample protein.[50] There's a good chance your grandparents ate liver. It's a popular meal in many cultures. Chopped liver is a traditional Jewish dish. Liver and onions is a quintessentially British meal. In Poland, they eat fried pork liver alongside fresh veggies. The French eat liver fried with butter and bacon. The Spanish eat it cooked in olive oil and garlic. And in Brazil, liver is served with potatoes or another starchy vegetable.

But in America, we've gotten out of the offal habit — that is, we prefer to eat muscle meat almost exclusively. One reason liver fell off the menu in America is that we were discouraged from eating it due to its high cholesterol content. Cholesterol after all is manufactured in the liver, and if we couldn't eat egg yolks because of their cholesterol, then liver was off-limits, too. But just as eating yolks will have a negligible impact on your blood cholesterol levels, so, too, will eating liver. Others may wonder if the liver stores toxins. It doesn't; it processes them. Most toxins are stored in muscle and fat tissues, including the brain. The organ's texture may be a turnoff for some people. But when it's properly prepared — thinly sliced and smothered in onions and a little organic bacon, for example — it can be a surprising delicacy and a great meal. Some people even eat it raw or blended in smoothies, but don't worry, I won't try to convince you to go that far! There's a simpler way to consume it. When I was a kid, my mother used to prepare sautéed chicken livers over rice, which everyone in my family considered a delicious treat. I can't recommend it highly enough.

Ideally, you should get your liver from grass-fed sources to ensure that it's good quality. And liver isn't the only organ that's good for you. More adventurous eaters should take advantage of the benefits of eating hearts, kidneys, tripe, sweetbreads, and so on. But dollar for dollar, liver is probably the single best concentrated source of nutrients you'll find.

8. How You Cook Meat Matters

When you fry, smoke, grill, or otherwise cook any meat at high temperatures, it leads to the creation of carcinogenic compounds called heterocyclic amines (HCAs) and polycyclic aromatic hydrocarbons (PAHs). For this reason, you should be careful not to burn or overcook any meat that you consume. But these compounds are also found in vegetables and grains![51] Those black grill marks on your steak or veggies might be mouthwatering—but that's where the hazardous by-products of grilling are most likely to be found. So focus on using low-temperature cooking methods like baking, roasting, and stewing.

GEEK ALERT: A LITTLE MORE SCIENCE ABOUT MEAT

But what about all the well-publicized scientific studies showing that meat eaters are in worse health than vegetarians and die sooner? Well, even that's not as simple as it seems. The findings may have something to do with *which* meat eaters are being studied. Generally speaking, people who eat a lot of meat also have unhealthy habits overall: They weigh more, drink more, smoke more, eat less produce and fiber, and are more sedentary than those who consume less meat, according to a study involving more than 600,000 subjects. So maybe it isn't the meat that's damaging carnivores' health—maybe it's everything else they are doing to damage their health. In an era when red meat was seen as bad, healthy people avoided it and unhealthy people didn't care and ate more meat. Another study was done of meat eaters and vegetarians who shop in health food stores and so are, presumably, pursuing healthy lifestyles. The result? Both groups were equally healthy, and they lived longer than those who don't pay so much attention to proper nutrition.[52] This is known as the "healthy eater effect"—and it explains why it's so difficult to tease out the influence of any individual food group or nutrient when we're trying to figure out how to eat healthy. Another large study, of 245,000 people, found no difference in mortality between vegetarians, pescatarians, and meat eaters.[53] Everything we eat (or avoid eating) adds up. Just as it's possible to be a sickly, overweight vegan, it's possible to be a healthy, well-nourished carnivore. You just have to eat smart.

DOES MEAT CONTRIBUTE TO GLOBAL WARMING?

It might sound funny, but intestinal methane gas produced by cattle accounts for almost *half* of agriculture's greenhouse gas pollution.[54] If there were a country populated solely by all the world's cows, it would rank third behind China and the United States as the biggest producers of gases responsible for global warming. On top of that, about 248 gallons of oil are required to produce the roughly 2,800 pounds of corn each conventionally raised cow will eat during its lifetime. Globally, one-fifth of all our energy consumption is used for industrial agriculture. That is more than is used for all our transportation—cars, trucks, planes, trains, boats—combined!

Livestock production also consumes about one-third of the world's fresh water. It takes 1,799 gallons of water to produce 1 pound of beef and 576 gallons to produce 1 pound of pork. To make matters worse, the cultivation of soybean and corn crops, which is what factory-farmed animals are fed, requires a massive amount of water.[55] Agricultural irrigation is draining the Ogllala Aquifer, the largest water supply in the United States, 1.3 gallons a year faster than rainfall is able to replenish it. However, most of this water is used to grow grains and feed for factory-farmed animals.

Can we do anything about all this? Early research has shown that regenerative farming may be the future of meat that is healthy for us as well as the environment, and humane for the animals, too. Well-managed grazing operations can actually offset or even completely compensate for methane and other greenhouse gases linked to beef production by trapping carbon in the soil. The grass soaks up and stores, or sequesters, carbon, preventing carbon dioxide from being released into the atmosphere. Soil farming will save us. Watch the movie or read the book

Kiss the Ground to learn how we can reduce carbon dioxide to preindustrial levels through regenerative farming.

These operations also involve regularly moving the animals to fresh pasture and keeping them away from streambeds, which can help prevent water pollution. For the most part, pasture-raised cattle do not rely on irrigated crops for feeding, which lessens the amount of water required to produce meat. By choosing grass-fed meat from small, sustainable farms, we also support the fair treatment of workers and livestock. If you want to learn more about this, check out the Savory Institute (www.savory.global) and our grass-fed meat resources page at www.foodthebook.com/resources.

SUMMING IT UP

When Buying, Look for These Labels

The following labels will help to ensure that you're buying meat that's humanely produced and sustainable, so do your best to choose them:

- Animal Welfare Approved
- Certified Humane
- Global Animal Partnership
- Food Alliance Certified

Go Grass-Fed!

I highly recommend you choose beef, bison, goat, lamb, and sheep that are certified by the American

Grassfed Association (AGA). To do that, look for the organization's green logo, which says "American Grassfed." Their certification ensures the following:

- **Diet:** All animals certified by the AGA are raised entirely on open grass pastures. This is important because some "grass-fed" animals are raised on grains and other crops for most of their lives and then "finished" on grass just before slaughter. The AGA certification forbids that practice.
- **Treatment:** The AGA certification ensures that animals are allowed to graze on grass without being forced into small feedlots or harsh confinements.
- **Antibiotics and hormones:** The AGA certification strictly forbids the use of antibiotics or growth hormones in animals.
- **Origin:** The AGA certification requires that animals be born and raised on family farms in America. No imported meat allowed.

You can find grass-fed meat at your local health food store and at some supermarkets. Just check with your butcher if there's any doubt. You can also use these resources to find grass-fed meat in your area:

- **The AGA Producer Profiles:** You can look for an AGA-approved producer on the group's website. You can browse by state and find the producers in

your area: http://www.americangrassfed.org/producer
-profiles/.

- **Eatwild:** You can go to Eatwild's directory of
pasture-based farms, which is one of the most comprehensive sources for grass-fed meat and dairy.
Click on your state to find your closest supplier:
http://www.eatwild.com/products/index.html.

- **Local Harvest:** This group helps consumers find
and purchase real food from local farmers. They
have a webpage devoted to grass-fed beef, where
you can type in your zip code to get a list of grass-
fed producers and CSAs in your area: http://www
.localharvest.org/beef.jsp.

- ***The Meat Eater's Guide to Climate Change and
Health:*** The Environmental Working Group published this guide to help provide consumers with
access to extensive research on labeling, certifications, and best practices for meat eaters. Check it
out to find more tips and advice on how to be a
responsible meat eater: http://www.ewg.org/meateat
ersguide/eat-smart/.

- Other resources include **Butcher Box** (www.butch
erbox.com) and **Walden Local Meat** (www.walden
localmeat.com) for online sales of grass-fed or
organic animal products. You can also participate
in cow shares—sharing a cow among a group of
people to lower the cost. For more information, see
www.eatwild.com/products/ and www.marksdaily
apple.com/where-to-buy-grass-fed-beef/.

When Grass-Fed Isn't an Option, Look for Organic

Grass-fed is best. But second best is USDA organic certified meat. It's cheaper than grass-fed and nearly comparable in price to conventional. Though USDA standards are not quite as stringent as the American Grassfed Association's, they're still far better than those applied to conventional meat. Buying USDA organic certified meat ensures the following:

- **Diet:** Unlike certified grass-fed beef, organic beef can be raised on a diet of grain and corn — but not exclusively. The USDA organic certification regulations require that animals be raised in living conditions that "accommodate their natural behaviors." So part of their lives must be spent grazing on grass.
- **Treatment:** The organic certification requires that cattle cannot be confined for extended periods of time.
- **Antibiotics and hormones:** To be certified organic, animals must not be subjected to harmful antibiotics or growth hormones, unlike conventional meat.
- **GMOs:** The organic certification requires that animals be fed 100 percent organic feed and forage. That means no GMO crops, synthetic contaminants, fertilizers, or artificial pesticides.

Watch the Amounts You Eat

The average adult in America consumes slightly more than a third of a pound of meat every day. Unless you're an athlete, that much probably isn't necessary. Remember, at least three-quarters of your plate should be vegetables, and the rest protein. I like the term "condi-meat"—a small amount of meat added to meals that are mostly vegetables. I've downsized my own consumption to no more than 4 to 6 ounces a day, which is a piece that's roughly the size of my palm. I eat mostly lamb, especially when I'm dining out, because it's almost all pasture-raised. Occasionally I'll eat grass-fed beef, bison, or venison.

Limit Processed Meats

As I've discussed, the evidence suggests that there may be some link between processed meats and cancer. However, that risk is small—an increase from an average population risk of 5 percent for colon cancer to a 6 percent risk if you eat processed meat every day. I know that most people can't live without bacon and sausage, so just think of it as a treat, not a staple. Here are some things to look for to reduce the risk from processed meats when you must have them.

- **Avoid preservatives:** Look for bacon, deli meats, ham, and sausages made from whole foods and not full of additives, fillers, preservatives, gluten, and high-fructose corn syrup. Some processed meats also contain nitrates, which are not carcinogenic, but when those nitrates get grilled, charred, or heated to high temperature (over 266°F), they turn into nitrosamines, which are carcinogenic. Slow, low-temperature cooking is best. Heat also creates two other toxic carcinogenic by-products — PAHs (polycyclic aromatic hydrocarbons) and HCAs (heterocyclic amines). Get organic or minimally processed meats. Try Applegate and Niman Ranch brands, which are often carried in most stores and supermarkets.

- **Buy local:** Buy your bacon, sausages, and other processed meats from local farmers. You can find them at your nearest farmers' market, where you can ask about which ingredients or preservatives (if any) they use.
- **Read the label:** Before you buy deli meat or bacon from your local store, read the label to make sure it doesn't contain any of the following: added sugar, high-fructose corn syrup, artificial ingredients, or MSG.
- **Uncured:** Look for processed meat labels that say "uncured." This helps ensure that you're not getting any nasty preservatives or chemicals.
- **Say no to hot dogs:** If there's any meat product you should avoid at all costs, it's hot dogs. They're often loaded with salt and chemicals and made from a combination of animal parts. It's just too

hard to know what you're getting when you buy a hot dog. So, avoid them.

Avoid Charred Meats

Grilled meat may be as American as apple pie. But grilling over an open flame or at very high temperatures can lead to the creation of heterocyclic amines and other carcinogenic compounds. Here are some tips to reduce your exposure:

- **Don't burn it:** Avoid eating burgers and other types of meat that are charred or very well done.
- **Marinate it:** Marinating your meat before you cook it helps reduce the production of toxic compounds. The healthiest, best-tasting marinades contain garlic, onion, and lemon juice.
- **Use rosemary:** A study in the *Journal of Food Science* found that adding rosemary extracts to beef patties before cooking them at high temperatures significantly reduced the production of heterocyclic amines (in some cases by more than 90 percent).[56] Add rosemary to your meat before you cook it.
- **The more spices, the better:** If you're not a fan of rosemary, try other spices. Studies suggest that the antioxidants in many spices help reduce toxin production.[57] That may be why rosemary works. Some other antioxidant-rich spices you can add to your meat before cooking are oregano, basil, paprika, cayenne pepper, turmeric, ginger, and chili.

MEAT: WHAT THE HECK SHOULD I EAT?

- Grass-fed beef
- Grass-fed lamb
- Pasture-raised pork
- Bison
- Venison
- Elk
- Small amounts of high-quality, organic, nitrate-, additive-, and sugar-free bacon, ham, turkey, salami, and sausages

MEAT: WHAT THE HECK SHOULD I AVOID?

- Conventionally raised beef, lamb, or pork (do your best)
- Deli ham and other processed meats
- Hot dogs (if not 100 percent beef or pork)
- Conventional sausage
- Conventionally made bacon
- Conventionally made salami

POULTRY AND EGGS

True or False?

1. It's better to eat chicken than red meat.
2. You should limit your egg intake because the high cholesterol content increases your risk of heart attack.
3. The best type of chicken you can eat is free-range.
4. It's better to eat egg white omelets than whole egg omelets.
5. You shouldn't eat chicken skin because it's bad for you.
6. Pastured eggs are better for you than conventional eggs.

Answers

1. False: The fat composition of grass-fed beef is actually more nutritious. Chickens eat grains and have higher levels of omega-6 fats, which are generally too abundant in our diets to begin with.

2. False: Eating cholesterol doesn't necessarily raise your blood cholesterol levels, and study after study has shown that eating eggs doesn't cause heart attacks.[1]

3. False: The term "free-range" is often misleading and doesn't mean the birds spend much time outdoors. You want to eat 100 percent "pasture-raised."

4. False: The yolk is the most nutritious part of the egg—it contains all the nutrients needed to create a new life. Plus, whole eggs taste better and are more filling. And cholesterol has been exonerated. It doesn't cause heart attacks.

5. True: Chicken skin is unhealthy if it's been cooked to a crisp, which creates harmful chemicals. The skin on baked poultry, however, is okay to eat.

6. True: Pastured chickens eat a healthier diet and live under less stress than conventionally raised birds. When chickens forage and eat insects, it dramatically increases the quality and amount of the nutrients in their eggs.

Get a new food fact and weekly recipe directly from my kitchen. Sign up for free at www.food thebook.com.

In the 1960s, the average American ate almost 65 pounds of beef, 60 pounds of pork, and 35 pounds of poultry every year.[2] But today, America's love of red meat has given way to an obsession with chicken. The average adult now consumes 92 pounds of chicken each year—a 200 percent increase since the Kennedy administration. That's a lot of birds! Meanwhile, the amount of pork and beef on our dinner plates has plunged, with Americans consuming just 56 pounds of beef and 51 pounds of pork annually. So, what happened?

Beef may have been what's for dinner decades ago. But the federal government's dietary guidelines changed all that with the demonization of saturated fat. Beef, veal, lamb, and other types of red meat were cast aside by the nutrition establishment, which began exalting white meat as a healthier alternative. But unfortunately, the USDA's misguided advice unintentionally created an increased demand for poultry that radically transformed the chickens we eat—and not for the better. Industrial tampering has morphed today's chickens from tiny barnyard critters into cheap raw materials for the masses, like coal or lumber. As a result, their meat is neither as nutritious nor as safe as it once was. And as the demand for chickens rose, the quality of their signature product — eggs — also took a nosedive, thanks in part to government fearmongering about cholesterol. The same dietary guidelines that told us to avoid fat and replace it with bread and pasta also told us that egg yolks would raise our cholesterol and give us heart attacks. That advice led generations of Americans to trade in their scrambled eggs and sausages for egg white omelets and potatoes. But those recommendations were wrong. Neither the chicken nor the egg deserved their bad reputations.

THE SCIENCE OF POULTRY

Poultry is a good source of some crucial nutrients: protein (4 ounces of chicken delivers around 30 grams, more than half the recommended daily allowance), B vitamins, choline, and minerals such as selenium, phosphorus, sulfur, and iron. Poultry contains the same amount of monounsaturated fat as olive oil and is a source of palmitoleic acid, which is antimicrobial and fights infection. (And you probably thought "Jewish penicillin" — also known as chicken soup — was a myth!) But today's chicken is nothing like it used to be. Factory farming, which drives down the price of poultry at a steep cost to its quality, reduces the amounts of many of these vitamins, minerals, and nutritious fats to near-negligible levels.

Your great-grandparents probably wouldn't recog-

nize the lean cuts of packaged chicken sold in supermarkets today. The chicken they ate was quite a
different bird. It was often sold in poultry stores that
slaughtered, plucked, and gutted on the spot. That's
about as fresh as it gets. My grandmother used to pluck
chickens in New York City for a nickel apiece and use
that money to go to the movies. Chickens didn't come
with labels telling us what they ate or how they were
raised because they all lived on real farms and ate as
nature intended—omnivorously, mostly on grass,
weeds, bugs, and seeds. So, it's no surprise that the
pasture-raised chickens of yesteryear were nutritionally vastly superior to the conventional birds of today,
which are fed a steady diet of grains, corn, soy, and
antibiotics to fatten them up as quickly as possible,
and raised in unbelievably cramped spaces known
as concentrated animal feeding operations, or CAFOs.
These cruel conditions are not just bad for the birds and
the environment, but bad for you, too. Studies show
that today's chickens have fewer anti-inflammatory
omega-3 fatty acids, more inflammatory omega-6 fatty
acids, and substantially fewer vitamins and minerals.[3]
That leaves you, the consumer, with only one option.
For the sake of your health, the environment, and
animal welfare, you should minimize your dependence on conventionally raised poultry. It's not always
easy. You'll have to make a special effort and, in
some cases, pay a little extra if you want to eat chicken
that is as natural and as wholesome as the birds our

great-grandmothers consumed. Later in this chapter I'll show you how.

WHAT THE EXPERTS GOT RIGHT

Chicken is generally lower in calories and fat than beef, as the food police told us, yet it still delivers the benefits of animal-based nutrition. The thing is, we now know that weight gain and heart disease are not related to calories or fat, but to the quality of calories and the type of fat. As far as eggs go, the authorities were wisest long ago when they made sunny-side ups a breakfast staple. Those eggs were a whole lot better for us than the bagels, muffins, croissants, cereals, and pancakes that took their place.

WHAT THEY GOT WRONG

The experts told us to eat chicken instead of beef because red meat contains saturated fat. Chicken is indeed leaner than red meat. But it still contains saturated fat and cholesterol (neither of which is actually bad for you), just like red meat and every other animal food. In fact, here's how they stack up: The fat in beef is roughly 37 percent saturated; chicken fat is 29 percent saturated; and brook trout fat is 26 percent saturated. The differences are so small that a randomized controlled trial published in the *British Journal of Nutrition* found that red meat and chicken have pretty much the same impact on cholesterol and triglyceride levels in consumers.[4]

As for eggs, what the experts got wrong is one of the biggest nutritional blunders of the past half century. Starting in the 1970s, they told us to limit our daily intake of cholesterol to roughly the amount contained in a single egg. That's right—eat an egg for breakfast and then you're a vegan for the rest of the day. That advice began to wobble a couple of decades later when the American Medical Association published a study involving 118,000 people that found no association between egg consumption and heart disease.[5] Even more striking, the researchers discovered that people who ate half a dozen eggs a week had a lower risk of heart disease than those who ate less than one. A number of other recent studies have also confirmed that the experts who slandered eggs got it wrong. A rigorous, randomized controlled trial published in the *American Journal of Clinical Nutrition* found that eating a dozen eggs per week had almost no effect on cholesterol levels.[6] And another study in *BMJ* found no link between consumption of eggs and heart attacks or strokes.[7]

In 2015, after decades of suggesting that people should throw away the yolk every time they crack open an egg, the panel of experts that shapes the USDA's dietary guidelines finally acknowledged that their recommendation against dietary cholesterol was not supported by scientific evidence.[8] The cholesterol warning, they said, should be dropped from the dietary guidelines. In a stunning revelation, one of the experts involved in creating the recommendations, Alice H. Lichtenstein of Tufts

University, explained that the cholesterol advice had been included in the guidelines for decades without much scrutiny. "For many years, the cholesterol recommendation has been carried forward, but the data just doesn't support it," she told the *New York Times*.[9]

If all that isn't persuasive enough, consider the case of Emma Morano, a 117-year-old Italian woman who, when she died in 2017, held the record for the world's oldest person. A century earlier, a doctor told Morano, who was then twenty, that she was anemic and should eat three eggs a day. She followed her doctor's advice dutifully, eating two to three eggs every day for the next 90 years—a habit she later credited for her remarkable longevity. "Assuming she has been true to her word," the *New York Times* wrote, "Ms. Morano would have consumed around 100,000 eggs in her lifetime, give or take a thousand, cholesterol be damned."[10]

While there is no way to know for sure whether all those eggs had anything to do with Morano's reaching such a ripe and astounding age, it seems pretty clear that eating 100,000 eggs over the course of her lifetime didn't hurt her!

WHAT WE STILL DON'T KNOW FOR SURE

Now that the dietary cholesterol–heart disease link has been debunked, some researchers are warning of another possible danger—a connection between choline, a vitamin contained in egg yolks (and other animal foods), and heart disease. The theory suggests that bacteria in our guts metabolize nutrients in animal foods, such as choline, into a compound called trimethylamine-N-oxide, or TMAO, which may promote atherosclerosis.[11] But that association hasn't been proven, and the theory has some pretty big holes in it. For one thing, the correlation between TMAO and atherosclerosis is based largely on research conducted on mice.[12] And studies show that the foods that create the biggest rise in TMAO in the bloodstream — even bigger than eggs and red meat — are fish. In fact, a randomized controlled trial by researchers at Cornell University found that people had substantially greater increases in TMAO when they ate six ounces of cod than when they ate six ounces of beef or three hard-boiled eggs.[13] Since we know for a fact that eating seafood is protective against heart disease, then it's possible that TMAO levels are not as meaningful as some scientists suspect. "TMAO-rich seafood, which is an important source of protein and vitamins in the Mediterranean diet, has been considered beneficial for the circulatory system," one group of scientists pointed out in the journal *Nutrition*.[14]

For now, we know for sure that choline is a valuable nutrient, important for a healthy liver, proper nerve function, normal brain function, and healthy energy levels. So, while the jury might be out on TMAO, you shouldn't worry about eating foods with choline.

Keep in mind that some opponents of animal-based

foods such as poultry and eggs will never stop claiming that these foods are deadly. They also claim, for example, that eating poultry increases the risk of some cancers. But the best research shows that eating poultry actually reduces your risk.[15] That includes a large systematic review and meta-analysis published in the *American Journal of Clinical Nutrition* in 2010, which showed that higher consumptions of poultry and fish, in particular, were strongly protective against cancer.[16] In another study, published in *Cancer Prevention Research*, scientists at the National Institutes of Health concluded that consuming too much factory-farmed red meat (which is not the same as grass-fed) could increase your disease risk. But replacing it with poultry and seafood had the opposite effect. For every 10-gram increase in fish or poultry intake per day, the risk of liver, colon, esophageal, rectal, lung, and several other types of cancers fell by up to 20 percent.[17]

FIVE THINGS YOU NEED TO KNOW ABOUT POULTRY AND EGGS

1. The Word "Natural" on Chicken Labels Is Meaningless

Shopping for healthy poultry and eggs is among the most complicated, confusing adventures you can embark upon in the grocery store. On its website, the USDA has a glossary of terms appearing on labels that is twenty items long.[18] Here's a partial list, along with some translations into plain English:

- "Natural" is meaningless—of course these animals are natural.
- "Fresh" means only that the poultry was never frozen. It has nothing to do with how recently it was slaughtered.
- "Cage-free" doesn't apply to birds raised for meat, only those raised for eggs. The chickens we eat don't live in cages (though they may still be raised in nightmarish CAFO settings).
- "Free-range" suggests that the animals had some access to the outdoors but doesn't say for how many hours each day or even whether they actually went outside or not. This also doesn't address what the birds were fed.
- "Antibiotic-free" is important, meaning the birds weren't given unnecessary antibiotics or similar drugs just to make them plump. But this label says nothing else about the animals' living conditions *or* what they ate.
- "Arsenic-free," like "antibiotic-free," is good—believe it or not, chickens are fed arsenic to fatten them faster—but this also doesn't tell us anything more.
- "Hormone-free" is totally meaningless because it's illegal to give hormones to poultry (not the case for other animals we eat, however).

- "Vegetarian" is deceptive because it sounds healthy—except that chickens aren't vegetarians. They're supposed to get some insect protein in their diet in the form of worms, bugs, and grubs, which they find outdoors by pecking in the dirt.

- Certified "organic" is the best commonly found label because it guarantees the birds didn't eat grain dosed with pesticides or GMOs and weren't given antibiotics or arsenic to promote fast growth. It also means they may have had some access to the outdoors.

- "Certified humane" or similar labels mean—in theory—that some animal-welfare organization has inspected how the birds are treated and deemed it acceptable. But there have been reports of lax oversight, so it's hard to be sure.

- "Pastured," though not an official designation, is ideal because—if it's accurate—it means that the birds were free to roam outdoors on dirt when they wanted and eat what they liked. Of course, pastured chickens are hardest to find, and usually most costly—easily double the price of conventionally raised chicken.

- The absence of any of the above terminology means that the poultry was conventionally raised, fed an unnatural diet (possibly including arsenic and antibiotics), and treated cruelly. The meat will contain the least amount of nutrients. Due to overcrowded living conditions, the birds will also have been at higher risk of infection. The methods used to grow them and dispose of their manure will also have caused the greatest amount of environmental damage. These, no surprise, will also be the cheapest chickens you can buy. But they're still a terrible bargain.

In January 2017, the federal Office of Management and Budget announced that it had approved a new set of rules called the Organic Livestock and Poultry Practices (OLPP), which set tougher animal-welfare standards for organic farming.[19] This set of measures — the only comprehensive federal law that would regulate the welfare of animals raised for food — aimed to greatly improve the living conditions, health care, transport, and slaughtering process of organic livestock — especially poultry. Among other things, the measures established minimum indoor and outdoor space requirements for chickens. The rules were supposed to go into effect by March 20, 2018. But in February 2017, less than a month after taking office, the Trump administration froze the implementation of the measures. The administration has insisted that it put the rules on hold so it could have time to properly review them,[20] but advocates say the OLPP is now in jeopardy and may not be implemented at all. Let's hope that doesn't happen. If these rules go into effect, as they should, they will not only make life substantially better for all animals raised for food but greatly improve the quality of meat sold to consumers as well.

2. Don't Be Fooled by Misleading Claims on Egg Cartons

Walk into the refrigerated dairy section at any grocery store and you'll see all sorts of labels on the cartons of eggs. Many of them are confusing and hard to decipher. But the labeling system for eggs, while not identical, is fairly similar to the label claims that are slapped on poultry. Here's a rundown:

- "Natural" is meaningless.
- "Fresh" is meaningless.
- "Pure" is not only meaningless; it's laughable.
- "Cage-free" means only that the birds weren't imprisoned for all of their lives, not that they got outside. And it says nothing about their feed or whether they were dosed with antibiotics or arsenic to make them grow.
- "Free-range," the same as "cage-free."
- "Antibiotic-free" is good, as is "arsenic-free," but it says nothing about living conditions.
- "Vegetarian" is bogus since birds are supposed to eat bugs.
- "Hormone-free" is nothing to brag about since hormones in poultry are illegal.
- "Gluten-free"—I actually saw that on an egg carton—is just plain absurd. All eggs are gluten-free, no matter what the chicken ate.

- "Raised on shady porches" — another common label — is misleading because it sounds so homey and old-fashioned. But in poultry farming, a "porch" is an indoor space with a fixed roof but open sides. Not exactly a barnyard.
- "Organic" is the best you can expect to come across, especially given the new OLPP rules I mentioned previously.
- "Pastured" eggs are even better, if you can find them. But unless you're buying your eggs directly from the farmer, these are not so easy to get your hands on.
- Omega-3 eggs are actually good for you. The chickens are fed omega-3-rich flaxseeds.
- If the label says nothing, then the eggs are coming straight from a nightmare farm where thousands of birds are housed in cages so tight that they can't turn around, their beaks are snipped off so they don't peck one another to death, and the manure gathers all around them creating a stench that words can't describe. The eggs aren't so great either.

3. Don't Throw Away the Yolk!

If you're like most people, by now you've probably come to regret all those tasteless egg white omelets and scrambles you ate over the years in your efforts to safeguard your cholesterol levels. Sorry to say it was a wasted effort. You got the protein that egg whites contain, but none of the many other nutrients found in the yolk. That means none of the minerals (calcium, zinc, and phosphorus), vitamins (A, D, E, K, and B complex), antioxidants (like glutathione), or anti-inflammatory omega-3 fats.

Many people still ask: Is it okay to eat the yolks? And the answer is a resounding *YES*. Eat the whole egg, as Mother Nature intended. But if for some reason you still insist on using only egg-white products, you should carefully read the ingredients on the carton. Some brands are 100 percent egg whites, while others contain flavorings, dyes, and thickeners in order to mask the unappetizing taste, color, and consistency of the whites. Haven't you wondered how all those slimy egg whites got so yellow and creamy?

4. Most Poultry Contains Nasty Bacteria

No matter what diet you follow, you're occasionally going to come across some foods that are tainted with harmful bacteria. Even fruits and vegetables are often contaminated with *E. coli* and other nasty bugs. But poultry, across the board, may be the worst offender. In part, this is due to rampant overcrowding at industrial farms. And when chickens are slaughtered in factory-farm conditions, their feces can sometimes come into contact with their skin. Furthermore, the antibiotics that are fed to many chickens (and to other animals we eat) create strains of food-borne bacteria that drugs can't kill. In fact, the use of pharmaceuticals in agriculture is so routine and widespread that more antibiotics are sold nationally for food-producing animals than for people.[21] According to the Food and Drug Administration, 80 percent of antibiotics are used for preventing infection in animals raised in confined conditions and enhancing animal growth (yes, antibiotics make you fat).[22] That leaves 20 percent of all antibiotics for humans. The consequences are dire.

Consumer Reports examined more than 300 raw chicken breasts purchased at stores across the country and discovered that 97 percent tested positive for six harmful bacteria, including *Salmonella, Enterococcus,* and *E. coli.*[23] All the major brands that were tested, including Perdue, Tyson, and Sanderson Farms, contained worrisome bacteria. So did the smaller brands. Most troubling, half of all the chicken breasts tested contained at least one bacterium that was resistant to three or more common families of antibiotics. All those bacteria could potentially cause sickness, hospitalization, and in some cases even death. So, what can you do about it?

First, buy organic poultry whenever possible. Because organic birds aren't fed antibiotics, their meat is less likely to harbor drug-resistant bacteria. Second, always make sure to cook your poultry thoroughly, to at least 165°F internally, which is hot enough to kill off germs.

For similar reasons, eggs are another prime suspect for food poisoning. In fact, eggs are the number two cause — right after leafy greens — of reported outbreaks of food-borne illness.[24] One report by the Center for Science in the Public Interest, a consumer advocacy group, found that between 1990 and 2006 more than 11,000 people fell ill from *Salmonella* poisoning after eating tainted eggs.[25] Eggs are typically contaminated either when the chickens that produce them carry harmful bacteria or when bacteria-laden feces come into contact with the eggshells. So, another precaution you should follow is to make sure that any eggs you eat are clean before you crack them (gently wash them under warm water).

5. Chicken McNuggets Are a Chicken McNightmare

Chickens have wings, not fingers, and they don't have nuggets either — they have flesh. So, it should be obvious that when we say chicken is good to eat, we mean intact chicken meat — not meat that has been processed and turned into something unrecognizable. But a lot of chicken ends up that way, in fast-food joints and restaurants and the frozen-food section of your supermarket. Here's the partial ingredients list from a national brand of frozen chicken nuggets: ground chicken meat, water, soy flour, isolated soy protein, a seasoning blend that includes a long list of ingredients, among them sodium tripolyphosphate (a chemical preservative also used in detergent[26]), and sugar (of course). And that doesn't include what's in the breading and the batter. Earlier, I mentioned the USDA glossary of terms describing various forms of poultry in our food. On that list is this one, which you will find throughout your supermarket if you study ingredients labels: "mechanically separated poultry," which is defined as "a paste-like and batter-like poultry product produced by forcing bones with attached edible tissue through a sieve or similar device under high pressure to separate bone from the edible tissue." In other words, chicken paste. Yum!

I went to Haiti after the earthquake in 2010 to provide medical care, and after days of no food, the military showed up with MREs (meals ready to eat). I asked for one, and they gave me chicken and dumplings. As I was heating it up, I read the label: no chicken! It was a "chicken-like substance." Clearly, not like the chicken Grandma used to make.

The standard-bearer of weirdly manipulated poultry products, the Chicken McNugget, is made of all white meat, McDonald's boasts on its website, and no longer has artificial preservatives. But it continues to contain chemicals like sodium aluminum phosphate, sodium acid pyrophosphate, calcium lactate, monocalcium phosphate—all supposedly safe for human consumption. So far.

GEEK ALERT: A LITTLE MORE SCIENCE ABOUT POULTRY

Why would anyone feed arsenic to a chicken? Because it makes the birds gain weight faster, turns their flesh a little rosier, and kills parasites. Unless the poultry you buy is labeled organic, it almost certainly has been treated with arsenic. Of course, the arsenic the birds are fed doesn't kill them—it's the organic kind, which is harmless. But once they eat it, it can be converted in the chicken's digestive tract to the inorganic kind,[27] which the World Health Organization classifies as a carcinogen.[28]

What does that mean for you? In 2013, researchers at Johns Hopkins University found that conventionally raised chicken from stores all over the country contained inorganic arsenic levels of about two parts per billion. Organic chicken, for comparison, was found to contain an inorganic arsenic level of about half a part per billion. According to federal standards, both levels are below the amounts that could harm us. But the authors of the study took issue with the federal standards. They estimated that the higher arsenic exposure causes an additional 124 annual deaths from lung and bladder cancer. In a country of 300 million people, that's not a huge deal. But do *you* want to be one of those cases?[29] And since there's no benefit from ingesting arsenic at any level, you should minimize your exposure by choosing organic poultry whenever possible.

BIG FOOD COMPANIES CAUSE BIG PROBLEMS

The eco-advocacy group Environment America reported that Tyson Foods is responsible for dumping more waste into US waterways than almost any other company in this country. Between 2010 and 2014, Tyson and its subsidiaries dumped 104 million pounds of pollutants into America's waters—the second-largest toxic discharge reported during those years, behind only AK Steel Holding Corporation.[30] This pollution creates "dead zones" and contaminates drinking water. Another major producer, Perdue Farms, was also on Environment America's top ten list of water polluters. Between 2010 and 2014, the famous chicken firm dumped 31 million pounds of pollutants into rivers, streams, and other waterways.

Chickens raised in these factory farms are often kept in tiny, cramped cages and exposed to very little sunlight. In fact, fewer than 9 percent of hens in the United States are raised without cages, according to United Egg Producers. In 2014, a former Perdue factory worker released a video explaining the true horrors of factory-farmed poultry. It shows USDA certified (not organic) chickens restricted to spaces smaller than a square foot, as well as birds, obviously in pain, walking around with open sores and other deformities.[31] These concentrated animal feeding operations (CAFOs) are also hotbeds for bacterial infections like *Salmonella*, in part because there's no mandate to control such infections on the farms or in hatcheries.

SUMMING IT UP

Whenever possible, you should eat pasture-raised chicken that's been fed an appropriate diet; that means organic but not vegetarian. This chicken meat will be tastiest and most nutritious. Plus, you can feel relatively confident that pasture-raised birds were not subjected to cruel and unsanitary conditions or treated with arsenic or antibiotics. Eating pasture-raised chicken also lessens the risk of food poisoning due to contamination with harmful, potentially deadly bacteria.

Ideally, you should find a trustworthy local source of chicken rather than just buying whatever's available at the supermarket or even the health food store. Most farmers' markets these days include a poultry seller. You should start there. You can even shop for pastured, organic chicken online.

As for eggs, don't be put off by the decades of misinformation. You should eat eggs freely—they're great for you and certainly don't cause heart disease. But you should observe the same rules for eggs as you do for chickens. You want eggs from pastured hens that were fed an organic diet, and you want them as fresh as possible. You can even get omega-3-rich eggs from chickens fed flaxseeds and other omega-3-rich foods. And if you're lucky enough to come across weird eggs—like ones with a bluish shell, or eggs from ducks or turkeys—you should give them a try, just to keep things interesting.

How to Shop for Eggs and Poultry

Buying the best poultry and eggs can be challenging. But fortunately, there are plenty of resources dedicated to helping you find the most sustainable, humane, and nutritious options. If possible, I recommend purchasing your meat from smaller, local farms. These farms create better environments for the chickens and produce less waste than huge slaughterhouses. To find local meat and eggs, visit the following websites:

- **Local Harvest:** This is one of my favorite sites. Go here to find all the farmers' markets, family farms, and other sources of local poultry and eggs in your area: http://www.localharvest.org.
- **Eatwild:** This website is the leading clearinghouse for information about pasture-based farming. It has a state-by-state directory that you can use to find local farmers who sell pasture-raised poultry in your neck of the woods: http://eatwild.com.
- **Eat Well Guide:** You can use this free and excellent online directory to find sustainably raised poultry and eggs from supermarkets, stores, farms, restaurants, and all sorts of retail websites: http://www.eatwellguide.org/.
- **Farmers' markets:** The USDA maintains a national listing of farmers' markets on its website: https://www.ams.usda.gov/services/local-regional.

- **ButcherBox:** This is an online source of organic and grass-fed animal foods: www.butcherbox.com/drhyman-fans/.
- **Walden Meats:** This is an online source of organic, grass-fed meat in New England and parts of New York State: www.waldenlocalmeat.com.

How to Prepare Your Poultry

Here are some guidelines to keep in mind.

- **Don't burn it:** Take care not to char or deep-fry your poultry, which creates unhealthy substances. That means no grilling over high heat to get crispy skin.
- **Baked is better:** Baking, braising, stewing, or sautéing your chicken is your best option. But you have to make sure you cook it all the way through. Use a food thermometer to ensure that your poultry's internal temperature reaches 165°F.
- **Beware of bacteria:** Raw poultry should never touch other food or even sit uncovered in the fridge or on a counter. The plastic wrap should be trashed immediately, and utensils such as knives should be cleaned thoroughly before they're used on anything else.
- **Clean it well:** Consider using a separate cutting board for raw poultry, or spray the board with a mixture of water and a touch of hydrogen peroxide when cleaning it. If you have a good dishwasher, be

sure to rinse the cutting board and put it directly in the machine.

■ **Wash thoroughly:** Always wash your hands after preparing raw chicken. Don't worry about using antibacterial soap. Plain soap and hot water work just fine.

What About Duck and Turkey?

Other poultry are fine (and duck, in particular, is very nutritious), as long as you follow the chicken rules — pastured, organic, and, if possible, from a known source. Use the resources provided for chicken to guide you to local, pasture-raised, or organic duck and turkey.

How to Cook Your Eggs

There are people who eat (or drink) their eggs raw, for maximum nutrition, something I would never do unless I was *extremely* confident that the eggs had been handled safely. It's smarter to soft-boil, poach, or otherwise lightly cook your eggs in grass-fed butter, ghee, or organic coconut oil so that the yolk is still runny. If it gets too hot, you risk oxidizing precious fats. Liquid yolks also retain their nutrients much better.

Is It Okay to Eat Egg Whites?

Sure — along with the yolk. Buying cartons of separated egg whites unnecessarily increases your processed food intake. And eating egg white omelets deprives you of good-tasting, nutritious meals for no good reason.

POULTRY: WHAT THE HECK SHOULD I EAT?

- Organic or pasture-raised whole chicken
- Organic or pasture-raised turkey or duck
- Pasture-raised, organic, or omega-3 whole eggs

POULTRY: WHAT THE HECK SHOULD I AVOID?

- Conventionally raised chicken, turkey, or duck
- All processed poultry
- Eggs from conventionally raised poultry
- Egg whites

AND WHAT ABOUT CHICKEN NUGGETS?

Do you really have to ask?

MILK AND DAIRY

NUTRITION IQ QUIZ

True or False?

1. Low-fat milk is better for you than whole milk.
2. Children need to drink milk to build strong bones and teeth.
3. Dairy is a great source of vitamin D.
4. Butter causes heart disease.
5. Yogurt is a health food.
6. Lactose intolerance affects most adults.
7. Butter can help prevent diabetes and has no effect on the risk of heart disease.

Answers

1. False: Fat is among the healthiest things in milk. In fact, low-fat milk has been linked to higher rates of obesity in children and many other health problems.[1]
2. False: Vegetables are actually a much better source of calcium. And despite the "conventional wisdom,"

also known as dairy industry propaganda, high intakes of milk are linked to *higher* rates of osteoporosis.[2]

3. False: Skim milk naturally has no vitamin D, and whole milk contains only trace amounts. Milk is "fortified" with vitamin D. Mushrooms and liver are better sources, as is sunlight.

4. False: Butter, at worst, has a neutral effect on our cardiovascular system. Real butter is healthier than all butter substitutes, including margarine and vegetable oil spreads (except olive oil).

5. Maybe: Yogurt can be healthy, depending on how you eat it, but most of it is little better than junk food. Your morning Yoplait yogurt has the same amount of sugar per ounce as Coke. It's a dessert, not a breakfast! Grass-fed sheep, goat, or cow yogurt, unsweetened and with live cultures, can be part of a healthy diet for those of us who are not sensitive or allergic to dairy.

6. True: Most adults can't properly metabolize lactose. About 70 percent of the world's population can't digest dairy, and for many others it can cause cancer, autoimmune disease, and acne.

7. True: A study that followed 3,000 people for more than 15 years found a 30 to 40 percent reduction in the rate of type 2 diabetes among those who had the highest levels of butterfat in

their blood, and there was no link found between butter and heart disease.[3]

Get a new food fact and weekly recipe directly from my kitchen. Sign up for free at www.food thebook.com.

If someone handed you a beverage that you knew would cause you weight gain, bloating, acne, gas, allergies, eczema, brittle bones, and possibly even cancer, would you drink it? Would you chug 3 cups of that liquid daily and give 2 cups of it to your children?

Probably not.

Yet the federal government tells us that milk is a perfect food that Americans should lap up daily—in spite of a large (and growing) body of research showing its lack of benefits and awful side effects. Humans are the only species that continues to drink milk after weaning. And the milk we drink today is not what our grandparents drank. Nowadays, cows' milk contains dozens of reproductive hormones, allergenic proteins, antibiotics, and growth factors, some of which are known to promote cancer, such as IGF-1 (insulin-like growth factor).[4]

Thanks to bad science, the food lobby, and the junk-food industry's influence on research, Americans have been fed a lot of lies and misinformation about their food. But only dairy has inspired wrong advice from all sides. The government's dietary guidelines say that adults should drink at least 3 cups of milk daily and that children should drink at least 2, so we can all get plenty of calcium and other nutrients that protect our bones and our health. But as we'll see, the evidence just isn't there. In fact, studies show that milk may actually make our bones weaker. On top of that, there are plenty of better, richer, healthier sources of calcium in food.

At the other end of the spectrum are the scientists and nutritionists who warned us against full-fat dairy products under the premise that saturated fat causes heart disease. They were wrong about that, too. And their bad advice has resulted in a generation of kids growing up on sugary, fat-free chocolate milk, which is worse than whole milk in every single way. In fact, low-fat sweetened milk makes kids hungrier and more likely to become obese. It's not the fat in milk that's the problem; studies show it's not connected to heart disease.[5] It's all the other bad stuff in there that we need to worry about.

Most people can't even stomach milk: As mentioned in the answers to this chapter's Nutrition IQ Quiz, about 70 percent of the world's population suffers from milk-induced digestive distress because of lactose intolerance.[6] One of milk's main proteins has been linked to cancer of the prostate.[7] Dairy causes problems in people who have irritable bowel syndrome and leaky gut.[8] Milk allergies are common, especially among children.

Got milk? I sure hope not.

THE SCIENCE OF DAIRY

Milk and other dairy products contain some good things—vitamins A, B_6, B_{12}, and D (but only because it is added), plus calcium, magnesium, niacin, riboflavin, selenium, and zinc. They also have a substantial amount of fatty acids, both the saturated and unsaturated kinds, some of which are extremely healthy. But all milk has one purpose: to make living things grow. So why would adults consume it? In most people, the production of lactase, the enzyme that digests dairy, begins to plummet around age two. That fact alone should tell you how our bodies feel about consuming dairy beyond childhood.[9]

But milk tastes good, and to people in parts of the world with few options, it's a nutrient-rich food. Masai tribesmen in Africa, for example, have historically lived largely on a diet of grass-fed milk, meat, and blood without suffering any ill effects. Humans have been consuming dairy in some form or another pretty much everywhere on earth over the course of millennia, mostly in traditional, wholesome forms. If you couldn't afford meat, dairy was the next best thing— instead of slaughtering a cow once, you could milk it for years. But the "heirloom" cows of yesteryear are not the breeds of today. Now we have genetically "improved" varieties that produce proteins our bodies don't recognize. Cows' milk is one of the first and most common causes of food allergy in early childhood.[10] Scientists have identified several different milk allergens,[11] most notably the casein proteins, which can induce inflammation that leads to eczema,[12] ear infections,[13] congestion, and sinus problems.[14]

While a big, cold glass of milk has long been America's national beverage, many people are rightfully becoming doubtful about dairy. In fact, annual US consumption of fluid milk dropped from 247 pounds per person in 1975 to 155 pounds in 2015. During that same period, ice cream consumption declined from 18.2 pounds to 13.1. Considering all the pitfalls of modern, industrialized dairy production and consumption, those trends are a good thing.

WHAT THE EXPERTS GOT RIGHT

Nothing, honestly. All the pro-milk advice was mainly intended to benefit the health of the dairy industry, not the public. In fact, a huge initiative by our own government (the USDA) created the National Dairy Promotion and Research Board, which funded, in partnership with the industry lobby group the National Dairy Council, many of the pro-dairy ads, public health campaigns, and dietary guidelines. Remember that famous ad slogan, "Milk: It does a body good"? Well, it doesn't.

WHAT THEY GOT WRONG

They told us milk was good for our bones. They were wrong. They said we should drink low-fat milk. Once again, dead wrong. Most people are allergic to the proteins in dairy or have trouble digesting them. But, as we'll see, the rest of us have plenty of other reasons to avoid milk, too.

WHAT WE STILL DON'T KNOW FOR SURE

By now the science is pretty much settled. There may be some benefits from modest amounts of yogurt and kefir, and butter and cheese, as well. Other than that, however, milk's halo is probably gone for good. Yet our government's dietary guidelines still recommend that we consume lots of dairy, specifically low-fat dairy, both ideas unsupported by the science but promoted by the dairy lobby. Sadly, science does not inform policy when money pollutes politics.

EIGHT THINGS YOU NEED TO KNOW ABOUT DAIRY

1. Big Dairy Is Behind the Guidelines

On the website for its MyPlate initiative, the Department of Agriculture asks Americans: "Got Your Dairy Today?" What follows are ten tips intended "to help you eat and drink more fat-free or low-fat dairy foods." The agency even encourages parents to drink milk to set an example for their children.

"Parents who drink milk and eat dairy foods show

their kids that it is important," the USDA says.[15] "Dairy foods are especially important to build the growing bones of kids and teens. Eat or drink low-fat or fat-free dairy foods with meals and snacks—for everyone's benefit."

But it wasn't always that way. When the federal government published its Dietary Goals for the United States—MyPlate's predecessor—in 1977, milk did not receive special status or any mention to increase dairy products. The report wasn't explicitly anti-milk, but it did not include dairy products in its final recommendations. That report was not viewed favorably by the dairy industry, which lobbied Congress to include a more full-throated endorsement in future guidelines. Congress obliged by creating a dairy promotion board and the dairy "check off" program, which funds dairy research and pays for milk ads, including the famous "Got Milk" campaign. The industry stepped up its spending in Washington and pressured the USDA, pushing it to reverse its stance on milk. By the time the government released its first food pyramid recommendations in 1992, it had done a one-eighty, recommending that adults drink at least 2 cups of milk each day. When they finally replaced the outdated food pyramid with MyPlate, the milk recommendation for adults was cemented at 3 cups per day.

Today, the $47-billion-a-year dairy industry[16] is one of the most influential food lobbies on Capitol Hill.

According to the Center for Responsive Politics, a nonpartisan group that tracks money in politics, the dairy industry gave nearly $46 million to politicians between 1990 and 2016.[17] And it's not just Congress that is feeding on the dairy udder. In 2015, the committee of scientific experts that shapes US dietary guidelines included not one but two different members with financial ties to Big Dairy. One was a paid scientific consultant to the national Milk Processor Education Program, and the other was a member of the Dannon Institute Scientific Council.[18] Furthermore, the dairy industry has spent millions of dollars funding studies that claim that milk offers benefits like weight loss, improved health, and stronger bones. An analysis in the journal *PLOS Medicine* found that nutrition studies funded by Big Dairy were eight times more likely to find health benefits associated with drinking milk than studies that received no industry funding.[19] Now, about those health claims...

2. You Don't Need Milk for Strong Bones

Let's start with the basics. Everyone knows you need calcium for stronger bones, right? Without it, children wouldn't grow up to be big and strong. Adults would easily suffer fractures. And many elderly would be riddled with osteoporosis and their bones would be crumbling to dust.

But there's just no evidence that we need milk to strengthen our bones. For one thing, countries with the lowest milk consumption have the lowest rates of osteo-porosis and fractures, while those with the highest dairy consumption and calcium intake have the highest rates of fractures—a phenomenon called the calcium para-dox.[20] In a large meta-analysis published in 2011,[21] scien-tists compiled data from nine different studies and found that milk consumption did not lower the risk of hip frac-tures in men or women. In another exhaustive meta-analysis that included a dozen prospective studies and nine rigorous clinical trials, researchers found that a higher calcium intake offered no protection against frac-tures; in fact it was linked to a higher risk.[22] The Har-vard Nurses' Health Study[23] and another prospective study in Sweden[24] also found no link between high dairy consumption and decreased risk of fractures.

But surely drinking milk must have some ability to build strong bones in children, right? Otherwise, why would the government mandate that public schools in America serve milk at every meal? That's right, schools can't get their federal lunch money unless they give every kid milk! But again, the evidence shows no ben-efit. A meta-analysis published in the journal *BMJ* combined nineteen randomized controlled trials that looked at calcium intake in more than 2,800 children, and it found that higher levels did not protect against fractures.[25] A large analysis published in *Pediatrics* also assessed the impact of calcium and dairy intake on bone health in children and adolescents. After review-ing fifty-eight studies and clinical trials, the researchers concluded there was "scant evidence" supporting the claim that increased dairy or calcium intake promotes stronger bones.[26] The Penn State Young Women's Health Study followed women between the ages of twelve and eighteen and found that the amount of calcium they consumed had no impact on their bone mineral density as young adults.[27] But physical activity did. The more exercise they got as adolescents and teenagers, the greater their bone mineral density on their eighteenth birthdays. This suggests that when it comes to promoting strong bones in children, encouraging them to play sports is wiser than telling them to drink chocolate milk.

3. Sources of Calcium Without the Added Junk

The studies are clear. There is nothing special about dairy and bone health. The amount of calcium the average person needs is likely far less than the levels recommended in the United States.[28] It's not total calcium intake that matters, but how much calcium you hold on to. These days, we pee out huge amounts of calcium—cigarette smoke, sugar, phosphoric acid in sodas, stress, and caffeine all make us lose the mineral. But we can get adequate levels of calcium from many foods besides milk. Some sources contain even more than dairy, minus the hormones, allergens, and other baggage. The FDA advises Americans to consume 1,000 milligrams of calcium each day. If it's a mineral you're lacking, there are better ways to get it than from dairy. Here's how some common food sources stack up[29]:

- Sesame seeds, ¼ cup: 351 milligrams
- Sardines (with bones), 3¾-ounce can: 351 milligrams
- Tofu, 3½ ounces: 350 milligrams
- Yogurt, 1 cup: 296 milligrams
- Collard greens, 1 cup: 268 milligrams
- Spinach, 1 cup: 245 milligrams
- Cheese, 1 ounce: 204 milligrams
- Turnip greens, 1 cup: 197 milligrams
- Canned sockeye salmon (with bones), 3 ounces: 188 milligrams
- Blackstrap molasses, 1 tablespoon: 180 milligrams
- Mustard greens, 1 cup: 165 milligrams
- Beet greens, 1 cup: 164 milligrams
- Bok choy, 1 cup: 158 milligrams
- Almonds, dry roasted, 2 ounces: 150 milligrams
- Cows' milk, 8 ounces: 276 milligrams

Furthermore, there's even evidence that it's vitamin D, not calcium, that truly strengthens our bones.[30]

4. Milk Increases Your Risk for Cancer

It's not often that the country's top health experts join forces to bring down one of America's most cherished foods. But in an editorial published in *JAMA Pediatrics* in 2013, two of the nation's leading nutrition scientists from Harvard, David Ludwig and Walter Willett, called out the federal government for advising 3 daily cups of low-fat milk for most Americans.[31] Their argument: The milk recommendations are not evidence-based and their potential harms could be severe.

As we saw earlier, milk does not promote bone health. But, as Ludwig and Willett noted, it turns out that it may promote cancer. That's because milk contains a witches' brew of hormones that act like Miracle-Gro for cancer cells. The average glass of milk has sixty different hormones in it. Many are anabolic hormones, which cause cells to grow. That's great for a newborn calf that needs to bulk up fast. But in an adult human, it's bad news. Today's industrial livestock practices keep dairy cows in a constant state of milk production. Cows are often milked while pregnant, so the milk we get from them is brimming with hormones.

The most troubling is IGF-1, a known cancer promoter that's also associated with chronic kidney disease,[32] diabetes,[33] and heart disease.[34] Some of the world's most prominent longevity researchers have found that people with reduced levels of IGF-1 live longer and have lower rates of cancer. But milk pushes your IGF-1 levels in the wrong direction. In a randomized controlled trial of 204 healthy men and women, researchers found that those assigned to follow the government's milk recommendations for twelve weeks had a 10 percent increase in their IGF-1 levels compared to those who drank no milk.[35]

In a report published in 2014, the World Cancer Research Fund compiled numerous studies indicating that men who consume a lot of dairy products have higher rates of cancer.[36] A large study in the *Journal of Nutrition*, for example, linked milk consumption — including skim and low-fat milk — to a higher risk of prostate cancer diagnoses and a greater risk of disease progression.[37] It's possible that men who consume a lot of dairy share other habits that might explain their increased cancer rates. Perhaps they eat a lot of sugar or drink more alcohol. They may also exercise less. But considering what we know about all the cancer-promoting hormones in milk and the dairy proteins that cause allergies and inflammation, why risk it?

5. Dairy Fat Is Not the Problem

The government's dietary guidelines strongly encourage Americans to drink milk. But they specifically recommend low-fat or fat-free versions because of long-standing (misguided) concerns that saturated fat causes heart disease. As I've mentioned, there are plenty of reasons not to eat dairy — but its fat content isn't one of them. In fact, it may be its one redeeming quality.

A landmark review and meta-analysis published in the *Annals of Internal Medicine* in 2014 examined seventy-two of the most rigorous studies on dietary fat and heart disease, including two dozen randomized controlled trials, and concluded that saturated fat and total fat consumption have little effect on heart disease.[38] In fact, the researchers found that consuming margaric acid, a type of saturated fat found in dairy, actually lowers cardiovascular disease risk. A number of other studies have also shown that the fats in dairy help protect against cardiovascular and other diseases. One study published in *Circulation* in 2016 measured the blood levels of different fats in 3,300 adults and found that those who had the highest concentrations of dairy fat in their bloodstreams were 30 to 40 percent less likely to develop type 2 diabetes.[39] That's right, butter in the blood protected against type 2 diabetes. And grass-fed butter and ghee (butter with the often-allergenic casein and whey removed) don't have most of the problems of milk.

When we remove the fat from dairy, we make it less satiating and promote overeating. Studies have shown that children and adults who drink low-fat milk gain more weight than those who drink whole milk.[40] As Dr. Ludwig wrote in his *JAMA* editorial, "People compensate or overcompensate for the lower calorie content of reduced-fat milk by eating more of other foods."

What's worse is stripping the fat from milk and then replacing it with sugar and artificial flavors to get kids to drink it. Many schools encourage kids to drink chocolate milk loaded with sweeteners under the premise that it's still better than soda. But that's a terrible idea.

Whether it comes from Coca-Cola (39 grams of sugar per 12 ounces) or chocolate milk (29 grams per 12 ounces), sugar drives obesity and undermines health.

If you've ever bought skim or 2 percent milk, you may have noticed that it's supplemented with vitamins A and D. This is required under federal law because removing the fat simultaneously removes these two important vitamins.[41] Whole milk, on the other hand, needs no such supplementation — another reason the fat in dairy is so beneficial. Adding fat-soluble vitamins like A and D back into fat-free milk is also pointless because you need fat to digest these vitamins.

6. Yes, Butter Is Back

As my good friend Dr. Ludwig advises, if you're offered bread and butter, skip the former and eat the latter. The same goes for baked potatoes, muffins, bagels, pancakes, and other foods we commonly pair with a little butter. (One exception: buttered vegetables, because we need fat to properly digest some of the fat-soluble vitamins in plants.) It's only butter combined with starchy carbs or sugar that's the problem.

Butter has had a terrible reputation because it is pure animal fat, much of it saturated, which is precisely the kind the federal government has warned us not to eat. In fact, about 60 percent of the fats in butter are saturated. Roughly 20 percent are monounsaturated (the predominant kind in olive oil) and the rest are polyunsaturated. But, as I've said before, we now know that saturated fat is not the dietary villain it was made out to be. Even better, butter has all of the natural fats found in dairy, with little or none of the problematic proteins and sugars such as casein and lactose.

Butter consumption in the United States has dropped precipitously since the nutrition establishment began its war on fat half a century ago. But with experts now waking up to the realization that carbs and sugar have been responsible for the obesity crisis all along, butter is on the rebound. In 2016 a group of leading scientists did an analysis of nine of the best studies on butter and health, which included consumption data on 636,000 people over many years (6.5 million person-years to be exact), and concluded that there was no link between butter and heart disease. They also found that butter is protective against diabetes.[42]

That doesn't mean you should eat butter with abandon. But it's fine to eat it like our grandparents did. They all ate grass-fed butter (there was no other kind at the time), and you should too because it has fewer toxins, better fats, and more antioxidants. In fact, grass-fed butter is one of the best sources of conjugated linoleic acid (CLA), which boosts your metabolism and helps prevent cancer and heart disease. Feel free to cook your eggs in butter. Melt a little on your veggies. Or slap a pat on your broiled fish. Butter adds texture, flavor, and moisture to your food. There's a reason chefs love it.

7. Grass-Fed Dairy Is the Kind You Should Eat

As we will discuss in the chapter on fats, Americans are consuming a diet that's too rich in inflammatory omega-6 fats and too low in healthy omega-3s. When the ratio of these two fats is lopsided, it sets the stage for chronic inflammation and disease. But the old adage that you are what you eat applies not only to humans but to cattle as well. Cows that graze on their natural diet of grass produce milk (and meat) with a better composition of fats and nutrients than cows that are fed corn, soy, and grains.

If you're going to consume butter or other dairy products, remember that grass-fed is best. The milk these cows produce has an omega-6 to omega-3 ratio of 1:1,[43] which is optimal. Conventionally raised cows eat grains and other crops that make their fatty-acid profiles more inflammatory. The milk they produce—and as a result the butter and cheese made from it—is heavily skewed toward omega-6 fats.[44] Organic dairy is somewhere in the middle. These products come from cows that are given some access to pasture. The rest of their diet comes from organic grains and feed that are free of pesticides, herbicides, and antibiotics. As a result, the milk they produce has a better ratio of fats than conventional dairy. But grass-fed is still best. It contains not only the best ratio of the essential fatty acids, but also the highest levels of carotene, vitamin A, and CLA, which has beneficial effects on metabolism.

I also recommend probiotic-rich dairy like kefir and yogurt (as long as they're grass-fed and not full of added sugar). I like clarified butter, which has all the water and milk solids removed (which means it can be used by those who are allergic to dairy). I also like organic, grass-fed ghee, the traditional Indian form of butter. It has all the great nutrients and fatty acids, but a higher smoking point, which makes it ideal for high-heat cooking and searing.

For a lot of people, it's hard to live without cheese—and you don't necessarily have to. It's okay to eat good-quality, locally sourced cheeses or, better yet, goats' and sheep's cheeses like Feta, Manchego, and Pecorino, and look for Humboldt Fog brand cheeses. Just be sure to avoid the industrially processed types, like prepackaged Swiss, cheddar, and American, which are full of hormones, allergens, and additives. If your great-grandmother didn't eat it, then you shouldn't either. Take, for example, Kraft American "cheese": Government regulations don't allow it to be called cheese because it is less than 51 percent cheese. It has to be called a "pasteurized prepared cheese product." Yuck!

8. Goats' Milk Is Different from Cows' Milk

You might be wondering about other forms of milk, such as goats' milk. For many, cows' milk is very inflammatory, causing gut issues, allergies, eczema, and acne. That's because modern cows have been bred to have high levels of A1 casein, which is much more inflammatory than A2 casein, which was present in cows of yesteryear. The good news is that goats' milk has only A2 casein and is not inflammatory. It is also easier to digest and doesn't cause stomach discomfort for most. Additionally, it has high levels of medium-chain triglycerides (MCTs), which boost metabolism and brain function, and higher levels of vitamin A, which is good for your skin. Studies have found that people who consume milk with A2 casein avoid the gastrointestinal symptoms, reduce inflammatory bio-markers, and improve cognitive function (likely from the MCTs in goats' milk).[45] So goats' milk can be a good alternative to cows' milk.

Also, A2 milk boosts the powerful detoxifying antioxidant compound called glutathione. Regular milk, with A1 casein, forms *caseomorphins*, which act like addictive morphine-like peptides that have negative consequences for your brain and behavior (especially in the case of ADHD and autism).[46] Ever wonder why people binge on dairy products or don't want to give them up? The A1 casein also seems to be a trigger for autoimmunity and diabetes, while the A2 casein doesn't have the same negative effect.[47]

GEEK ALERT: A LITTLE MORE SCIENCE AND THE POLITICS OF DAIRY

It's one of the hottest battlegrounds in food today—the debate over whether it's a good idea to consume products made with milk that has not been pasteurized—in other words, raw milk. On the one hand, as we've said throughout this book, it's healthiest to eat whole foods that have been processed as little as possible. But do the benefits of raw milk outweigh the risks? It depends on whom you ask. The conventional wisdom says beware: The federal government makes it a crime to sell unpasteurized dairy across state lines, and, as of 2016, twenty states have outlawed all sales of raw milk. In seventeen states, raw milk is legal, but only if you buy it on the farm where it was produced; in thirteen states you can also buy it in stores; and in eight states it's legal only if purchased through a "cow share" agreement.[48] But the laws are always changing due to food activist efforts. All this caution is understandable, since people do get sick and even die from consuming raw milk that's contaminated with *E. coli*, *Salmonella*, listeria, campylobacter, parasites, and viruses, all of which are eliminated by pasteurization. Studies show that between 2007 and 2012, the number of disease outbreaks caused by raw milk consumption in the United States almost doubled.[49]

But, raw-dairy advocates argue, serious and even fatal outbreaks of food poisoning are caused by *everything* we eat—vegetables, fruit, poultry, eggs, meat, the works. So why single out dairy? The case in favor of unpasteurized dairy goes like this[50]: Heating milk kills some of the vitamin content. That's true. Some people say they have difficulty digesting pasteurized milk, but no such problems with raw. That may also be true, even if it's hard to prove. And it's virtually certain that raw milk comes from pastured, grass-fed cows, which is a definite improvement over conventionally raised dairy.

In the end, this fight is as much about the freedom to choose the foods we want, without government interference, as it is about nutrition or health. Raw milk usually comes from small farm operations, a plus in the eyes of some conscientious eaters who shun anything that comes from Big Agriculture or Big Dairy. But the bottom line is that adults shouldn't be consuming very much milk at all, of any kind. We can get all the nutrients it contains from safer sources.

Cheese made with raw milk is a slightly different story: It's allowed in the United States as long as it's been aged for sixty days or more. Most connoisseurs today favor artisanal varieties made with raw dairy. But we should go easy on cheese, too — it's a "sometimes" treat.

THE ENVIRONMENTAL AND ETHICAL IMPACT OF DAIRY

Dairy is terrible for the environment. Roughly 19 percent of the water used in animal agriculture is consumed by dairy farming.[51] In the United States alone, there are about 9 million dairy cows. The cows need to stay hydrated; the farm floors and walls need to be washed;

growing feed requires water. According to One Green Planet, "When you add up the water used for growing food, drinking water, and cleaning the facility, the average dairy cow uses 4,954 gallons of water per day."[52] Additionally, when it comes to food production, cheese making generates the third-highest amount of greenhouse gas emissions, behind only meat and poultry. How can that be? Well, it takes about 10 pounds of milk (1 gallon) to produce 1 pound of cheese. It takes 2 gallons of milk to make a pound of butter. Dairy-cow manure emits a lot of methane gas and nitrous oxide, and with all the resources used to create feed for the cows, the footprint adds up. There are less dense cheeses that require less milk, like ricotta, cottage cheese, and mozzarella. So, if you're worried about the carbon footprint of your food but you still love cheese, these options might leave you feeling a bit better. As far as butter, stick to the grass-fed variety, which is healthier and helps cut down on emissions from feed production.

The dairy industry wants us to believe that their cows are happily producing milk and grazing through green pastures, but for the most part, that couldn't be further from the truth. In fact, dairy cows are often denied access to pastures, and they live in small, filthy quarters while they are pumped for more and more milk. Calves are quickly taken from their mothers and fed cheap powdered milk filled with antibiotics so farmers can sell every drop their mothers produce.

The only animals meant to drink cows' milk are the ones denied access to it.

Unlike cows, goats and sheep are not typically found on mega-farms, so their milk is generally more ethically produced than cows'. Goats and sheep also produce less methane gas than cows, and since they are smaller, they require fewer resources.

When buying a dairy product, you should look for one of the following certifications on the label to ensure that it was produced in an ethical manner:

- Animal Welfare Approved
- Certified Humane
- American Humane Certified
- Food Alliance Certified
- Global Animal Partnership

Smaller local farms that actually allow their cows to roam on the pasture are better for the environment and better for the animals. And although dairy products from such farms are better for you, most humans are prone to health troubles from eating dairy, so go easy. And if you have any chronic illness or symptoms, getting off dairy for two to three weeks can help you see if it is contributing.

- For a directory of local dairy farms and grass-fed products, visit: http://www.eatwild.com/.

- For pasture-fed, unprocessed, full-fat milk in your area, visit: http://www.realmilk.com/real-milk-finder/.
- For information about whether your favorite milk is ethical and sustainable, look up its rating here: https://www.cornucopia.org/dairysurvey/index.html.

SUMMING IT UP

If you're lactose intolerant or sensitive to dairy, then you should avoid it at all costs. But even if you are tolerant, it shouldn't be a major part of your diet. Milk from conventionally raised cows is full of hormones, chemicals, and inflammatory compounds. Stay away from it, and reduce your intake of all other industrially produced cheeses or dairy products.

If you suffer from digestive issues; autoimmune disease; weight gain; type 2 diabetes; PMS; infertility; heavy menstrual bleeding; skin disorders like acne, eczema, or psoriasis; allergies; sinusitis; or any chronic disease, you should avoid dairy, or at least do the Blood Sugar Solution 10-Day Detox Diet and then add dairy back in to see how it affects you.

That being said, dairy does not have to be completely off-limits. It's fine to have some grass-fed milk, cheese, and butter from time to time—as long as they're full-fat, free of additives, and ethically and sustainably produced. Try sheep or goat products. They are less inflammatory and easier to digest. Use the resources provided in this section to help you find the best, most responsibly produced options in your area.

DAIRY: WHAT THE HECK SHOULD I EAT?

- Grass-fed whole milk in very small amounts—a splash in your coffee is okay; ideally, use goats' milk
- Grass-fed, full fat, unsweetened yogurt that contains milk and live cultures and nothing else; ideally, use goat or sheep yogurt
- Kefir (fermented cows' milk), following the same rules as for yogurt
- Whole-milk, grass-fed cheese made with no additives
- Butter or ghee, grass-fed, of course
- All these products made with goats' milk or sheep's milk when you can find them, but still in small amounts

Note: Consume these products only if you have no dairy allergies or sensitivities.

DAIRY: WHAT THE HECK SHOULD I AVOID?

- Dairy from conventionally raised cows
- Skim, 1 percent, or 2 percent milk
- Low-fat or nonfat yogurt
- Yogurt that contains fruit, sweetener, additives, or anything extra

- Cheese made from skim milk or reduced-fat milk
- Processed cheese that contains preservatives, additives, flavorings, or anything unnatural sounding (added herbs, pepper, fruit, truffles, etc., are all fine to eat)
- Cheese that comes in a spray can

FISH AND SEAFOOD

NUTRITION IQ QUIZ

True or False?

1. You shouldn't eat shrimp because it contains a lot of cholesterol.
2. Swordfish has the least amount of mercury of any fish.
3. Sushi is a health food.
4. Eating farmed fish is better for you.
5. Sardines are a better source of calcium than milk.
6. White-fleshed fish is more nutritious than dark.

Answers

1. False: Shrimp does contain a lot of cholesterol, but it has little or no impact on your blood cholesterol or your risk of heart attack.
2. False: Swordfish is ranked second in mercury contamination, right behind tilefish. The bigger the fish, the more pollutants it contains.

3. False: Mainly because of the white rice, which is loaded with starch but stripped of all its fiber. Once you take away the rice and the seaweed, there's not much fish in there either.

4. False: Farmed fish are fed soy, grains, and other foods they shouldn't eat. They're forced to swim in their own feces and they're often infested with parasites. And farmed fish contain high levels of dioxin, PCBs, and mercury.[1]

5. True: Wild-caught sardines are great sources of calcium, omega-3 fats, and choline needed for a healthy brain and liver.

6. False: You need to eat dark, fatty fish such as sardines, mackerel, herring, and anchovies to get all the benefits of seafood. Tuna is full of omega-3 fats, but also very high in mercury. Whitefish generally contains lower omega-3 fats, except for halibut and Chilean sea bass. The only problem is that both of those are high in mercury.

Get a new food fact and weekly recipe directly from my kitchen. Sign up for free at www.food thebook.com.

Perhaps it's possible to be a healthy person who doesn't eat fish—but it isn't easy. We've known for a long time that eating seafood is a wise idea. Anthropologists say one reason the earliest human settlements sprang up near coastlines and large bodies of water is that fish consumption helped our ancestors develop larger brains.[2]

The notion that fish is brain food is not just an old wives' tale. Our brains are more than half fat, and even developing fetuses need the omega-3 fats found in fish.[3] In addition to benefiting our brains, nervous systems, hearts, and cardiovascular systems,[4] large studies have found that omega-3 fats also protect against type 2 diabetes,[5] inflammation, autoimmune disease,[6] and even depression.[7] But fish are almost too nutritious for their own good. Global demand has grown so rapidly that we're depleting the oceans, turning fishing into an unsustainable practice. As a result, countries across the globe are increasingly relying on factory-farmed fish operations. That may seem like a good solution to the problem of overfishing, but in reality, it brings a whole new set of health and environmental challenges to the dinner table.

Half of the seafood Americans consume comes from farms. According to researchers at Johns Hopkins, it's the fastest-growing food-animal sector, ahead of even the beef and poultry industries.[8] Aquaculture production has nearly tripled in the last two decades, bringing with it a significant increase in the use of antibiotics to quell diseases and infections that run rampant in overcrowded factory fish farms.[9] Traditionally, farmed fish were raised on manufactured feed mostly composed of fishmeal and fish oil derived from wild fish, which is similar to their natural diets (carnivorous fish eat smaller guys in the wild). But feeding the growing numbers of farmed fish high-quality food has become unsustainable. So instead, many farmed fish are now given manufactured feed that consists of corn, wheat, soy, and vegetable oils like canola — none of which are found in their natural diets — or meal that can contain toxic chemicals.[10]

Eating wild fish is best. But even then, you're not entirely in the clear because there is still the very real problem of pollution. The coal and gas industries have spent decades dumping mercury and other contaminants into our oceans and rivers, and although we can't see these chemicals, they're absorbed by fish and then by those who eat them (translation: you and me!). All of which means that eating seafood these days has become a balancing act. As you'll see in this chapter, it's possible to get all the benefits of fish while minimizing any potential downsides. You'll need to do your homework, but don't worry, I am here to help!

THE SCIENCE OF FISH

Seafood is one of the best dietary sources of protein around, and it's chock-full of nutrients like iodine, selenium, and vitamins D and B_{12}. But the biggest health benefits of fish come from the two omega-3 fatty acids that we get from them and nowhere else. It's these polyunsaturated fats—docosahexaenoic acid and eicosapentaenoic acid, better known as DHA and EPA, respectively—that make fish the flesh of choice for healthy eaters. Some of the primary benefits of DHA and EPA are cardiovascular. Eating salmon twice a week is enough to cut your risk of a heart attack, arrhythmia, stroke, high blood pressure, and high triglycerides.[11] Similar benefits come from eating other fish high in omega-3s, especially small baitfish such as sardines, herring, mackerel, trout, and anchovies.

The omega-3 fatty acids are so special that virtually every health authority agrees that they belong in your diet. They're a big part of the reason fish consumption lowers the risk of cancer, type 2 diabetes, rheumatoid arthritis, and other autoimmune diseases,[12] as well as depression and inflammation. In a landmark study of omega-3 fats published in the *Lancet*, 11,000 people who had recently suffered a heart attack were randomly assigned to consume either 300 milligrams of vitamin E or 1 gram of omega-3 fats daily. The study found that taking vitamin E showed no apparent benefits. But the people assigned to consume more omega-3s had a 20 percent reduction in mortality.[13] In another study published in the *Lancet*, researchers recruited thousands of heart patients who were on statins, antiplatelet drugs, and other medications, and assigned one group to start taking daily fish oil supplements in addition to their medication. Compared to a control group, the group that took the fish oil experienced a 19 percent reduction in heart attacks and other major coronary events.[14]

It is true, as my vegan friends point out, that walnuts, flaxseeds, and a few other plant foods contain a third type of fatty acid, ALA, that our bodies can convert into DHA and EPA. But the conversion rate is extremely low—we access less than 10 percent of it, which is far from enough. One study published in the *American Journal of Clinical Nutrition* reviewed the effects of omega-3s on blood clots, LDL cholesterol, triglycerides, colitis, and other conditions and concluded that "[omega-3 fats] should be included in the diets of all humans."[15] As we'll see in the chapter on fats and oils, a big concern in nutrition today is the ratio of omega-3 to omega-6 fats in your diet. We're getting too little of the former and too much of the latter, and this is causing widespread chronic inflammation, the underlying cause of today's most prevalent deadly diseases. This imbalance has even been blamed for mental health problems, like violent behavior, including homicide and suicide as well as depression.[16]

The omega-6s come from ultraprocessed junk foods made with refined grains and processed oils—while the best sources of omega-3s come straight from the sea or wild or grass-fed animals.

WHAT THE EXPERTS GOT RIGHT

Has there ever been a time when we weren't advised to eat fish? I don't think so, even though many Americans wound up eating seafood in ways that are nutritionally less than optimal. We gravitated toward the wrong kinds: fish sticks, fish and chips, or deep-fried fish fillet sandwiches from McDonald's. There are also federal guidelines cautioning pregnant women and children to limit consumption of tuna and other mercury-containing fish.

WHAT THEY GOT WRONG

For more than 35 years the federal government's US Dietary Guidelines told us to limit our intake of foods rich in dietary cholesterol, including shrimp, because of the mistaken belief that eating it would promote heart disease.[17] That was wrong. It's now clear that for most people the cholesterol in shellfish and eggs does not elevate the amount of cholesterol in their blood or increase the risk of heart attacks. After reviewing all the current research on the link between dietary cholesterol and heart disease, the 2015 Dietary Guidelines eliminated any restriction on dietary cholesterol, quietly declaring that it is "no longer a nutrient of concern." The government assumed (and so did nearly all nutritionists and doctors) that if blood cholesterol is bad, dietary cholesterol must be bad too. Except it was never proven and is not true. Beyond the cholesterol issue, government guidelines did encourage us to eat fish but failed to explain that not all varieties are created equal. All seafood contains omega-3 fats, but some more than others, and some are more sustainable and less likely to carry toxins.

EIGHT THINGS YOU SHOULD KNOW ABOUT FISH

1. Small Fish Are the Best Fish!

Much like our preference for vegetables, the fish that Americans love the most tend to be the kinds that are the least nutritious, like tilapia and farmed catfish. Americans often opt for the pale, mild-tasting varieties that are lowest in omega-3s, rather than the dark, oily, stronger-tasting fish that are better for you. The lists that follow show which fish are highest and lowest in omega-3s, as well as which fish are most popular with consumers. The best fish to eat are small wild salmon and smaller, toxin-free kinds such as sardines, herring, anchovies, and mackerel, which are brimming with omega-3s. I call them the SMASH fish (salmon, mackerel, anchovies, sardines, and herring). I always tell people that if you can fit the entire fish in your pan, then it's probably a good choice. Larger fish are higher on the oceanic food chain, and as a result they accumulate more mercury, PCBs, and other toxins. That's why you should stay away from swordfish, Chilean sea bass, halibut, and tuna. The toxins these big fish accumulate outweigh the benefits from their omega-3s.

These are the varieties of seafood that are highest in omega-3s[18]:

- Sardines (canned or fresh)
- Herring (especially wild-caught)
- Salmon (wild-caught)
- Mackerel (Atlantic or Pacific, not king)
- Trout (especially farmed rainbow trout)
- Oysters
- Mussels
- Tuna (canned or fresh)*
- Swordfish*

These varieties are relatively low in omega-3s:

- Sole
- Tilapia

---

* These last two should be eaten infrequently because of mercury contamination. In fact, I would never eat swordfish. Limit tuna to once a month.

- Flounder
- Cod
- Snapper
- Lobster
- Scallops
- Shrimp
- Crab

2. Fish Goes to Your Head

Need more proof that fish is brain food? There's evidence that DHA and EPA are more effective than psychotherapy and antidepressants in treating depression.[19] Researchers at the Yale Child Study Center found that the fats in fish can improve symptoms of attention deficit hyperactivity disorder in children.[20] They have even been found to reduce acts of aggression and rule breaking among prisoners.[21] And in a major study published in the *Journal of Clinical Psychiatry*, scientists at the National Institutes of Health found that members of the US military who have the lowest omega-3 levels also have the highest risk of committing suicide.[22] "The findings add to an extensive body of research that points to a fundamental role for DHA and other omega-3 fatty acids in protecting against mental health problems and suicide risks," said the lead author of the study, Dr. Joseph Hibbeln, a military researcher.[23] In his decades of research on fats and brain health, Dr. Hibbeln has found that diets low in omega-3 fats and heavy in omega-6 fats are linked to higher rates of violent crime, psychosis, suicide, and even homicide.[24]

3. But Pregnant Women Aren't Getting Enough

Our brains are largely made of fat, primarily the omega-3 fatty acid DHA. This is the main reason the Food and Drug Administration advises pregnant women to eat two to three servings (roughly 8 to 12 ounces) of low-mercury fish[25] per week: It makes their babies smarter. In a study published in the *American Journal of Epidemiology*, children born to mothers who regularly ate low-mercury fish scored 2 to 6 points higher on intelligence tests than children whose mothers consumed little or no fish. The authors concluded, "Higher fish intake was associated with better child cognitive test performance, and higher mercury levels with poorer test scores."[26] But according to an FDA analysis of fish consumption among pregnant women,[27] "21 percent of them ate no fish in the previous month, and those who ate fish ate far less than the Dietary Guidelines for Americans recommends."

For the sake of their babies, pregnant women should consume at a minimum 8 ounces and ideally 12 ounces of fish per week, preferably wild salmon, sardines, herring, mackerel, and anchovies. Better yet, they should take fish oil supplements. Omega-3s are important during breastfeeding, too. A study in the *American Journal of Clinical Nutrition* compared infants whose diets were supplemented with omega-3 fats to those whose diets were not. The study then tested them when they were between three and five years old and found that the group that consumed omega-3 fats as infants did better on some mental tasks.[28] To totally prevent any exposure to mercury or toxins, I recommend that women eat only sardines or herring and take fish oil supplements.

4. Your Fish Could Be Fake!

As demand for fish has increased, so, too, has fraud. As we see with extra virgin olive oil, the stakes are too high for crooks to resist. In 2016 the nonprofit conservation group Oceana published a review of 200 published studies from fifty-five countries, which found that as many as one in five samples of fish were intentionally mislabeled.[29] In the United States alone, the figure may be as high as 28 percent. The motive is economic—fish that are cheaper, endangered, or unsafe to eat because of contamination are being substituted for the costlier, safer varieties that consumers are paying for. The Oceana report found that 87 percent of snapper sampled nationwide was mislabeled. Is this a health hazard? It certainly could be—any time you don't know what you're eating, you're vulnerable. In other cases, consumers have been duped into eating endangered species. In one instance, a pair of sushi chefs at a restaurant in Santa Monica disguised meat from endangered whales as fatty tuna and sold it to their customers.[30] You can improve your odds of actually getting what you want by buying from fish sellers who are knowledgeable and trustworthy. Another way to tell: If the price of that wild salmon you're thinking of buying at the grocery store seems too good to be true, then it probably is.

5. Canned Fish Is Okay, but Not Every Kind

Americans love canned tuna—it's convenient, it's affordable, kids will eat it, and it can be stored for months. It has lots of omega-3s, protein, and other nutrients. But like all tuna, it also contains significant levels of mercury. The albacore "white" tuna is highest in pollutants. "Light" canned tuna has fewer pollutants, but also less healthy fat. (The fat tends to be where the contaminants are stored.) The fact that kids will eat tuna is a double-edged sword—it means they're getting mercury along with their nutrition. If you want canned fish, you're better off eating other varieties, such as Alaskan salmon (which is always wild-caught), sardines, anchovies, herring, mackerel, or shellfish including clams and oysters, all of which are usually safe (taking care that the cans aren't lined with BPA). Fish packed in olive oil is better than the kind packed in water, since the oil preserves the nutrients. Also, the softened bones in canned fish are edible and will provide you with a highly absorbable form of calcium.[31] A final advantage of canned: It tends to have less mercury (unless it's tuna) because it is generally made of smaller fish (salmon, sardines, herring, mackerel).

6. Sushi Is Health Food? Not So Fast

Sushi sounds like it should be good for you — eating fish raw means you're not missing out on enzymes or nutrients that would have been destroyed during cooking. The exceptional cardiac health and longevity of the Japanese are often ascribed to the raw fish in their diet. But it's not that simple. First, there's the mercury contamination. A study by researchers at Rutgers University found that sushi-grade tuna had *three to ten times* more mercury than eel, crab, salmon, and kelp.[32] Interestingly, the tuna served at some of the best sushi restaurants had the highest mercury concentrations of all, whereas the inexpensive tuna in supermarket sushi had less. The study found that the 10 percent of respondents who ate the most sushi took in around three times the recommended daily limit for mercury. And that's not the only reason to avoid sushi: The refined white rice and sugary preparation of the fish add unnecessary starches to the meal. Next time you order sushi, try this: Take one piece apart and see how much of what you're eating is actually fish. Most of what you're getting is starchy white rice. Next time you order sushi — watch how much rice (which is also made with added sugar) goes into a sushi roll. Or just unroll your sushi and pile up the rice — you will be surprised. You are better off just ordering sashimi, which doesn't come buried in a giant ball of carbs.

7. Forget Farmed. Go Wild!

The majority of the salmon we eat is farmed. Many people prefer it because the price of wild-caught salmon can be excessive: up to $30 per pound, which is about three times the price of farmed. Unfortunately, some of the same issues that plague feedlot livestock—low-quality food with too many grains, overcrowding, and unsanitary conditions—diminish the quality of farmed fish. Salmon in the wild don't eat corn or grains. But that's what they're fed when they're farmed. By the time they reach your dinner table, they contain more omega-6 fatty acids (which you don't need) and less omega-3s (which you do), a combination that creates the same inflammatory effect caused by processed oils and junk foods. A study published in the *Journal of the American Dietetic Association* analyzed thirty samples of commonly consumed fish sold at supermarkets throughout the United States and found that some farmed fish contained nearly undetectable levels of omega-3s. The same study also found that two of the most popular farmed fish on the market, tilapia and catfish, were among the worst offenders when it came to their ratio of omega fatty acids. "These data reveal that marked changes in the fishing industry during the past decade have produced widely eaten fish that have fatty acid characteristics that are generally accepted to be inflammatory by the health care community," the researchers concluded.[33]

Farmed fish also contains higher levels of persistent organic pollutants (POPs) than their wild brethren, including chlorinated pesticides and polychlorinated biphenyls (PCBs)[34] (more on that later). According to the Monterey Bay Aquarium, an authority on aquatic sustainability, the only kind of salmon we should be eating is wild-caught Alaskan—because the fishing methods are environmentally friendly and the fish are full of omega-3 fatty acids and low in contaminants.[35] However, there are brands of organic sustainably farmed fish that are good to eat. Check out www .cleanfish.com to learn more.

8. Farmed Salmon Could Lead to Diabetes

Ideally you should eat a variety of seafood so you're not at risk of getting too much of any one toxin or pollutant. The main thing you need to look out for is mercury, which comes largely from the coal that's burned in electricity-generating power plants. The pollutants from these factories fall into our rivers, lakes, and seas, and then into the fish, and into us. Almost all seafood is tainted to some degree. So, the best thing you can do is to keep your mercury exposure low enough that you avoid any real damage to your health.[36] According to the FDA,[37] the ten types of seafood lowest in mercury contamination are, in order:

1. Scallops
2. Canned salmon
3. Clams
4. Shrimp
5. Oysters
6. Sardines
7. Tilapia
8. Anchovies
9. Wild salmon
10. Squid

And the highest in mercury contamination, in order:

1. Tilefish
2. Swordfish
3. Shark
4. King mackerel
5. Bigeye tuna
6. Orange roughy
7. Marlin
8. Spanish mackerel
9. Grouper
10. Tuna

Mercury isn't the only concern. Many fish also contain dioxins, carcinogenic pollutants that come from pesticide use and other industrial manufacturing. Dioxins linger in the environment and are stored in fat tissue, so exposure can come from meat, dairy, and eggs as well as from fish. Studies suggest they are linked to type 2 diabetes and metabolic syndrome. One group of researchers found that high consumption of farmed Atlantic salmon was tied to high blood sugar levels, though it's not clear from the correlation if there are other factors involved.[38] Fortunately, cooking your fish and removing some of its skin — which is where toxins tend to concentrate — can reduce the levels of dioxins.[39] In case you're wondering, studies have found that cooking beef and other meat significantly reduces the levels of dioxins they contain as well.[40]

GEEK ALERT: A LITTLE MORE SCIENCE ABOUT FISH

As important as omega-3s are to every cell in our bodies, we're not going to eat salmon and sardines every day. Some of us won't eat those dark, oily fish *ever*. So, we supplement with fish oil. It's a good idea, with a few caveats. For most of us, taking a supplement of 1–2 grams a day is wise. It protects your cardiovascular system and reduces inflammation.[41] But you have to be careful about the source. You can find fish oil capsules in all kinds of stores, at every price point, but there's no way to tell which is responsibly sourced, tested, and handled, and which is not. If the fish have been contaminated with toxins and pollutants, so has their oil. If the oils have been mishandled, they may be oxidized. However, there are companies that produce fish oil that has been filtered, distilled, or purified to remove all toxins and mercury. See www.food thebook.com to learn more about the best brands of fish oil and other supplements.

Krill oil is an alternative. The tiny crustaceans it's made from eat plankton, which means they're extremely low on the food chain and, as a result, low in mercury, dioxins, and PCBs. Krill oil contains the same levels of DHA and EPA as fish oil.[42] However, I worry about depleting the main food source for much of marine life. As we discussed earlier, the ALA in plant foods like walnuts or flaxseeds is a poor source of omega-3s, but that's not true of at least one plant-based supplement: algae, which contains preformed DHA, an omega-3 that is critical for your brain. For people who are vegan or vegetarian, algae is a much better source of omega-3s than other plant-based fats like walnuts and flaxseed oil.[43]

HOW TO EAT SAFE AND SUSTAINABLE SEAFOOD

To make better fish and seafood choices, we have to investigate where our food is coming from, and fortunately there are a lot of great resources for finding fish and seafood that have been harvested sustainably. Here are some:

- To find fresh, local, low-impact seafood, you can join a community-supported fishery. To locate one in your area, visit www.localcatch.org.
- The Natural Resources Defense Council, or NRDC, publishes a guide to buying fish that's healthy for you *and* the environment: https://www.nrdc.org/stories/smart-seafood-buying-guide.
- The Monterey Bay Aquarium Seafood Watch program helps consumers choose seafood that is sourced in ways that support a healthy ocean: http://www.montereybayaquarium.org/conservation-and-science/our-programs/seafood-watch.
- The Monterey Bay Aquarium also has a great app that you can use to make sure you're buying fish that has been caught sustainably: http://www.seafoodwatch.org/seafood-recommendations/our-app.
- The Environmental Working Group publishes an easy-to-use consumer guide to seafood that helps people determine what is safe to eat and what contains too many contaminants. It's a quick, consumer-friendly read that I highly recommend: http://www.ewg.org/research/ewgs-good-seafood-guide/executive-summary.

Don't Be Duped: Look for These Labels to Avoid Fraud

Fish fraud is widespread, so you have to be careful. Look for logos from third-party organizations certifying that the seafood you're purchasing at your local market is authentic. Here are some tips that can help you:

- Look for logos from third-party certifiers like the Marine Stewardship Council or another organization called Gulf Wild.
- When you're buying wild salmon, you can look for the Wild Alaska Pure logo, which appears only on Alaskan salmon. Or better yet, buy your fish from a local fishmonger you know and trust.

If Wild Salmon Is Too Pricey or Hard to Find, Try This…

I'm generally against farmed fish for health and environmental reasons. But I know wild salmon can be expensive or simply unavailable depending on where you live. If farmed fish is your only option, here are some resources that can guide you to the best choices. Also included are guidelines for safe and sustainably harvested fish.

- Look for the Global Aquaculture Alliance Best Practices symbol. This organization promotes responsible aquaculture practices and strictly forbids the abuse of antibiotics in fish farming.
- Go to cleanfish.com, which can connect you to farmed fish that has no antibiotics or hormones, low mercury levels, and lots of omega-3s. Clean

Fish promotes farmed fish that are sustainably harvested and not overfished and sustainably farmed.

- Check out fishwise.org to learn about retailers in
your area that are working to ensure that the seafood they sell is sustainable and traceable.

- Seafood Watch (www.seafoodwatch.org) recommends a number of eco-certification organizations
for farmed and wild-caught seafood. I suggest you
look for these certifications: ASC (Aquaculture
Stewardship Council), Best Aquaculture Practices,
Naturland, Friend of the Sea, Canada Organic,
Certified Sustainable Seafood (MSC, or Marine
Stewardship Council). Or check out www.clean
fish.com for fish brands that are sustainably raised
or farmed.

SUMMING IT UP

You should eat seafood at least three times a week. The
best fish are sustainably sourced, chock-full of omega-3s,
low in contaminants and omega-6s, and certified
authentic. But stay the heck away from farmed seafood
(unless it is organic) or wild fish that contains a lot of
toxins. Bigger fish are higher on the oceanic food chain
and therefore accumulate more mercury. Farmed fish
can also contain a lot of antibiotics and toxins such as
PCBs, but not the sustainably raised or organic farmed
fish.

What If I'm Pregnant?

If you're pregnant, you should definitely eat seafood, but you have to be especially careful about your choices. Follow the guidelines provided in this section, but strictly avoid all farmed seafood and large fish — it's not worth the risk of exposure to even small levels of contaminants. The omega-3s in seafood are critical for fetal brain health. So prioritize the fish that are highest in omega-3s — like sardines, herring, mackerel, anchovies, and wild salmon — and eat two or three servings (or roughly 12 ounces) per week.

SEAFOOD: WHAT THE HECK SHOULD I EAT?

- Wild salmon, either canned or fresh, or salmon labeled Alaskan (since all salmon from Alaska is wild).
- Small, toxin-free fish (the smaller the better) such as sardines, anchovies, herring, and mackerel.
- Clams, scallops, mussels, and oysters, which are loaded with beneficial zinc. You should eat shrimp, too, if it comes from the Gulf of Mexico.
- When in doubt, you can find and download a handy wallet card from the Natural Resources Defense Council listing fish with the lowest mercury levels at: www.nrdc.org/health/effects/mercury/walletcard.pdf.

SEAFOOD: WHAT THE HECK SHOULD I AVOID?

- Big fish such as shark, swordfish, Chilean sea bass, king mackerel, marlin, grouper, halibut, tilefish, and orange roughy.
- Most farmed fish, with rare exceptions. Use the resources provided in this chapter to find the best types of farmed fish when it's your only option.
- Tuna.
- Sushi.
- Imported shrimp.

It just so happens that many of these fish are also on the brink of extinction due to overfishing. Unsustainable demand for the most popular fish is a huge problem that can be solved only by diversifying your fish choices and choosing seafood from truly renewable sources.

VEGETABLES

NUTRITION IQ QUIZ

True or False?

1. Alfalfa sprouts are a health food.
2. Potatoes contain complex carbs, which are better for you than simple carbs like sugar.
3. The benefits of organic vegetables are overstated because studies show they're no healthier than conventionally grown food.
4. White button mushrooms are relatively low in nutrition.
5. Tomatoes can create inflammation in the body.
6. Arugula is just another kind of lettuce, like iceberg.
7. Some of the most nutritious vegetables are weird ones, like seaweed.

Answers

1. False: *Salmonella* contamination is a big problem with alfalfa sprouts, and they contain toxins such as canavanine, which can cause cancer.

2. False: Most potatoes are not much better than white bread. The old distinction of simple and complex carbs is pretty much useless. Fingerling or Peruvian potatoes are better than most because they have a lower glycemic index and more nutrients.

3. False: Unless you like having lethal chemicals inside your body, go organic. The one study showing no difference between organic and conventional was funded by the food and agriculture industry. Many other studies have linked organic vegetables to a decrease in negative effects from pesticides and have found that organic vegetables contain more nutrients and phytochemicals than conventional ones.[1]

4. True: They are surprisingly short on vitamins and contain cancer-causing toxins when eaten raw, as many people do in salads.

5. True: Some people react badly to nightshades (potatoes, tomatoes, peppers, eggplant). Negative effects include pain, inflammation, and arthritis.

6. False: Unlike lettuce, arugula is in the cruciferous vegetable family. It is more like broccoli than lettuce and contains all sorts of nutrients like calcium and phytochemicals that help with detoxification of environmental chemicals and prevent cancer.

7. True: We should all make an effort to eat them more often. In fact, the best way to get more nutrient-dense food is to eat organic foods, wild foods, or unusual plants such as purslane, dande-

lion greens, or kohlrabi, for example. They are not staple foods so are less likely to be genetically altered (as long as they're not starchy either).

Get a new food fact and weekly recipe directly from my kitchen. Sign up for free at www.food thebook.com.

You know you have to eat your veggies. You've heard it a thousand times. But here's a good question: *Why* should you eat your veggies?

After all, plants don't contain all the vitamins and minerals that you need to be healthy. And in some cases, they provide surprisingly little. Beef liver has several times more vitamin A than any plant, including carrots, which, though noted for that particular nutrient, actually only contain beta-carotene, which has to be converted by the body into vitamin A. Oranges might come to mind when you think of vitamin C, but you can also get that from organ meats. Seafood is the best source of the essential omega-3 fatty acids that you need to survive and thrive. You can't get them from veggies, except algae and purslane. We all know how crucial vitamin D is for health, yet plants deliver virtually none (except for certain mushrooms, like porcini). The same is true of the B vitamins, especially B_{12}, which comes from animal foods like meat, eggs, and wild salmon. Vegans must supplement with vitamin B_{12} to avoid becoming deficient.

Plants do contain some protein, and some, like kale and black beans, even have significant amounts. But plant protein is poor quality compared to animal protein. There's nearly seven times as much protein in ground beef as in spinach, for example. This is where my vegan and vegetarian friends run into trouble—without eating meat or fish, they're more likely to end up with nutritional deficiencies of iron, calcium, vitamin K, omega-3 fats, B_{12}, and fat-soluble vitamins such as A and D.[2] I've seen it in many vegan and vegetarian patients in my practice.

However, vegetables do contain carbs, a source of energy. In fact, the majority of your diet should be carbs: not bread, potatoes, sugar, beans, or grains, but vegetables. Veggies don't spike blood sugar (except the starchy ones) and they are critical for health. But it's worth noting that carbs are not a nutritional necessity. Although there are essential amino acids (protein) and essential fats (omega-3 and omega-6), most people don't realize that there is no such thing as essential carbs. We do not need any carbs for our survival. Nonetheless, we need vegetables because they contain many vitamins, minerals, and powerful disease-fighting, health-promoting compounds called phytonutrients.

THE SCIENCE OF VEGETABLES

Though they cannot deliver pristine health on their own, there are very compelling reasons to make vegetables the bulk of your diet. Plants are our only source of fiber, which is fertilizer for the good bacteria that make up the internal garden in your gut. Fiber keeps digested food moving smoothly through your system.

It prevents cancer and heart disease.[3] It helps you lose weight. And the average person doesn't even come close to getting enough. Our hunter-gatherer ancestors ate 100 to 150 grams of fiber each day. Today? The typical American eats a paltry 8 to 15 grams daily.[4]

And here's another important reason you should eat your veggies: They're our only source of phytonutrients (*phyto* meaning plants), a group of chemicals essential to vibrant health that protect us from cancer, inflammation, infection, heart disease, autoimmune disease, and a long list of other chronic ailments.[5] Plants are living *farm*acies that dispense natural substances with medicinal powers. Many pharmaceutical drugs and nutritional supplements have their origins in plants. The other great thing about vegetables is that if you eat enough of them, you won't have any room left over for all the ultraprocessed Frankenfoods that are slowly killing millions of Americans.

But here's the rub. Most of what we've been told about which veggies to eat is wrong. The ones that turn up on America's plates most often are sorely lacking in phytochemicals, loaded with fast-acting carbs, and sprayed with pesticides. Let's discover some amazing facts about veggies and some ground rules that will help you choose wisely. But first...

WHAT THE EXPERTS GOT RIGHT

On this one, all the experts—from the scientific and medical communities to your mother—got it at least partly right: You can't go wrong heeding the age-old "eat your vegetables" advice. It just doesn't go far enough. The idea of dinner as a big slab of conventionally raised meat accompanied by two side dishes—one vegetable, usually overcooked, and one potato—should be turned around completely. You shouldn't just eat your veggies. You should aim to eat them at every meal. Nonstarchy vegetables like spinach, asparagus, broccoli, and kale should make up 50 to 75 percent of your plate with a small portion of animal protein as "condi-meat." Think of this as the 3-to-1 rule.

WHAT THEY GOT WRONG

They told us to eat our veggies, but they didn't really specify which ones and why. Maybe that's the reason some of the least beneficial vegetables are America's favorites. According to the USDA, potatoes, especially big, white Idaho potatoes, are the number one most consumed "vegetable"—they're tubers, technically—in America. Unfortunately, they are so full of fast-acting carbs that they'll rapidly raise your blood sugar and insulin. And most potatoes are consumed as French fries after they've been cooked in toxic oil.

Physiologically speaking, you might as well be eating sugar. The combo of heated, refined vegetable oils and starch is toxic. The number two vegetable in the Western diet is the tomato, which, as we've said, may be an inflammatory food for some. Most of them are tasteless, sold unripe and designed to fit stacked in a box. And the rest are usually found in ketchup or tomato sauce that's loaded with sugar. Right behind tomatoes comes sweet corn, which is not only a starchy carb, but another common allergen. Onions are number four, but they are actually quite good for you. Finally, rounding out the inglorious list of America's top five favorite vegetables is the all-too-common iceberg lettuce, which is little more than water with a touch of fiber and vitamin A. It has some of the lowest nutritional values of any vegetable known.

Meanwhile, the nutritional powerhouses, such as kale, Brussels sprouts, radishes, artichokes, and collard greens, are all clustered together near the bottom of the USDA's list of veggies, inhabiting the "least popular" group. You should flip that list upside down. Eat all the strange, weird, and unpopular veggies instead of the boring, all-too-common ones. This is where you'll find the highest levels of healing phytochemicals that pack the greatest nutritional punch.

Seek out wild or heirloom varieties of veggies. These are old-fashioned strains that have been grown and handed down through generations. They're open-pollinated by wind or insects, meaning they have not been altered by human intervention or genetic modification. The sad reality is that for more than a hundred years we've deliberately bred our produce to be sweeter, less colorful, and less nutritious. The most potent phytonutrients are what give veggies their bitter and astringent tastes and deep colors. We've taken our wild plants—vegetables *and* fruit—and stripped them of their best qualities.

A wild crabapple, for example, has one hundred times more cancer- and inflammation-fighting anthocyanins than the Golden Delicious variety found in supermarkets. Purple carrots contain twenty times more phytonutrients than their more common orange brethren. Wild blueberries have dozens of times more phytonutrients than domesticated berries. And the heirloom purple corn that you've probably never seen or tasted has sixty times more anthocyanins than the sweet white corn so ubiquitous in America.[6]

WHAT WE STILL DON'T KNOW FOR SURE

We're just beginning to understand the role of food as medicine, and how exactly the chemicals in plants interact with our own cells and those in our microbiome. We've all been told that our genes are our destiny. But that's not entirely true. Studies show that your genes can be turned on or off by the foods you eat. This is referred to as the science of nutrigenomics. There's evidence that plant RNA may regulate RNA,[7] an extraordinary thing to contemplate. It means that there may come a time when you'll know precisely which plants you need to eat to maximize your health and protect against disease.

SEVEN THINGS YOU NEED TO KNOW ABOUT VEGETABLES

1. Eat the Rainbow

Vegetables and fruits use their colors to signal which beneficial substances they contain. Red means one thing, yellow another, purple something else. The colors attract the insects and animals that will disperse the plant's seeds; these are the same chemicals—phytonutrients—that give flowers their colors. It's the language of the plant kingdom, and we would do well to learn it because each color represents a different group of healing compounds.

Did you know that our hunter-gatherer ancestors ate more than 800 varieties of plants? That's how they got so much fiber each day. Because they foraged far and wide, they typically ate a range of wild plants of all different colors. In other words, they ate the rainbow, and you should too. Think of that the next time someone hands you a plate of pale, white mashed potatoes or iceberg lettuce salad.

Our ancestors didn't have drugs or pills. They ate their medicine in the form of plants. In general, the more colors you eat when it comes to plants, the more anti-inflammatory, detoxifying, healing compounds from the phytonutrients you'll soak up. Some of these colors even work together synergistically to have a more powerful effect, which is another reason you should eat a diverse array of veggies. Though these are not "essential" like vitamins and minerals, without them you will age and die faster.

Some of these medicinal plant nutrients are familiar, such as resveratrol in red wine or grapes. Others are more obscure, like compounds that are anti-inflammatory and detoxifying, or the vast array of antioxidants that protect us from the damage caused by free radicals (or rusting) that are part of every chronic disease—things like the detoxifying and anti-cancer compounds in broccoli called glucosinolates, or cancer-preventing lycopene in tomatoes, or the anti-inflammatory curcumin in turmeric, the Indian spice in curry.

So, what do all those colorful nutrients mean? Here's how to read the rainbow:

Red	Indicates the carotenoid lycopene in tomatoes, bell peppers, and carrots.[8] Lycopene protects against heart disease and genetic damage that may cause cancer.
Blue-purple	Is caused by anthocyanins in eggplant, beets, red cabbage, and purple potatoes. Anthocyanins prevent blood clots, delay cell aging, and may slow Alzheimer's onset.

Green	Is found in the brassicas—broccoli, Brussels sprouts, bok choy, cabbage, cauliflower, kale, collards, arugula, and others—and indicates phytochemicals, sulforaphane, isocyanates, and indoles, which inhibit carcinogens and boost detoxification.
Pale green-white	Appears in garlic, onions, leeks, and other vegetables and alliums and is caused by allicins, which have powerful anticancer, antitumor, immune-boosting, and antimicrobial properties. These vegetables also contain antioxidant flavonoids like quercetin and kaempferol.
Orange	Represents alpha-carotene and beta-carotene in carrots, pumpkin, acorn and winter squash, and sweet potatoes. Alpha-carotene protects against cancer and benefits skin and vision.
Yellow-green	Signals the carotenoids lutein and zeaxanthin, which benefit our eyes and safeguard our hearts against atherosclerosis. Vegetables in this group may not always appear yellowish to the eye: They include spinach, collard, mustard, and turnip greens, yellow corn, peas, and even avocado.

2. When You Should Eat Organic

For most of human history, all agriculture was pesticide-free. But that changed dramatically after World War II, when companies that produced chemical weapons for the war began to sell their toxins (former biological weapons such as poison nerve gas) to farmers to kill off weevils, wireworms, beetles, and other agricultural pests. By the 1950s, American farmers were regularly spraying their crops with vast quantities of DDT, an endocrine disruptor and carcinogen. In the 1970s, DDT's harmful side effects in humans and wildlife became widely known thanks to Rachel Carson's book *Silent Spring.* Public outrage led to a nationwide ban on its use in agriculture in 1972, but by then scientists had already developed whole new classes of chemicals to spray on produce. Today, more than 5 billion pounds of pesticides are used in farming each year—a quarter of it in the United States alone.[9]

Pesticides became a mainstay as a way to increase the yield and profitability of farming. But there's plenty of evidence that they're neurotoxic and carcinogenic for those of us who eat them. A large meta-analysis in the journal *Neurotoxicology* found that chronic exposure to some common pesticides significantly increased the risk of Parkinson's disease.[10] Farming is one of the most dangerous occupations because of that. Studies in adults and children have also linked pesticide exposure to kidney, pancreatic, prostate, breast, and stomach cancers,[11] as well as respiratory problems and depression.[12] Wind and runoff carry these harmful chemicals from farms into rivers and surrounding areas, affecting even those of us who don't consume them in our food. And they linger in the environment—and our bodies—for decades. In a 2005 report, the Environmental Working Group found DDT in the umbilical cords of babies before they even took their first breath. These toxic chemicals stick around for dozens or sometimes hundreds of years, even after their use is banned or stopped.

But you can greatly lower your exposure to pesticides by eating organic. A 2015 study funded by the EPA found that consumers who often or always bought organic had significantly less insecticide in their urine, even though they ate 70 percent more produce than people who bought only conventionally grown fruits and vegetables.[13]

As you've no doubt noticed, organic is often costlier, which can be an obstacle for many people. Is it worth it? In some cases, *absolutely*. The Environmental Working Group ranks the fruits and vegetables that are most contaminated with pesticide residue. That list, known as the Dirty Dozen, can tell you which foods you must buy organic. The EWG also keeps a list of the foods that have the least amount of pesticide residues, known as the Clean Fifteen. You can go to EWG.org for the lists and background report in its entirety. The EWG research turned up some interesting information:

■ The average potato has more pesticides by weight than any other produce.

- A single sweet bell pepper sample contained fifteen different pesticides.
- Kale, collard greens, other leafy greens, and hot peppers are not among the Dirty Dozen, but they are "of particular concern" because residue tests conducted by the USDA found especially toxic pesticides, "including organophosphate and carbamate insecticides. These are no longer detected widely on other produce, either because of binding legal restrictions or voluntary phase-outs." My advice: Buy these organic.

Half of the foods on the EWG Dirty Dozen list—the ones that contain the highest pesticide residues—are vegetables. (The rest are fruits, which we'll discuss in another chapter.) Here are the vegetables we should buy organic when possible:[14]

- Celery
- Spinach
- Tomatoes
- Bell peppers
- Cherry tomatoes
- Cucumbers
- Kale
- Collard greens
- Other leafy greens
- Hot peppers

Here are the ones you can more safely buy nonorganic when your options are limited:

- Cabbage
- Frozen sweet peas
- Onions
- Asparagus
- Eggplant
- Cauliflower

3. How You Prepare Your Vegetables Makes a Big Difference

Here's a little-known fact: If you crush garlic and chop broccoli and then let them rest before you cook them, you significantly increase their power to fight cancer and heart disease. Crushing or chopping garlic and letting it sit a few minutes releases antiplatelet enzymes that help prevent coronary artery blockages. But whole garlic cloves, once they've been cooked, offer no heart benefit at all. Neither does garlic that's been microwaved.[15] A similar phenomenon occurs with broccoli. Studies show that chopping it up, then letting it sit for forty minutes before cooking, releases the cancer-fighting compound sulforaphane, which would otherwise have been destroyed by cooking.[16] Using precut, frozen raw broccoli is just as beneficial. Of course, eating garlic or broccoli raw is the best way to get all the nutrients intact, but raw garlic and broccoli aren't appetizing to everyone. Better to eat a lot, deliciously cooked, than little or none raw.

This underscores the importance of properly preparing your veggies before eating them. Boiling vegetables is almost always a bad idea. Most of the nutrients are leached out into the water that you pour down the drain.

Let's run down a few more ground rules:

1. Always wash nonorganic produce thoroughly to rinse away as much pesticide as possible. Friction helps remove contaminants from the surface of your produce, so don't just rinse them. Rub them. You can use a vegetable brush. Some suggest washing in a dilute solution of 3 percent hydrogen peroxide. You can be less fastidious with organic.

2. Frozen vegetables are about as nutritious as fresh, and in some cases even more so. That's especially true if they were flash frozen right after picking, which locks in the vitamins, minerals, and phytonutrients, preventing them from degrading over time.[17] They are also cheaper.

3. The best way to cook most vegetables is to steam them for no more than 4 minutes. They should still be bright and crunchy.

4. Some veggies are best when cooked and allowed to cool before eating. In the chapter on grains, I will discuss how cooking rice and then cooling it overnight in the fridge slows the rate at which

your body absorbs the starch. The same is true of potatoes. If you're going to eat them, cook and cool them first. You can gently heat them up again before digging in. The cooking and cooling creates resistant starch, which is good for your gut bacteria, helps your metabolism, and lowers the glycemic index of the food.

5. If you prefer to sauté or roast your veggies, that's fine, too, as long as you don't overcook them into oblivion.

6. Don't deep-fry your veggies. You'll destroy their beneficial compounds and create harmful substances like acrylamide during the frying process. Good veggies are not deep-fried zucchini or cauliflower.

7. Microwaving your veggies, like boiling them, should be avoided. Too many of their nutrients will be lost. And microwaving creates AGEs— molecules that create inflammation and oxidative stress in the body. Not good.

8. Vitamins A, D, E, and K are fat-soluble, meaning you need to eat them with fats for your body to absorb them. Good sources of plant fats like olive oil, coconut oil, avocado, nuts, and seeds (or healthy animal fats like grass-fed meat and wild seafood) should be a part of every meal. Never use fat-free or low-fat dressings on your salads; make your own with olive oil and vinegar.

9. The cancer-fighting lycopene in tomatoes is released when they're heated, so look for ways to enjoy tomato sauce without having to load up on pasta.

4. White Potatoes Are Like Wonder Bread

Technically, *all* vegetables are considered carbohydrates, which is part of the reason nutrition can be so confusing. So, how can you know which are fine to eat abundantly and which you need to consume in moderation? When choosing veggies, you should follow a simple principle: Pick the ones that won't cause a quick spike in your blood sugar. Most kinds — the healthiest ones, like leafy greens, broccoli, peppers, and many other varieties — will barely increase your blood sugar at all. We call these slow carbs. Others — the starchy ones, like potatoes, corn, beets, pumpkin, winter squash, parsnips — *do* cause a quick rise in blood sugar. We call these fast-absorbing carbs. All foods are ranked by their effect on our blood sugar when we measure their glycemic index and glycemic load. We'll discuss this in detail later in this chapter, in the "Geek Alert" section.[18]

5. Some Veggies Can Make You Fat and Sick

Remember Michael Pollan's famous advice? "Eat food. Not too much. Mostly plants." Well, you should eat plants — but not *all* plants. Some vegetables are trouble because they act as allergens that cause chronic inflammation. When you think of food allergies you probably think of someone eating a peanut and having an acute, life-threatening reaction. But some provoke a delayed, low-grade allergic reaction that you may not even notice. They're more like sensitivities than true allergies. But over time, with repeated exposure to the offending foods, along with other insults that damage your gut, you can end up in a chronically inflamed state that leads to weight gain, irritable bowel syndrome, headaches, fluid retention, depression, joint pain, and sinus problems—or worse. Millions of people have these reactions and have no idea. But in my practice, I see the scope of this silent epidemic of chronic food allergies or sensitivities firsthand.

A blood test can help determine when you're producing antibodies to certain foods, and an elimination diet can allow you to pinpoint the troublesome ones. You may know of some common food allergens, such as gluten, dairy, nuts, and soy. But another one most people don't know about is nightshades—tomatoes, bell peppers, potatoes, and eggplant. Everyone is different, but for some, these particular plants are difficult to digest and metabolize, which leads to bloating and other manifestations of chronic inflammation. Uncontrolled inflammation is a smoldering fire that can lead to insulin resistance, which sets the stage for many chronic diseases. If you suspect you're allergic to nightshades, the best thing you can do is to drop them from your diet for one week and see if you notice any improvements. People with arthritis or autoimmune disorders are often so sensitive to nightshades that they should just avoid them altogether.[19] My book *The Blood Sugar Solution 10-Day Detox Diet* (minus the nightshades) is a good place to start with an elimination diet.

6. One of the World's Best Veggies Doesn't Grow on Farms

You probably ignore seaweed when you think of vegetables. But that's a mistake. As the Japanese know, it's one of the most nutrient-rich foods you can eat, containing minerals that are hard to come by in the American diet, like manganese and thyroid-boosting iodine.[20] Seaweed is rich in vitamin C and iron. It fights cancer and inflammation and strengthens the immune system. It contains important nutrients and antioxidants not found in land vegetables. So, if the only time you eat seaweed is when you're having sushi—it's the thin black sheet wrapped around the rice—then you're missing out. The most common varieties of seaweed in the United States are wakame, kombu, and nori. I recommend using them in salads, stews, and soups. One of my favorite recipes is my Ultrabroth, which I make with chopped radishes, greens, cilantro, carrots, celery, fresh ginger, and seaweed. You can find the recipe on my website www.foodthebook.com. Or you can just munch on seaweed as a snack. Many health food stores sell packs of roasted and lightly salted or flavored seaweed. It beats potato chips! Stay away from hijiki, though — it contains high levels of arsenic.

7. Fermentation Performs a Kind of Magic on Our Food

Humans have been fermenting foods since Neolithic times. Studies of ancient pots and jars uncovered in China show that they were used to hold mixtures of fermented foods that carried social, religious, and medical significance.[21] The practice of fermenting veggies was historically common in many countries. But in today's fast-food culture most people eat just a handful of fermented foods, like pickles, soy sauce, yogurt, and sour cream — and of course beer.

That's a shame. Many traditional fermented veggies offer myriad health benefits. Researchers at Michigan State University noticed that the breast cancer rate among Polish women rises threefold when they emigrate to the United States. Though they are not sure why, one reason, they suspect, is the change in their diet. Polish women in Poland eat fermented cabbage — better known to us as sauerkraut — daily, up to 30 pounds of it a year.[22] But after they move to America, where fermented cabbage is little more than a condiment, their sauerkraut consumption drops significantly. Of course, the research on these women is observational, which means it can only show a correlation, not cause and effect. But cabbage, like broccoli and other cruciferous vegetables, contains the enzyme myrosinase and compounds known as glucosinolates, which are detoxifying and play a role in cancer prevention. There's some evidence that fermentation makes these compounds more bioactive.[23]

Their anticancer potential aside, there are other reasons to love fermented veggies. Fermented foods like kimchi, kombucha, tempeh, miso, and sauerkraut are dietary sources of beneficial bugs that help you maintain a healthy gut. If you have irritable bowel syndrome, these probiotic-rich foods may be a good way to repopulate your gut with good bacteria. Probiotic supplements are another option. But eating fermented foods is better.[24] If you're adventurous, you can ferment almost anything you like, vegetable or fruit, fairly easily at home. All you need is a jar, water, salt, some spices or herbs, and a little time. Some people use a starter culture as a shortcut, which is fine. But never use vinegar — as food companies tend to do with sauerkraut and other dishes — because it kills the live bacteria, defeating the purpose of fermentation. When you buy fermented foods, make sure they were prepared naturally, without the use of vinegar.

GEEK ALERT: A LITTLE MORE SCIENCE ABOUT VEGETABLES

The glycemic index is a useful tool in nutritional science for measuring how much a particular food will raise a person's blood sugar. But the amount of food

you eat matters too. For example, carrots have a reputation as being high in starch, and their glycemic index
number, 68, is in fact pretty far up the scale—higher
than those of some ice creams. But the glycemic load
(which accounts for the actual amount of the food you
would typically eat) for an average 80-gram serving of
carrots is just 3. So unless you plan on eating a couple
of pounds at a time, you can eat carrots fearlessly. As
we've said, most vegetables don't even register on the
glycemic load scale, meaning it's virtually impossible to eat enough of them to significantly raise your
blood sugar.[25] Feel free to consume as much as you
like of:

- Salad greens
- Spinach
- Broccoli
- Kale
- Asparagus
- Cabbage
- Bok choy
- Tomatoes
- Peppers
- Eggplant
- Celery
- Cucumbers
- Mushrooms
- Herbs
- Seaweed

On the other hand, there are vegetables that *do* rank high on the glycemic load list. These tend to be the starchier ones, as you'd expect. But even here there is a big range of GL numbers:

- Pumpkin: 3
- Sweet corn: 11
- Japanese sweet potato: 11
- Parsnip: 12
- Baked russet potato: 26
- Microwavable potato: 27

Our goal should be to stick with foods that have a glycemic load of 11 or lower.

ORGANIC AND LOCAL ARE BEST FOR THE ENVIRONMENT

We've already established why organic produce is better for our health, so it shouldn't come as a surprise that it's also better for our environment. Growing vegetables organically helps eliminate water, air, and soil toxicity, and it promotes biodiversity. The farther food has to travel, the greater its environmental burden. The best way to find fresh, local food is to grow it yourself. If that's not an option, you can buy a share in a nearby farm's output by joining a CSA (community supported agriculture) organization. Barring that, you can shop at the nearest farmers' market. Visit either of these two sites for help finding one:

- Local Harvest: Community Supported Agriculture: http://www.localharvest.org/csa
- USDA: Local Food Directories: National Farmers Market Directory: https://www.ams.usda.gov/local -food-directories/farmersmarkets

Waste Not

The Natural Resources Defense Council estimates that 40 percent of all food in the United States is thrown out. That includes millions of pounds of fresh fruits and vegetables that farmers discard due to over-production or that supermarkets can't sell because of minor cosmetic imperfections. The USDA estimates that supermarkets lose $15 billion annually in unsold fruits and vegetables that in many cases are perfectly edible. To combat this waste, a number of organizations have begun collecting these unwanted fruits and vegetables and selling them to consumers at low cost. A new company called WTRMLN WTR takes advantage of 800 million pounds of ugly, misshapen, and sun-bleached watermelon and turns it into a delicious, healthy, low-sugar drink.

You should take advantage of these services to get cheap, organic produce while fighting food waste. Try the following:

- Imperfect Produce is a California-based company that works with local farmers to recover perfectly edible "ugly" produce that supermarkets won't buy. Then it sells it at a deeply discounted rate to consumers. For as little as $12 a week, the company will deliver a box of fruits and veggies to your door: http://www.imperfectproduce.com/#ugly-produce-delivered.

- Hungry Harvest is a community-supported agriculture program that recovers surplus produce and sells it at discount prices to consumers. Each time you buy a box of their fruits and vegetables, they donate a second box to a needy household: http://www.hungryharvest.net/#how-it-works.

SUMMING IT UP

Your guiding principle should be this: Eat locally grown, organic vegetables whenever possible. Seek out veggies that haven't been denatured, bastardized, and tamed by the industrial food complex or genetically altered. Many vegetables are bred for high yield, profitability, high sugar content (this is true of fruits too), and hardiness for shipping. Many of the veggies consumed in America today are genetically modified, deficient in nutrients, and lacking in biodiversity. A study in *Molecular Metabolism* concluded that of the 250,000 to 300,000 known edible plant species, humans consume only between 150 and 200. Roughly three-quarters of the world's food is generated from only twelve plant and five animal species, which is sad and astonishing.[26]

Our ancestors consumed a diverse array of veggies and plants, and you should too. Eat at least seven to nine servings of vegetables daily, or roughly 4 cups' worth, with a focus on the slow-burning, low-glycemic veggies that pack the most nutrition.

You should also go out of your way to eat as many weird vegetables as you can find. If you come across a strange sea vegetable from Japan that you never knew existed, or a traditional fermented veggie that you've never had before, eat it. Search for heirloom varieties of other veggies—in other words, go wild. If you eat this way you'll be less likely to consume GMO foods or pesticide-laden plants. Weird varieties tend to be grown by smaller farmers who are dedicated to sound agricultural principles.

Meanwhile, the most commonly consumed vegetables in America are some of the least beneficial. They tend to be either low in nutrients, high in starch, or both. Since there's a limit to how many vegetables you will consume on an average day, you can safely ignore the boring ones.

VEGGIES: WHAT THE HECK SHOULD I EAT?

- Broccoli, kale, cabbage, Brussels sprouts, and the other members of the cruciferous family
- Dark leafy greens like arugula (which is also a crucifer), spinach, Swiss chard, and collard greens (also a crucifer)
- Alliums such as garlic, shallots, and onions
- High-fiber veggies like celery and asparagus
- Shiitake, oyster, and cremini mushrooms
- Radishes, turnip greens, and beet greens
- Cucumbers, escarole, and watercress
- Zucchini and okra
- Sweet potatoes and winter squash (they're starchy but packed with nutrients, so enjoy 1 cup a few times a week but don't binge)
- Dandelion greens
- Mustard greens
- Broccoli sprouts (they have much more nutrition than even broccoli)
- Kabocha or pumpkin squash
- Sea vegetables such as seaweed
- Purple or red or white fingerling potatoes
- Japanese eggplants
- Red, yellow, or purple carrots
- Sorrel
- Jerusalem artichokes (also called sunchokes)
- Kohlrabi

VEGGIES: WHAT THE HECK SHOULD I AVOID?

- Iceberg lettuce
- White potatoes
- Raw white button mushrooms
- Alfalfa sprouts
- Most supermarket tomatoes, bell peppers, eggplant, and other nightshades (if you have arthritis or inflammation)
- Vegetables with a high glycemic load, as listed earlier in this chapter in our "Geek Alert" section
- Ketchup and tomato sauce, unless you make it yourself or buy the kind made without sugar (yes, Congress once declared tomato paste a vegetable, which, under pressure from the biggest pizza maker for schools, the Schwan Food Company, qualified pizza as a healthy food for school lunches)

FRUIT

NUTRITION IQ QUIZ

True or False?

1. Bananas are the best natural source of potassium.
2. Frozen berries are better for you than fresh.
3. You should eat at least five servings of fruit each day.
4. Juicing is a great way to get plenty of fruit into your diet.
5. Pomegranates are one of the best fruits you can eat.
6. Buying organic is a waste of money.
7. Apples are the most nutritious fruit. One a day keeps the doctor away.

Answers

1. False: We get more potassium from avocados and other plant foods without the sugar.
2. True: Believe it or not, frozen berries have high levels of nutrients because they are picked ripe

and frozen right away. Fresh fruit is often picked too soon, transported long distances, and stored.

3. False: That's too much. Although fruit contains fiber, vitamins, and phytonutrients, it can spike blood sugar. Grapes, pineapples, and most melons are the worst offenders.

4. False: Juice delivers all the sugar, or fructose, of fruit, which your body quickly absorbs, and none of the fiber. Fructose can cause insulin resistance and weight gain. It also stimulates lipogenesis, the process of making fat and dangerous types of cholesterol and triglycerides in your liver, which can lead to fatty liver disease, obesity, type 2 diabetes, heart disease, cancer, and dementia.

5. True: They're a superfruit because of all the antioxidants they contain.

6. False: Eat organic apples, berries, and other fruit to minimize your exposure to toxic pesticides. Check out the Environmental Working Group's list of the Dirty Dozen for more info.

7. False: Apples are fine, but there are other fruits that are much more nutrient- and phytonutrient-rich, such as blackberries, blueberries, and raspberries.

Get a new food fact and weekly recipe directly from my kitchen. Sign up for free at www.food thebook.com.

You've probably been told to "eat your fruits and veggies" ever since you were a kid. But this advice gives the false impression that fruits and vegetables should occupy equal space in your diet. It's easy to see why most people would welcome that conclusion—fruit is by far the sweeter of the two, and more convenient. But fruit's sugary profile is also its main drawback: Some varieties are sweet enough to be a disaster for people with weight or blood sugar issues. Roughly 70 percent of Americans are overweight or obese,[1] and 115 million are either diabetic or pre-diabetic,[2] so a lot of us need to go easy on our fruit intake. I have seen many people give up cookies and candy only to start binging on pineapples and grapes, replacing one sugar addiction with another. Some studies show that fruit consumers have a lower incidence of type 2 diabetes, but that may be because fruit eaters generally make healthier life choices and are not bingeing on sheet cakes. Patients of mine with type 1 or type 2 diabetes report that fruit often spikes their blood sugar.

THE SCIENCE OF FRUIT

In the pre-agriculture, pre-Twinkie era of human existence, wild fruit satisfied our sweet tooth. But back then fruit was quite a bit different from what we find today in the supermarket aisle, or even the farmer's roadside stand. Modern horticulture's ability to satisfy the strong consumer preference for sweetness has essentially wiped out fruit as nature originally intended it. There were once roughly 15,000 varieties of apples grown in the United States. Today, there are usually no more than a dozen you can find in most stores, unless you go to a specialty shop or farmers' market at the end of the summer. The most popular variety is the Golden Delicious—the sweetest apple, but also among the least nutritious. Wild fruits, especially berries, still exist and still possess the antioxidant, anti-cancer, antimicrobial, and anti-inflammatory properties that make them such potent natural medicines.[3] We often call them superfoods these days. For instance, the legendary baobab tree in Madagascar and other parts of Africa, sometimes known as the "tree of life," bears fruit that contains several times more vitamins, minerals, and other phytochemicals than almost any other produce.[4] While you won't see the fruits of the baobab tree at your local market, you can find it in powdered form online or at health food stores. The top antioxidant fruits you can buy pretty easily are berries, especially dried goji berries from the Himalayas, frozen wild blueberries, elderberries, cranberries, and blackberries.

WHAT THE EXPERTS GOT RIGHT

Fruits, much like vegetables, are universally and justifiably revered in the nutrition world. Americans have long been advised to eat multiple servings per day because fruits deliver fiber, antioxidants, and vitamins in one sweet little package. Although most of the data we have on fruit and its health benefits comes from observational research, the best studies have virtually all reached the conclusion that eating fruit prevents cancer, diabetes, and heart disease and lowers your overall mortality risk.[5]

WHAT THEY GOT WRONG

The government's dietary recommendations, which tell us to eat between five and nine servings of fruits and vegetables per day, are too vague and misleading. You're better off eating a minimum of ten servings of plant foods each day: seven or eight servings of veggies and no more than two or three servings of fruit. Sadly, most Americans skimp on fruit, and when they do eat it, they pick the least nutritious options. According to nationwide studies, the number one "fruit" Americans consume is orange juice, which is almost pure sugar, lacks some key nutrients found in whole fruits,[6] and has been linked to weight gain and diabetes.[7] Next on the list are bananas, which are high in sugar and ideally best consumed as an occasional treat. Another top ten "fruit" consumed in America? Apple juice. Unfortunately, the American understanding of what constitutes healthy fruit consumption is skewed.

SIX THINGS YOU NEED TO KNOW ABOUT FRUIT

1. Fructose with Fiber Is Not a Problem

Fructose, or "fruit sugar," has pronounced effects on your body when you digest it. It is processed almost entirely in the liver, where it's metabolized into fat. Clinical studies show that consuming fructose spikes your levels of triglycerides, a type of fat in the blood that causes heart disease and plays a role in metabolic syndrome (pre-diabetes).[8] Fructose occurs naturally in fruit, but it is also used as an industrial-strength sweetener that can be found in countless processed foods. When you encounter a product with high-fructose corn syrup (or even just the word "fructose") on its ingredients label, you should put that "food-like substance" back on the shelf.

In a study published in the *American Journal of Clinical Nutrition*, researchers assigned people to drink two servings per day of soda, diet beverages, milk, or water for six months.[9] In Mexico soda is sweetened with sugar. In the United States and most of the world it is sweetened with high-fructose corn syrup. At the end of the study, the soda drinkers had increased liver fat, muscle fat, triglycerides, and visceral or belly fat in their abdomens. In other words, the soda had produced the hallmarks of fatty liver disease and metabolic syndrome in just six months. Thanks to soda, now even kids have fatty liver and need liver transplants. Another study published in the *Journal of Nutrition* found that such changes could occur after as little as ten weeks of consuming a fructose-containing beverage daily.[10] Because of its powerful ability to stimulate fat production, fructose has a direct impact on your waistline. A meta-analysis of randomized controlled trials published in the journal *BMJ* showed that as your sugar intake rises, so too does your body weight. But reducing the amount of sugar in your diet causes weight to fall off.[11]

The fructose that occurs naturally in fruit — with some exceptions — does not belong in that category of substances to be avoided at all costs. Fructose in whole fruit is accompanied by soluble fiber, a type of cellular scaffolding that delivers many benefits. When you bite into a nectarine, its fiber slows your body's absorption of its fructose and gives your liver more time to metabolize it.[12] The fiber in fruit also feeds the friendly flora in your gut and cleans your intestines. Randomized controlled trials have found that consuming fruit does not have the same adverse effects on weight, blood pressure, insulin, and triglycerides that consuming fructose from highly processed foods does.[13] Large observational studies also show no evidence that increased fruit consumption raises your risk of coronary heart disease. In fact, a large meta-analysis of studies published in the *Journal of Human Hypertension* found the opposite: Test subjects who regularly consumed fruit had a 17 percent reduction in heart disease risk.[14]

Fruit can be a healthy addition to your diet. But that doesn't mean you should go crazy. Fruit is great—in moderation. If you are overweight or have pre-diabetes or diabetes, you shouldn't have more than a cup a day of fruit, and ideally you'll pick lower glycemic fruits like berries.

2. All Fruits Are Not Created Equal

You don't have to be a nutritionist to know that fruit is a health food. A study in the *British Journal of Nutrition* found that middle-aged and elderly people who regularly consumed high amounts of fruits and vegetables were less likely to develop signs of cognitive decline as they aged.[15] In a meta-analysis of rigorous studies in the *Lancet* that included more than 250,000 subjects, researchers found an inverse correlation between daily consumption of fruits and veggies and risk of stroke.[16] A meta-analysis of studies carried out by researchers at the prestigious Imperial College London found a similar relationship between fruit intake and breast cancer risk.[17]

Clearly, we need to eat fruit, but which fruit is best? In the vegetable chapter, we discussed why veggies containing "slow" carbs—meaning foods that release their carbs into your bloodstream gradually—are better than varieties that contain carbs that our bodies absorb quickly. The same applies to fruit.[18] To get the best results, you have to understand two concepts: glycemic index and glycemic load.

Glycemic index, or GI, is a scale that measures how much a particular food raises your blood sugar. (We discuss this in detail in the "Geek Alert" section of the chapter on vegetables.) The lower the glycemic index, the smaller the effect a food has on your insulin output, which is especially important if weight control is an issue, because insulin is the fat-storage hormone. The GI number is useful for comparing one food to another. But because it doesn't take serving size into account, it's not a perfect yardstick.

In 1997, scientists at Harvard developed the glycemic load, which is a more useful way to measure a food's actual impact on your blood sugar and insulin response.[19] Basically, glycemic load measures how much a typical serving of a food will raise your blood sugar. Watermelon, for example, is high in sugar, with a glycemic index of 72 (100 is pure glucose). But because watermelons contain mostly water, you don't get a huge hit of sugar per serving, so its glycemic load is low—at 4.

When you're choosing which fruits to eat, you should let the glycemic load be your guide. Below, you'll find the GL figures for some popular fruits. To give you a point of comparison, the GL of a slice of Betty Crocker chocolate cake with frosting is 20, or about five times that of a typical serving of watermelon. As a general rule, you should stick to eating fruit that has a glycemic load of no more than 11. Lower is even better.

- Apricots: 3
- Oranges: 3
- Watermelons: 4
- Nectarines: 4
- Wild blueberries: 5
- Golden Delicious apples: 6
- Pineapples: 6
- Kiwis: 7
- Mangoes: 8
- Cherries: 9
- Black grapes: 11
- Bananas: 16
- Dried figs: 16
- Raisins: 28

3. Berries May Be Best

Among all the nutrients contained in plant foods, antioxidants are most prized because they help prevent cancer, heart disease, diabetes, dementia, and arthritis. You've almost certainly never had the fruit with the highest measured antioxidant content: the Indian gooseberry, or amla berry. In India, the tree is worshipped, and its berry is considered the number one food for rejuvenation. How has this gem escaped us? Maybe because its taste has been described as "sour and astringent." Doesn't sound like something you're going to pack in your lunchbox! If you go online, you can find it easily — in powdered form, which is convenient for adding to shakes and smoothies that mask its bitter taste. But don't expect to find it in the supermarket produce aisle.

If you're looking to get antioxidants from produce — and you absolutely should be — berries, across the board, have more per calorie than any other fruit. So, you should resolve to eat plenty of them, whether fresh or frozen. Here's a list of some of the best, in descending order of antioxidant content[20]:

- Goji berries
- Black raspberries (which aren't all that easy to find)
- Wild blueberries
- Blackberries
- Raspberries
- Elderberries
- Cranberries
- Strawberries
- Cultivated blueberries

As we've already said, the key with fruit is striking a healthy balance between nutrient intake and sugar intake. The non-berry fruits with most antioxidants per calorie are, in descending order:

- Plums
- Cherries
- Red Delicious apples
- Figs
- Granny Smith apples
- Pears

4. Dirty (or Clean) Makes a Difference

Every year the US Department of Agriculture tests more than 6,900 kinds of produce for pesticide residue—and finds it on about three-quarters of the samples. According to the Environmental Working Group,[21] which compiles these statistics, 146 different pesticides can be found on fruit and vegetables, sometimes even after they have been washed and peeled. Does this matter? According to the USDA, every chemical used on the crops we eat has been evaluated, and none pose a threat to our health.[22] Unsurprisingly, many scientists disagree, and a lot of research backs them up. According to an EWG report,[23] among the pesticides most commonly used on our fruit are:

- Carbendazim, a fungicide that damages the male reproductive system and is banned by the European Union

- Bifenthrin, an insecticide that California has designated a "possible human carcinogen"
- Malathion, a "probable carcinogen" that is toxic to the nervous system

And there are 143 more we could list, many of them just as scary. How can you protect yourself? The obvious answer is to buy organic produce only. That way there's no danger of toxic chemicals on your food. It's also a guarantee that you won't get any genetically modified produce, and that your fruits and vegetables are grown in ways that maintain the health of the soil. Of course, that gets expensive, especially if you're trying to eat a lot of produce every day. A less reliable solution is to buy conventionally grown fruit and carefully wash off the chemical residue (but beware, this doesn't always work). Or you could heed the EWG's Dirty Dozen and Clean Fifteen lists—the fruits and vegetables found to have the most and least pesticide residue, respectively—and buy organic selectively. There's quite a disparity: More than 98 percent of strawberries, apples, nectarines, and peaches tested positive for at least four different pesticides, according to the EWG, while just 1 percent of avocados had any residue.

Here are the fruits on the EWG list, ranked from most to least contaminated:

- Strawberries
- Apples

- Nectarines
- Peaches
- Grapes
- Cherries
- Domestic blueberries
- Imported blueberries
- Plums
- Pears
- Raspberries
- Tangerines
- Bananas
- Oranges
- Watermelons
- Cantaloupes
- Grapefruits
- Honeydew melons
- Kiwis
- Papayas
- Mangoes
- Pineapples
- Avocados

It's no coincidence that the cleanest fruits are also the ones with the thickest, toughest skins. They keep the chemicals from reaching the edible parts. My advice would be to buy organic everything down through raspberries. Below that, you're probably okay with conventionally grown. But remember that pesticides are stubborn: Traces of Monsanto's bestselling weed killer, glyphosate, are found even on highly pro-cessed grain-based foods, everything from Cheerios to Oreos to Doritos.[24]

5. Fresh Fruit Isn't Always the Best Choice

Would you rather buy fresh fruit or frozen? How about canned? Hold on before you decide. This may be a no-brainer when it comes to fruits that are cheap and plentiful at supermarkets year-round, like bananas, apples, and oranges. But for other fruits, like berries, that's not always the case. In fact, sometimes frozen varieties offer not only more convenience, but more nutrition as well.

To keep fruit from rotting on its long, often overseas journey from the farm to your supermarket, it is often picked unripe. As a result, its nutrients don't have a chance to fully develop. That's where frozen fruit has an advantage. The produce is flash frozen right as its nutrient content peaks. And because it remains frozen until you thaw and eat it, there's no need to worry about the nutrition content degrading during shipping. Researchers have found that frozen produce retains its phytochemicals and other nutrients far better than fresh produce. And it is cheaper!

In a study published by the *Journal of Agricultural and Food Chemistry*, researchers harvested, processed, and then analyzed the vitamin and nutrient contents of eight different types of produce, including fruits like blueberries and strawberries, before and after they were frozen. Tests showed that after ten days in the freezer, their levels of key nutrients like vitamin C had remained stable. In some cases they'd even increased. The frozen produce was tested again after ninety days; its nutrient levels had risen even higher.[25]

So, what can you do with frozen berries? Turns out you have plenty of options. I love adding them to my smoothies. But cooking with them or gently thawing them for use in salads and other recipes may be even better. That's because heating them does not deplete all of their nutrients. In fact, a study in the *Journal of Agricultural and Food Chemistry* found that heating blueberries actually *boosted* some of their antioxidant levels.[26]

I eat blueberries every chance I get — and for good reason. In a clinical trial published in the *American Journal of Clinical Nutrition*, researchers recruited twenty-one healthy men and examined their arterial function after feeding them either a serving of blueberries or a vitamin-rich beverage.[27] They found that their vascular function improved after eating the blueberries, but not the placebo. The results suggest that the beneficial compounds in the blueberries reduce blood levels of harmful enzymes like NADPH oxidase, which plays a role in causing heart disease. All of this means that if it weren't for the sugar and refined carbs, blueberry pie might actually be health food! For now, though, avoid the pie and stick to eating your berries in smoothies, in salads, or on their own as a heart-healthy snack. You can watch a video of me making my favorite blueberry smoothie at www.food thebook.com.

6. Don't Drink Your Fruit; Eat It

As I mentioned, the number one "fruit" consumed in America according to surveys is orange juice. But as you probably know by now, juice is the absolute worst way to consume fruit because you get all the sugar with little or none of the fiber. The glycemic load of an orange is 3, while the GL of orange juice is 12—four times higher, which means it raises your blood sugar much faster and higher than eating an orange in its natural state. The other problem: When you drink your fruit, it doesn't create the sensation of fullness you get when eating it. Also, your brain doesn't recognize calories you drink the same way it does those you eat. As a result of those two factors, you end up consuming more calories drinking juice or any sugar-sweetened beverages than you do when eating whole fruit.[28]

Does this mean you should swear off fruit juice altogether? Well, that depends. If you're overweight or insulin resistant or have type 2 diabetes, then you should avoid all fruit juice. Under those circumstances the last thing you need is another source of liquid sugar. But even if you don't have an issue with your weight or blood sugar, you should go easy on fruit juice. Try to avoid it if you didn't squeeze it yourself or get it straight from a juicer. That's because the phytonutrients in commercial varieties of fruit juice are destroyed during pasteurization, leaving behind nothing but a whole lot of sugar. Clear apple juice (the kind you find in the supermarket) can have as little as 6 percent of the phytonutrients found in the apples themselves.

You're better off replacing fruit juice with smoothies. But even then, you have to be careful. You still get fiber from drinking blended fruit, but it's been substantially broken down, so you'll absorb the sugar faster than you would if you had just eaten the fruit whole. And as with juice, when you turn your fruit into a smoothie, you're more likely to consume larger quantities. The smoothies you get at the fancy organic juice bar or the Smoothie King kiosk at the mall will almost always be a heck of a lot bigger than any smoothie you'd make for yourself (after all, the stores have to justify their high price tags). Even worse, there's a good chance that sugar (or honey or syrup) will be added to your drink. If you're making smoothies at home, avoid adding sweeteners and stick to low-glycemic fruits like blueberries and strawberries along with other healthy produce like kale, spinach, ginger, avocado, celery, or cucumber. And watch out for "healthy" drinks like "green" juices, which can contain more sugar than a can of Coke or Pepsi.

ENVIRONMENTAL AND ETHICAL CONSIDERATIONS OF FRUIT

According to the USDA, about half of the fresh fruit consumed in the United States is imported.[29] Most of the bananas we find in North American supermarkets are shipped in from Peru, Ecuador, Honduras, and other South or Central American countries. The top pineapple producers include Costa Rica, Brazil, the Philippines, Thailand, and Indonesia. Most of our berries come from California or Florida, and the distance from Florida to New York, for example, is more than 1,000 miles—a long trek by any measure. According to a 2008 study published in *Environmental Science & Technology*, the transportation of fruit alone may account for half of its total carbon emissions.[30]

One of the trendiest fruits in America is avocado (yes, it's a fruit). But while our relatively newfound love of avocados means more income for Mexico—that's where we get 60 percent of them—it also means trouble. There isn't enough farmland available to meet the skyrocketing global demand, so some farmers are illegally cutting down forests to make room. Between 2001 and 2010, some regions of Mexico lost as many as 1,700 acres of forestland per year as a direct result of the growing demand for avocado production.[31] On top of that, gangs sometimes demand a cut of growers' profits, and those who refuse to pay face violence. Unfortunately, that guacamole you add to your burrito bowl may come with a high karmic price tag.

The agricultural regions of Colombia, Ecuador, and other countries are often unstable, violent environments. In 2007, Chiquita was fined for paying a notorious terrorist group in Colombia for protection. Dole, in 2009, came under fire for funding militia groups that murdered union leaders and used terror tactics to discourage workers from organizing. To ensure that you're not supporting these practices or the people who perpetrate them, you should look for bananas with "Equal Exchange" stickers, which mean that the fruit was produced in a safe way that's fair to workers. Whole Foods, Trader Joe's, and other health food stores offer organic fruit from smaller farms closer to home.

Going local, seasonal, and organic can reduce the environmental impact of fruit. Organic eliminates the many dangers that pesticides pose to your health, the environment, and farmworkers, and eating locally grown produce while it's in season reduces its carbon footprint.

You can also grow your own fruit, the safest and freshest choice of all. I just planted a mini-orchard of five fruit trees in my backyard. But if that's not an option, you can shop farmers' markets or join a CSA (community-supported agriculture). To find the nearest CSA or farmers' market, or to learn more about fair trade and farmer co-ops, check out the following resources:

- The Local Harvest website, which maintains a nationwide directory of small farms, farmers' markets, and other local food sources: http://www.loc alharvest.org/csa/
- The National Farmers Market Directory, maintained by the USDA: https://www.ams.usda.gov/ local-food-directories/farmersmarkets
- The website of Equal Exchange, which promotes fair trade and worker co-operatives that benefit farmers: http://equalexchange.coop/about

SUMMING IT UP

If you're like most Americans, the "fruits" you consume most often are juice. They are often as full of sugar as soda is, and they promote obesity, diabetes, and heart disease. An apple or orange without its fiber isn't fruit — it's sugar water with a few vitamins, and it's no substitute for eating whole fruit.

You should focus on the lower-sugar fruits, such as berries, apples, and pears, and use the others as treats in smaller quantities. The average serving is ½ cup or one piece of fruit. If you are overweight, diabetic, or have other blood sugar issues, then you need to be more careful; limit your fruit intake to ½ cup of berries or one piece of fruit per day.

When you think of fruit, fat is probably the last thing that comes to mind. But three of the best varieties are loaded with it. And the fats that they contain have some remarkable health benefits.

- Avocados are almost 80 percent fat, most of which is monounsaturated—the kind that's been shown to protect against heart disease and strokes.[32] They contain ample amounts of fiber, and even more potassium than bananas. During the low-fat craze, avocados were dismissed as "fattening" because of their fat and calorie content. But now we know better. Make sure you buy avocados grown in California. The ones from Mexico are often called "blood avocados" because of their connection to drug cartels.
- Coconuts are chock-full of special fats called medium-chain triglycerides, which are metabolized differently from other fats. Your body absorbs and utilizes them much more efficiently than it does other fats. They even help you burn fat, improve brain function, and boost your metabolism.[33]
- Olives are the fruit of the olive tree. The oil they produce is one of the most heart-healthy foods on the planet.[34] But the flesh of the olive fruit contains a lot of vitamin E and fiber, too. And olives are brimming with antioxidants—which is why they are naturally

bitter. They're cured and fermented to make them more palatable. Try snacking on olives as a healthy alternative to potato chips and other junk.

FRUIT: WHAT THE HECK SHOULD I EAT?

- Wild, organic, fresh blueberries, cherries, blackberries, and raspberries*
- Frozen organic berries, either thawed or in shakes or frozen desserts*
- Organic stone fruit like plums, peaches, nectarines, cherries, and others
- Organic oranges, grapefruits, tangerines, and other citrus fruit
- Pomegranates, kiwis, and papayas
- Weird fruit like goji berries, snake fruit, acai berries, gooseberries, mangosteen, or dragon fruit
- The "fat" fruits — avocados, coconut, and olives
- Lemons and limes — keep them in the kitchen and use them to flavor food and your drinking water

FRUIT: WHAT THE HECK SHOULD I AVOID (OR AT LEAST GO EASY ON)?

- Grapes are delicious and easy to overeat. But because they're sugary, eat in small quantities only.

---

* These are the fruits with lowest glycemic load.

- Bananas are quite starchy and high in sugar.
- Dried fruits like figs, dates, raisins, and currents are highest in sugar, and they sometimes contain added sugar or the preservative sulfite.
- Pineapples are a good source of an enzyme called bromelain, which helps alleviate inflammation and improve joint health. But they are very high in sugar. Have no more than 1 cup a day.
- Conventionally grown apples and strawberries are among the worst offenders when it comes to pesticides. Buy organic.
- Any and all fruit juice, especially any that you didn't squeeze yourself.

FATS AND OILS

NUTRITION IQ QUIZ

True or False?

1. Vegetable oils are better for your health than animal-based fats.
2. A salad with nonfat dressing or lemon juice is healthier than one drenched in oil.
3. The cholesterol from eggs clogs your arteries and causes heart disease.
4. Vegetable shortening is a better alternative than lard (pork fat) when cooking or baking.
5. Fats and oils make you gain weight because they contain more calories than carbs or protein.
6. The federal government's dietary guidelines now tell us there is no limit on the amount of fat you can eat and be healthy.

Answers

1. False: Refined vegetable oils promote inflammation and may increase the risk of heart disease, suicide, homicide, and violent behavior.[1]

2. False: You need to eat fat along with plant foods in order to absorb all their fat-soluble nutrients, like vitamin A. And olive oil has been shown to reduce the risk of heart disease, type 2 diabetes, and obesity.

3. False: Eating cholesterol-rich foods like eggs or shrimp has little to no effect on the cholesterol circulating in your bloodstream, and it is not linked to heart disease.

4. False: Shortening is highly processed and made from trans fats, which have been ruled non-GRAS, or not safe to eat, by the FDA. It is inferior to lard and other animal fats for baking.

5. False: Eating the right kinds of fats and oils can protect you against weight gain. In fact, in more than fifty-three randomized controlled trials, a high-fat diet beat out a low-fat diet for weight loss.[2] Eating the right fats burns body fat, boosts your metabolism, improves your HDL, lowers your triglycerides, and is associated with a significantly lower risk of heart disease, diabetes, and obesity.

6. True: Until 2015, the guidelines mistakenly urged us to limit fats and eat plenty of carbs. Now they have finally caught up with the science.

Get a new food fact and weekly recipe directly from my kitchen. Sign up for free at www.food thebook.com.

Fat is confusing. So many different kinds of fat—some, we are told, are good, some bad. What's true? And then there is the word "fat." We all were taught that eating dietary fat leads to accumulation of body fat—that fat that passes through your lips ends up on your hips. We were also told that fatty streaks in arteries causing heart attacks came from dietary fat and cholesterol. But it's not true. Far from it. Eating fat doesn't make you fat. Eating fat doesn't cause heart attacks. This is not only my opinion, but the consensus of the 2015 Dietary Guidelines Advisory Committee, a group of conservative scientists who finally eliminated any recommendations to limit dietary fat or dietary cholesterol.

Assumptions must be tested and proven in studies before we accept them as fact. But historically that hasn't always happened in nutrition science. And no assumption has been more catastrophic for our health than the one insisting that fat makes you fat and causes heart disease. It led the government to promote all the wrong foods. It enabled the profit-hungry food industry to sell billions of dollars' worth of low-fat junk as "health foods." And it caused millions of people around the world to become obese, sick, and diabetic and to die. All thanks to one seemingly commonsense assumption that was accepted with hardly any scientific scrutiny at all. So how did it all happen?

The lie that dietary fat is public health enemy number one was built on three bad ideas. The first was that body fat and dietary fat are one and the same, and that the fat we eat becomes fat in our bodies. The second was a simplistic view of human metabolism and weight gain—that "a calorie is a calorie"—which the experts drilled into our heads. The thinking went like this: A gram of carbohydrate has 4 calories and a gram of fat has 9 calories, so eating lots of carbs and reducing fats will keep you lean. That was dead wrong. In fact, a 2012 Harvard study found that a very-high-fat diet, compared to a very-low-fat diet, speeds up metabolism by 300 calories a day. Eating fat speeds up your metabolism and helps you lose weight.[3] That turns conventional wisdom on its head.

Finally, the medical community came to believe that eating saturated fat and its first cousin, cholesterol, creates roadblocks in our arteries and death by heart attack. Put all three of these falsehoods together and you get one big reason for health authorities to tell us all to throw away our butter, meat, and coconut oil. This is why, in 1980, the US Dietary Guidelines began recommending low-fat diets. As the years went on, their advice became more and more aggressive, leading to the Food Guide Pyramid in 1992 that told us to load up on bread, rice, cereal, and pasta, to avoid even fatty plant foods like nuts and avocado, and to eat fats and oils only sparingly.

But after 40 years of spreading this gospel, health authorities and nutrition experts are now finally confessing that what they told us was false. And it wasn't simply because they misunderstood the science, but because there was no good science to begin with. One of the consequences of the government's crusade against saturated fat was that Americans replaced animal fats like butter and lard with the industrially produced hydrogenated vegetable oils known as trans fats. Walter Willett, the chair of Harvard's nutrition department, estimates that the nationwide shift to trans fats caused up to 228,000 heart attacks in America every year.[4]

Today, every well-informed researcher, nutritionist, and clinician *should* know that eating fat doesn't make you fat or cause heart disease. But you could go online right this second and spend all day reading nutrition advice about fat that's outdated, inaccurate, and even deadly. The shift in our understanding of fats has been monumental. But like our ancestors slowly getting used to the idea that the earth revolves around the sun, it's going to take some time for the great big reveal about dietary fat to sink in.

We've been taught to think of fats and oils as a necessary evil—the unhealthy part of anything we eat and the stuff needed to keep food from sticking to the pot. Nothing could be further from the truth.

Fat is essential for health. Let's start there.

THE SCIENCE OF FATS

We burn two kinds of fuel for energy, carbs and fats (although we can burn protein when needed). Most people are more familiar with carbs in that role and know that sugar and bread give us energy. Fats are more mysterious. Most of the fats we eat are natural parts of foods like meat, fish, dairy, and nuts. And those fats are typically the good ones. Naturally occurring fats in our whole foods aren't the problem; refined, processed fats and oils that are added to our food by the food industry are.

Before we turn our attention to those bad fats, let's address a basic question: What exactly is the nutritional purpose of fats and oils anyway? They help us feel full and satiated. They increase our metabolism. Because fats (unlike carbs) don't contain glucose, they don't spike our blood sugar levels and trigger the release of insulin, which acts like fertilizer for our body's fat cells. They do the opposite. In a rigorous metabolic ward study published in the *Journal of the American Medical Association*, researchers compared the effects of high-fat, low-carb diets vs. high-carb, low-fat diets on metabolism.[5] A metabolic ward study is the most accurate type of nutrition study. Participants are confined to a locked ward and everything they eat is measured, as is their metabolic rate. So you know exactly how many calories are eaten and burned. One group was assigned to follow a diet that was 60 percent carbs, 20 percent proteins, and 20 percent fats for four weeks. The other subjects consumed 60 percent fats, 30 percent proteins, and 10 percent carbs. Then the high-fat-diet subjects were switched to the low-fat diet, and vice versa. This allowed the researchers to study and compare the effects of the two dramatically different diets on each subject's metabolism. The findings were astonishing. On the high-fat diet, the subjects burned 300 more calories per day than they did on the low-fat diet. That's like running an hour a day without getting off the couch. The high-fat diet also produced the biggest improvements in blood sugar, insulin, triglycerides, and HDL cholesterol and other cardiovascular markers.

In another study published in the *Annals of Internal Medicine,* researchers recruited 150 overweight people and assigned them to follow either a low-fat diet or a higher-fat diet for a year. At the end of the experiment, subjects in the high-fat group had lost an average of eight pounds more than those in the low-fat group, had greater reductions in body fat, and had maintained more lean muscle—even though neither group had changed its physical activity levels.[6] At the same time, the high-fat subjects saw their inflammation and triglyceride levels plunge, and their protective HDL cholesterol levels rise sharply. All this in spite of the fact that their saturated fat intake had been more than double the amount recommended by the American Heart Association.

Findings from all the relevant studies point in the

same direction. The prestigious Cochrane Collaboration published a systematic review that found that low-glycemic diets—which tend to be higher in fat—were superior for weight loss and overall health to high-glycemic diets, which tend to be lower in fat.[7] In 2015, another group of researchers published a systematic review and meta-analysis in the *Lancet Diabetes & Endocrinology* that examined fifty-three clinical trials that lasted a year or longer. They found that high-fat, low-carb diets led to the most weight loss.[8] And the more extreme the difference in fats and carbs, the more significant the weight loss. In other words, the more fats subjects ate, the more weight they lost.

The evidence in support of eating fats—traditional, unrefined fats from plants and animals—is overwhelming. The largest randomized controlled study comparing a high-fat diet to a low-fat diet, the PREDIMED study, showed that a high-fat diet reduces heart disease, diabetes, and obesity. We need fats for healthy cell membranes. We need them to make hormones (like testosterone and estrogen) and immune cells, to regulate inflammation and metabolism. We need fats because 60 percent of our brains are fat. That sounds pretty important, doesn't it?

WHAT THE EXPERTS GOT RIGHT

Nothing really. Except that we need omega-3 fats because they are "essential" for life. Recently, the 2015

US Dietary Guidelines removed any limits on total dietary fat and cholesterol. However, they still recommend limiting dietary saturated fat.

WHAT THEY GOT WRONG

"The biggest public health experiment in history."[9] Those are the words David Ludwig of Harvard Medical School uses to describe the intense efforts undertaken by the scientific establishment and the federal government to get us all to adopt low-fat diets. In the four decades that followed, Americans, and eventually people in many other Western countries, followed their advice faithfully. Unfortunately, the experiment was a failure, and a lot of people died from the very cardiovascular problems that those recommendations were meant to avert. According to the USDA, as the total amount of fat eaten by Americans fell by roughly 25 percent—from 40 percent of our calories to 30 percent—the number of calories we consumed from sugar and carbs rose dramatically. And so did the prevalence of obesity and type 2 diabetes. In fact, the nationwide rise in obesity rates began at exactly the same time we started weaning ourselves off fat. According to the CDC, obesity rates were relatively flat between 1960 and the mid-1970s. Then they suddenly took off, rising more than 8 percent between 1976 and 1994, and continuing on an upward trend until today.[10] Childhood obesity rates also tripled during the same period.[11] It's easy to see how the spike in obesity coincided with the federal government's release of the first Dietary Guidelines for Americans in 1980, which told us to restrict fat and eat carbs and starches.

By June of 2015, one of the country's top nutrition authorities, Dariush Mozaffarian, a cardiologist and dean of the Tufts school of nutrition science and policy, had seen enough. In an editorial published in the *Journal of the American Medical Association*,[12] he and coauthor David Ludwig called on the government to end their decades-long war on dietary fat and to promote consumption of healthful fat.

Healthful fat? What was once a contradiction is becoming the new gospel: Fat is good.

WHAT WE STILL DON'T KNOW FOR SURE

Saturated fats—which are found mainly in animal foods like dairy and meat, as well as in coconut oil and a few other plant foods—were once widely considered to be the reason that heart disease was our number one killer. All the research has done an about-face since then. We know now there is no monolithic saturated fat. There are many saturated fats, each with its own effects (mostly good). The saturated fat in coconut, for instance, is different from the saturated fat in butter. A lot of research remains to be done before we really understand everything about saturated fats, but study after study has failed to demonstrate a link between them and heart disease.

EIGHT THINGS YOU NEED TO KNOW ABOUT FATS AND OILS

1. Monounsaturated Fat Is Our Friend

Unless you plan on majoring in organic chemistry, there's really no reason to wade through the intricacies of the molecular makeup of fat. It's complicated. There are classifications within classifications, most having to do with the number and alignment of carbon and hydrogen atoms. It's a lot of science to think about every time you want to eat. And yet, the distinctions are important. They determine which fats are healthy and which are not. So, let's just focus on that and forget about the rest: We don't eat molecules, after all; we eat food.

Monounsaturated fatty acids—or MUFAs for short—are good for us. They come from plant and animal foods. They contain important nutrients and antioxidants, and they protect you against heart disease (and more). They've been shown to lower blood pressure, improve insulin sensitivity, and lower LDL cholesterol.[13] More important, when it comes to cholesterol, they've been shown to reduce the small, dense LDL particles that attack the walls of your arteries and accelerate atherosclerosis or hardening of the arteries.[14]

MUFAs constitute the main pillar of the Mediterranean diet. They're found in foods like olive oil, nuts and nut oils, avocados, and other plants. They are also present in animal foods, which is why butter, lard, beef tallow, chicken fat, and duck fat can be healthful when used in cooking. MUFAs are found in some unhealthy refined foods, though, like canola oil, which is refined and bleached with strong chemicals and high heat. It's so processed that it has to be deodorized before it can be sold. That's not an appetizing thought. And it's not good for the oils. When you expose mono-unsaturated or polyunsaturated fatty acids to high temperatures, they become oxidized, or damaged.[15] When that happens, the fat can turn rancid and harmful.

2. Polyunsaturated Fat…the Good, the Bad, and the Ugly

Scientists call some polyunsaturated fatty acids, or PUFAs, "essential," which means that we require them but our bodies can't make them. We need them in our diets because they deliver two necessities: linoleic acid and omega-3 fats (alpha-linolenic acid from plant sources, and EPA and DHA, which are found mostly in fish and wild game or grass-fed meat). Here are the details that matter: The two most critical polyunsaturated fats are omega-3 and omega-6 fatty acids. These guys are the yin and yang of polyunsaturated fats. You need them both. One is good, the other (as we mostly eat it in refined vegetable oils) is bad. One can be inflammatory (omega-6) and one is anti-inflammatory (omega-3), and they work together in different ways. It's all about balance.

Omega-3s are the better of the two. They're like powerful medicine without the side effects. They reduce inflammation, promote cardiovascular health, protect your brain, and help prevent metabolic syndrome and chronic diseases.[16] We know how important they are because of what happens when we don't get enough (and more than 90 percent of Americans are deficient in omega-3 fats). People who lack omega-3s in their diets are at greater risk of heart disease and chronic inflammation. Deficiencies have been linked to a higher prevalence of Alzheimer's disease and dementia, ADD, violence, depression, and even suicide.[17]

Omega-6s, on the other hand, can increase inflammation in the face of oxidative stress. When your body has too much omega-6 and not enough omega-3, the natural result is chronic inflammation, which promotes a variety of diseases.[18] A large randomized controlled trial, the Lyon Diet Heart Study, found that decreasing the amount of omega-6 fats people consumed while increasing their omega-3 fat intake reduced heart attacks by 70 percent, protected against cancer, and lowered mortality rates.[19] Omega-3s are abundant in a few natural whole foods like fatty fish, seafood, eggs, grass-fed meat, flaxseeds, algae, and walnuts. Omega-6s are mostly found in nuts, seeds, grains, beans, highly refined vegetable oils, and ultraprocessed packaged foods—exactly the things you shouldn't be eating (except small amounts of whole grains and beans). Whole nuts and seeds are the best source of omega-6 fats. In fact, according to the USDA, Americans now get almost 10 percent of their calories from refined soybean oil, which is one of the most abundant sources of omega-6 fatty acids.[20] Plus, it often contains high levels of glyphosate, or Roundup, the toxic herbicide used by Monsanto. It's not that Americans are drinking soybean oil by the cup; most people aren't even aware they're eating it. But it's lurking everywhere. If you eat fast food, grains, desserts, packaged snacks, potato chips, muffins, or conventionally raised meat, or buy almost anything cooked in oil at a cafeteria, diner, or restaurant, then you're almost certainly consuming lots of soybean oil and other oils rich in omega-6 fatty acids without even knowing it.

In prehistoric times, our ancestors consumed omega-3 and omega-6 fatty acids in the healthy ratio of 1:1. Since the advent of refined vegetable oils, however, most of us are eating far more omega-6s than we should.[21] The ratio can get up to 20:1 for people who eat a lot of processed foods. That's because as part of their war on saturated fat, the nutrition establishment has long advised Americans to replace butter, lard, coconut oil, and other saturated fats with canola oil, soybean oil, corn oil, margarine, and oils made from safflower and sunflower, supposedly to reduce the risk of heart disease. Of course, as we've seen, Americans obliged. But our health only got worse. In large clinical trials, people who reduced their saturated fat intake and ate foods cooked or prepared with omega-6-rich vegetable oils saw their mortality rates rise, not fall.[22]

The bottom line is that we absolutely need polyunsaturated fats—both omega-3 and omega-6. But we should get them from whole foods—things like fish (fatty, wild-caught varieties like salmon, sardines, herring, anchovies, and mackerel); meat (especially pastured, grass-fed animals that haven't been fed grains and other junk); pastured poultry and eggs; grass-fed dairy; and whole plant foods like avocados, walnuts, and other nuts and seeds (pumpkin, sesame, chia, hemp, and flax).

3. Saturated Fat Was Once the Enemy, but Not Anymore

Saturated fat kills, we were told (wrongly), end of story. But it's a lot more complex than that. For one thing, saturated fat comes in many forms. All told there are more than *thirty different* types,[23] such as lauric acid (found in coconuts and breast milk), margaric acid (in dairy), and palmitic acid (in palm oil and other foods), to name a few. But the saturated fats we eat are not related to the fats that are found in our blood and tissues.[24]

In fact—and this is going to sound paradoxical—rigorous studies show that eating carbohydrates increases the levels of some saturated fats in our bloodstream, particularly palmitoleic acid, a fatty acid that's strongly linked to metabolic syndrome, insulin resistance, and cardiovascular disease.[25] (Don't confuse palmitoleic acid with palmitic acid, which is mentioned in the previous paragraph—they're related but are not the same thing.)

This fundamental nutritional truth was demonstrated clearly in a landmark paper written by a team of prominent researchers from around the world and published in the *Annals of Internal Medicine* in 2014.[26] The study didn't just look at what people reportedly ate. It reviewed objective data from seventy-two studies, including observational data and rigorous, randomized controlled trials that manipulated the types of fat people ate and analyzed the fatty acids circulating in their bloodstreams and in their fat tissue. All together, their study incorporated data from more than a half million subjects. What they discovered is striking. The study showed that the fats in your blood that cause heart attacks—palmitic and stearic acid—are the ones that come from eating sugar and carbs, not fat. This occurs because your body literally turns carbohydrates to fat in a process known as *de novo lipogenesis*, which is most active when you consume lots of sugar and simple carbs.[27] Think of that the next time you're eating a bagel or a bowl of pasta. It may look like carbs, but when it hits your liver, a lot of it is converted straight to fat. The omega-6 fats from vegetable oils were also found to cause a slight bump in heart disease when studied alone (without being consumed along with omega-3 fats). The fats that reduced heart disease risk were the omega-3 fats and saturated fats that come from animal products, especially margaric acid, which we get from eating foods like dairy and butter.

Some of the study's authors had previously endorsed replacing saturated fats with polyunsaturated vegetable oils, and even they acknowledged that the evidence clearly exonerated saturated fat and undermined the government's recommendations against consuming it.

Critics may dismiss that study because it included population data that can't prove cause and effect. But another study can. It was conducted 40 years ago but wasn't published until 2016 because the results so contradicted the prevailing dogma that saturated fat was bad and that LDL cholesterol causes heart disease. This gold-standard study (a randomized controlled trial) couldn't be done now — and probably should have never been done — for ethical reasons, but the findings are interesting nonetheless. Researchers took 9,000 patients in mental hospitals and fed them either butter and saturated fats or corn oil (polyunsaturated vegetable oil, which the AHA report[28] says we should eat more of).[29] Guess what? The patients who ate the corn oil had more heart attacks and deaths despite lowering their LDL cholesterol. What? Really? Yes, it's true. In fact, for every 30-point drop in LDL, the risk of heart attack went up 22 percent. So much for LDL being bad and vegetable oil good.

Another recent, very large, impressive population study (the PURE study) found no link between total fat or saturated fat and heart disease. In fact, the fats were found to be protective.[30] And so was animal protein, by the way. The study examined more than 135,000 people from eighteen countries on five continents over ten years. Researchers found that carbohydrates increased the risk of heart disease and death, while total fat, saturated fat, monounsaturated fat, and polyunsaturated fat all reduced the risk of heart disease and death. This study cannot prove cause and effect, only correlation. And since there is no correlation between saturated fat or animal protein and disease, it can prove there is no correlation.

Not only is saturated fat not as dangerous as we've been told; it's actually beneficial for several reasons. Many saturated fats are necessary for proper hormone and immune system function. They suppress inflammation and even contain vitamins.[31] Mostly we get saturated fat from whole foods, though there is a line of artisanal animal fats for cooking — organic, humanely raised beef tallow, pork lard, and duck and chicken fat — aimed at hard-core foodies. The good news about saturated fat is spreading, but it's taking a long time to reach everyone. We're still getting bad advice even from the National Institutes of Health, which publishes on its website a chart of fats and oils ranked from those we should "choose more often" to the ones we should "choose less often."[32] Unsurprisingly, it continues to recommend that we cook and bake with highly processed unsaturated vegetable and seed oils like canola (which contains just 7 percent saturated fat), safflower (10 percent), corn (13 percent), soybean (15 percent), and tub margarine (17 percent), while telling us to steer clear of butter (68 percent saturated fat) and coconut oil (91 percent).

That is just the opposite of what all the latest and most credible research says is true.[33] And it's particularly bad advice for anyone who cooks. Remember earlier when I explained that some fats and oils do not hold up well when exposed to high temperatures? It's the unsaturated fats that are most vulnerable to oxidation. These oils are easily damaged and can turn into rancid, oxidized fats when overheated.[34] It's far better to cook or fry using saturated fats like butter, coconut oil, or ghee (clarified butter). Because the molecules in saturated fat contain strong double bonds, they're less likely to break down and turn into harmful oxidized fats. They're not only more nutritious and flavorful, but also more stable than refined vegetable oils. There's a reason our grandparents and their grandparents before them cooked and baked with butter and lard.

4. Trans Fats Were Never Our Friends

Margarine, Crisco vegetable shortening, fake-butter spreads—these are the hydrogenated trans fats we were advised to eat instead of butter and lard for the sake of our health. Bad advice, it turns out, because they're far more toxic than the saturated fats they were meant to replace.[35] This is a good example of what happens when scientists and food engineers decide they know better than nature. Trans fats came into being only around a century ago. Americans were encouraged to buy and cook with them long before they were ever actually studied, which means we adopted them without really knowing how they'd affect us. Originally, margarine (which was soybean oil with hydrogen added to make it solid) was invented due to a butter shortage. Before long, these "hydrogenated" oils, or trans fats, took the place of butter and lard in pastries, cakes, cookies, piecrusts, potato chips, French fries, and thousands of other processed foods. Trans fats were cheap to make and gave foods a long shelf life, making them perfect for industrial food production. It's why your Twinkie can last on the shelf for years. But these fats increase your small, dense LDL particles, which get under the lining of your arteries and cause blockages, and they contribute to chronic inflammation, diabetes, obesity, dementia, and even the risk of cancer. It wasn't until 2015 that the FDA finally took trans fats off the "generally recognized as safe" list and ordered food companies to gradually phase them out of their products.[36] Trans fats are supposed to be phased out by 2018, but it is not clear if they will be out of all foods. You may still find some processed foods that contain them lingering on store shelves. The key to avoiding them is to read ingredients labels and look for the word "hydrogenated." Trans fats show up as hydrogenated soybean or vegetable oil. Even if the label says "zero" trans fats, you can't be sure it's true thanks to a loophole given to the food industry by the FDA.

5. Fats and Veggies Are the Perfect Pairing

Think of all the times you've heard someone order a salad and say, "Dressing on the side, please!" Or how often you've chosen low-fat salad dressing from the supermarket shelf. Now think about what a waste all that sacrifice was. The reason is that some very important nutrients — such as vitamins A, D, E, and K — are fat-soluble, meaning our bodies can't absorb and use them unless fat is present. That's because fat stimulates the production of bile, which you need in order to absorb fat-soluble vitamins. Without it, the fat-soluble vitamins in vegetables, like vitamin A, won't be well absorbed.

A salad full of healthy raw vegetables without olive oil, or a plate of steamed broccoli with just a squeeze of lemon, will do you a lot less good than you imagined. And if you use low-fat dressing instead of olive oil, you not only reduce the bioavailability of the vitamins in your salads, but almost certainly get an unhealthy dose of refined oils, emulsifiers, artificial flavorings, and other nonfood ingredients, including high-fructose corn syrup. Studies have also shown that the flavonoids and other polyphenols in tomato sauce are enhanced if we add some extra virgin olive oil. In other words: Everything goes better with fat.[37]

6. But Even Olive Oil Can Be a Problem

As I alluded to earlier, many fats and oils are volatile. Even the healthy ones can go from good to bad depending on how they're handled. They can oxidize when exposed to heat or light. When cooked to the point where they smoke continuously—known as the "smoke point"—the fat molecules break down and release free radicals and other toxic substances. To be safe, you must select the appropriate oils for the cooking you're doing. Olive oil is practically a miracle food, as everybody knows, full of healthy fats, polyphenols, antioxidants, and anti-inflammatory compounds.[38] Just a couple of spoonfuls a day protect you from heart disease.

But it has its drawbacks. Olive oil has a relatively low smoke point: around 350°F. So, it's best when used raw, in dressings, or in sauces and gravies slow-cooked over low heat. Coconut oil has a higher smoke point, which makes it better for sautéing. Butter has a high smoke point, too. In fact, the smoke point of clarified butter (or ghee) is 450°F, so it's perfect for hotter cooking. At high temperatures, animal fats such as lard or tallow (beef fat) are also good choices. It's worth noting that refined "light" olive oil's smoke point, 465°F, is considerably higher than extra virgin's,[39] but the light olive oil has very little health benefit.

Even if you don't cook your olive oil, there's another potential problem: It may be fake. If you've seen the price of good imported extra virgin olive oil lately, you know why counterfeiters might be interested. An estimated 70 percent of what is sold in America as extra virgin olive oil has been adulterated, either with lesser-quality oil or something else altogether, like nut or soybean oil. This is nothing new. It's been happening since ancient times,[40] and it's a major source of income for criminal organizations in Italy. The phony olive oil trade is three times more profitable than the trafficking of cocaine.[41] Genuine extra virgin olive oil is dark green in color and tastes strongly of olives. It may even be peppery and slightly bitter. Try a spoonful. If it tastes bitter in the back of your throat, it is likely okay. Because many Americans don't have much experience using olive oil, counterfeiters dump a lot of their junk here. A report from the University of California, Davis, Olive Center found that domestic olive oil produced and bottled in California was more likely to be authentic than imported.[42]

7. Coconut Oil Has Gotten a Bad Rap

First, there is not a single study showing that coconut oil causes heart disease. Not one. Second, the whole case against coconut oil is founded on a hypothesis that has been proven wrong. It's the diet-heart hypothesis: Saturated fat raises LDL cholesterol; LDL cholesterol causes heart disease; anything that raises LDL cholesterol is bad; therefore, coconut oil is bad. The only problem is that the data does not support the hypothesis. But just as it took us a while to accept Copernicus's observation that the Earth revolves around the sun, it will take time for people to lose the false belief that low-fat and low-cholesterol diets can save us from heart disease. In fact, low-fat diets *cause* heart disease.

A 2017 *USA Today* article declared that "Coconut Oil Isn't Healthy. Never Been Healthy" based on a review of fat by the American Heart Association (AHA). The AHA has been at the vanguard of bad advice for decades since it first hooked onto the "fat is bad and will kill you" meme. It told us to eat very-low-fat, low-cholesterol diets and to eat tons of starchy carbs. (The AHA gets huge funding from cereal makers, who put their seal of approval on sugary cereals because they are "fat-free" but 75 percent sugar.) But now an overwhelming amount of research has proven that idea dead wrong. In fact, the AHA's recommendations have killed millions of people (no joke) from heart disease and diabetes. That's why the very conservative 2015 US Dietary Guidelines removed any upper limits on dietary fat and eliminated any restrictions on dietary cholesterol. If you are interested in the corruption of the AHA, how its funding is supported by the pharmaceutical industry, industrial food giants, including sugary cereal makers and industrial vegetable oil manufactures, then read Kevin Michael Geary's article on

Medium.com, entitled "Is the American Heart Association a Terrorist Organization?" The title is a bit inflammatory, but the content is accurate.

It's true we have had a coconut oil craze. So what's the deal? Broccoli is healthy, but if it was all you ate, you would get sick. Coconut oil is healthy, but only as part of an overall healthy diet, not as the main course. Coconut oil has been consumed by populations in the South Pacific for thousands of years without ill effect. It has many health benefits. Here's the short list: It raises the good cholesterol, HDL. It improves the quality and size and type of cholesterol. It lowers the total cholesterol–to–HDL ratio—a far better predictor of heart disease than LDL. And cultures with more than 60 percent of their diet as coconut oil have no heart disease.[43] There is a unique type of saturated fat in coconut oil called MCT, or medium-chain triglycerides, and it boosts metabolism, reverses insulin resistance, and improves cognitive function. Coconut oil is also antifungal and antimicrobial. MCTs are odd—they travel from the gut straight to the liver, meaning they're not stored in our fat cells. Instead, they convert easily into energy. Experiments have shown that when overweight subjects consume MCT oil, it speeds up their metabolisms and leads to weight loss and a better ratio of good to bad cholesterol.[44] And it contains lauric acid, which is great for immune function. The only other good source is breast milk. By the way, breast milk is 24 percent saturated fat—far higher than the 6 percent the AHA recommends. Who would you trust, nature/God or the American Heart Association? I am sorry that you have to be buffeted about by bad conclusions from insufficient outdated science and bad journalism. I take MCT oil derived from coconut oil just about every single day. It makes your brain sharper and clearer and is a great addition to exercise since it boosts your energy production.

8. Is the Hype About Ketogenic Diets and Intermittent Fasting True?

You may have heard that a ketogenic diet can be beneficial for your health—that it promotes weight loss, longevity, and enhanced cognitive function—and wondered if the hype is true. You may have also heard of "intermittent fasting" or "time-restricted feeding" and how it may have similar effects. Is there anything to these diets? Well, yes.

First, it's important to recognize that ketogenic diets have been around in medicine for a long time. We use them for treating intractable epilepsy when medications fail. Yes, that's right, when meds fail we use food. Now mounting research has found them to be effective in reversing type 2 diabetes, obesity, Alzheimer's, autism, and brain and other cancers, in addition to increasing life span, enhancing brain function, and more. So what is a ketogenic diet anyway?

Let's start with a little biology. The body has a backup energy storage system that it can use when faced with starvation. Ordinarily, we burn glucose (carbs) for energy, but, as a contingency plan, our bodies have the ability to burn fat as well. We have about 2,500 calories of carbohydrate (in the form of glycogen) stored in our muscles. But we each have about 40,000 calories of fat stored through our bodies (and some people have a lot more). When carbohydrates are scarce (back in our caveman and cavewoman days this was generally a result of food scarcity), fat gets mobilized as ketones, which are used as an alternative fuel source. They are a much cleaner-burning source of fuel and stimulate all sorts of good things in your body.

A ketogenic diet decreases the size of your organs, increases stem cell production, reduces visceral or dangerous belly fat, improves your gene expression, reduces cancer, increases the size of your brain's memory center (known as the hippocampus), improves immune function, improves mitochondrial function (your energy production), enhances cognitive function, and reduces inflammation and oxidative stress.[45] All good things that promote health and longevity. In fact, mice live 13 percent longer on a ketogenic diet without restricting calories.[46] That's about ten more years in human terms. Ketogenic diets mimic calorie restriction (which is a lot less fun than eating lots of fat), which is the only thing that has been proven to extend life expectancy, and it does so by up to 30 percent. This means the average person would live to 104 years old if they followed such a diet.

Why wouldn't everyone want to eat a ketogenic diet (about 70 percent fat, 20 percent protein, and 10 percent carbohydrates)? It's hard, and it's just not necessary for most people. If you have type 2 diabetes or Alzheimer's, you should seriously consider it. But for the average person, it's a level of sacrifice that isn't necessary.

However, there are two "hacks" that shortcut your biology and allow you to get almost all the benefits of a ketogenic diet without all the effort: intermittent fasting (or time-restricted eating, which involves fasting for fourteen to sixteen hours a day) and the coconut and MCT oil hack.[47] You can do one or both. Intermittent fasting simply means fasting overnight. It's what we always did as cavemen and cavewomen: Eat dinner before dark, and then don't eat again until the next morning (hence the name "break-fast"). But now most of us eat late and get up and eat early. Ideally you should finish dinner at six or seven p.m. and not eat again until eight or nine in the morning. That's it. It gives your body a chance to repair, heal, clean up metabolic waste in your body and brain, and more. And it stimulates weight loss.

The second option is to take 2 to 3 tablespoons of a 1:1 mixture of coconut oil and MCT oil three times a day. The MCT produces ketones quickly, and the coconut oil allows you to produce ketones over a longer period of time. This will keep your body producing low levels of ketones all day even if you don't restrict your carbohydrates. And it will provide many of the same benefits as a ketogenic diet or intermittent fasting. Yes, you still don't want to eat sugar and refined flour and other refined carbs (except as an occasional treat). But you can eat more starchy veggies and nuts and whole grains and beans.

Bottom line: Our bodies do better when we switch from carb burning to fat burning. And so do our brains.

ARE YOU HARMING THE ENVIRONMENT BY EATING FAT?

Palm oil, olive oil, coconut oil, avocado oil — it seems like just about anything can be turned into oil these days. And now that the war on fat is over — or at least nearing its end — many of us have been embracing fat with open arms. As a fat lover (see my previous book: *Eat Fat, Get Thin*), this makes me happy. But I also want everyone to understand that not all oils are created equal.

Palm Oil: Now that trans fats are on their way out of the food supply, palm oil is being used as a replacement in snack foods, baked goods, and other processed foods. But the production and sourcing of most of the palm oil in our food supply involves deforestation, disruption of ecosystems, and human rights violations.

In fact, surging demand has caused palm oil production to become the "largest cause of deforestation in Indonesia and other equatorial countries with dwindling expanses of tropical rainforest," according to *Scientific American*. This rain forest destruction contributes to global warming and has endangered vulnerable orangutan populations that rely on it as their natural habitat. If you purchase palm oil, look for the CSPO label (Certified Sustainable Palm Oil). When purchasing products containing palm oil, look for the RSPO trademark, which means that the palm oil used in the product was produced using sustainable practices.

Olive Oil: Intensive olive farming has led to widespread soil erosion and desertification (a process by which fertile land becomes desert) in Greece, Italy, Spain, and Portugal.[48] A report commissioned by the European Commission singled out irresponsible olive-farming practices as a severe environmental problem across European Union countries. In addition to destroying fertile lands, large olive producers rely on massive amounts of pesticides and other chemicals, which pollute waterways. Because olive production occurs on such a large scale to meet the growing demand for oil, it also puts a lot of pressure on local water supplies.

Coconut Oil: We've established how beneficial this once-vilified oil actually is, but there's a downside to its rise in popularity. An estimated 60 percent of small-scale coconut farmers live in poverty in the Philippines, a major source of the fruit. According to the nonprofit group Fair Trade USA, many coconut farmers in countries like the Philippines and Indonesia are among the poorest of the poor, which raises questions about the sustainability of coconut farming as a livelihood in these regions. Despite the soaring popularity of coconut products in America, there is a disparity between what consumers spend on it and what farmers earn. Americans might pay top dollar for fancy coconut waters and coconut oil beauty products, but farmers in Southeast Asia earn as little as 10 cents per coconut they produce. On top of that, coconuts are often grown as a mono-crop, and this lack of diversity can be detrimental to the environment.

How to Buy the Best Sustainable Fats and Oils

- **Truth in Olive Oil:** It would be great if we could all purchase from small farms with well-managed production practices, but that isn't always possible. I recommend checking out Tom Mueller's guide to buying better olive oil: www.truthinoliveoil.com/ great-oil/how-to-buy-great-olive-oil.
- **Buy California:** Here are some of the brands of extra virgin olive oil that studies have found to be authentic and top quality:
  1. California Olive Ranch
  2. McEvoy Ranch Organic
  3. Corto Olive
  4. Kirkland Organic
  5. Cobram Estate
  6. Bariani Olive Oil

- **Certified coconut oil:** Fair Trade USA has established a Community Development Premium in which coconut farmers earn a bonus for every "responsible" coconut they sell. You should be sure to use organic virgin coconut oil—other forms may not be healthy. Virgin coconut oil is rich in disease-fighting phytonutrients. Old studies that may have shown problems were done with coconut oil made from dried coconut, not fresh, and dried coconut has been deodorized, heated, and chemically processed. When purchasing coconut oil, look for certified Fair Trade organic labels, which you can learn more about here: http://fairtradeusa .org/press-room/press_release/fair-trade-usa-laun ches-fair-trade-certified-coconuts.
- **Grass-fed butter is best:** When buying butter, look for the American Grassfed logo. Or go to the group's website so you can find farmers in your area who produce and sell grass-fed butter: http://www .americangrassfed.org/.
- **Thrive Market:** Visit the website of Thrive Market, which carries a wide assortment of healthy oils and fats. You can find everything from grass-fed ghee to beef tallow, avocado oil, walnut oil, macadamia oil, organic Fair Trade coconut oil, almond oil, duck fat, and lard—just about any nutritious oil or fat you can think of: www.thrivemarket.com.

SUMMING IT UP

If there's anything you should take away from this chapter, it is this: Consuming lots of natural, whole-food-based, healthy fats, including saturated fats, is absolutely critical for good health. We've been conditioned to believe that unsaturated fats from vegetable and seed oils are best, and that butter, coconut oil, lard, ghee, and other saturated fats are toxic. But in fact, the reverse is true. Focus on eating the fats and oils that our ancestors ate, and banish the industrially produced, highly processed ones from your kitchen.

If you want to keep things really simple, limit yourself to these two: organic, cold-pressed, extra virgin olive oil and organic virgin coconut oil. Use olive oil liberally on your food but cook with it only at very low temperatures. Use coconut oil for cooking at higher temperatures. Scramble your eggs in it; use it when you bake; add it to smoothies or a veggie stir-fry. (It also works great as a skin or hair moisturizer.)

How Much Fat Should I Eat?

You should get most of your fats from meat, fish, poultry, eggs, grass-fed dairy, avocados, nuts, extra virgin olive oil, virgin coconut oil, and grass-fed butter. You should not live in fear of fats and oils — they make food taste better, offer many nutritional benefits, make you feel fuller, and help you lose weight. In the end, the kind of fat you eat is more important than how much. Americans are eating frightening amounts of refined vegetable oils, seed oils, and omega-6 fats, all of which contribute to inflammation and chronic diseases. My advice is to stay away from these oils completely. That should be pretty simple if you eat a diet of whole foods and avoid processed junk foods. The other absolutely key thing to remember is this: Fats combined with starch or sugar are like rocket fuel for weight gain. I call this "sweet fat." That combo also produces bad cholesterol. So, when it comes to French Fries, ice cream, buttered bread, and pasta with cream sauce — eat at your own peril!

How Often Should I Eat It?

Every day, and ideally at every meal.

FATS AND OILS: WHAT THE HECK SHOULD I EAT?

- Organic avocado oil
- Butter from pastured, grass-fed cows or goats
- Grass-fed ghee (clarified butter)
- Organic virgin coconut oil
- Organic, humanely raised tallow (beef fat)
- Organic, humanely raised lard (pork fat)
- Organic, humanely raised duck fat
- Organic, humanely raised chicken fat

Use these raw, on salads or other foods, but don't cook them:

- Organic extra virgin olive oil
- Walnut oil
- Almond oil
- Macadamia oil
- Sesame seed oil
- Tahini (sesame seed paste)
- Flax oil
- Hemp oil

FATS AND OILS: WHAT THE HECK SHOULD I AVOID?

- Soybean oil
- Canola oil
- Corn oil
- Safflower oil
- Sunflower oil
- Palm oil
- Peanut oil
- Vegetable oil
- Vegetable shortening
- Margarine and all other butter substitutes, including the newest ones, which actually include butter among the ingredients
- Anything that says "hydrogenated"; it's poison
- Anything else that looks fake

BEANS

NUTRITION IQ QUIZ

True or False?

1. Beans are a good source of protein.
2. Beans are the ultimate health food.
3. Prehistoric humans foraged for legumes, so they're part of the Paleo diet.
4. Beans contain toxins that can't be avoided.
5. You shouldn't eat beans if you have type 2 diabetes.
6. Soybeans are a superfood.

Answers

1. False: Ounce for ounce, beans have more carbs than animal protein. When it comes to protein content, a 6-ounce grass-fed steak equals nearly 2½ cups of kidney beans. But that amount of beans also contains roughly 100 grams of carbs. The steak has none.

2. False: Beans contain fiber and minerals and are a source of protein and carbohydrates for vegetarians. However, they also contain potentially inflammatory proteins that trigger inflammation for some with autoimmune disease.

3. False: Beans have been around since the advent of agriculture 10,000 years ago, which makes them a relatively new addition to the human diet.

4. True and false: Beans contain lectins and phytates, which can damage our intestinal lining and prevent us from absorbing all the nutrients we need. But there are ways to neutralize these substances.

5. True: Beans can be beneficial and nutritious for many people. But they contain a fair bit of starch, which can be a problem from those with prediabetes or type 1 or 2 diabetes.

6. True and false: Soybeans are often considered a health food. And there can be benefits to eating some forms of organic soy like tempeh or tofu. But GMO, non-organic soy is problematic. Despite Big Agriculture's insistence that GMO food is harmless, the research is mixed. Shouldn't we prove it's safe before we put it on our plates?

Get a new food fact and weekly recipe directly from my kitchen. Sign up for free at www.foodthebook.com.

At last, a food we can all agree on, one seemingly without a hint of controversy or concern. Seriously, who can argue with a bean? High levels of nutrients and, as plants go, unmatched amounts of protein. Plus, they're a tried-and-true traditional food, consumed for centuries on every continent: a cheap and plentiful source of fiber, vitamins, and minerals. The federal government's dietary guidelines recommend that Americans consume as much as 3 cups of beans per week. There are countless studies linking bean consumption with markers of good health like decreased blood pressure, low inflammation, proper body weight, and lower risk of cancer, diabetes, depression, suicide—even skin wrinkling. Dan Buettner, author of the bestselling books on the Blue Zones, has done longevity research showing that eating beans makes you less likely to die, which is about all you can ask of any food. Case closed—beans are totally good for us. Right?

If only it were that simple.

THE SCIENCE OF BEANS

Botanically speaking, beans (or legumes, if you prefer—they're the same thing) aren't vegetables at all. They're the dried seeds of a certain family of plants—that's why they're so rich in nutrients. A seed's job, after all, is to contain everything necessary for new life. Legumes are also unique in their ability to absorb nitrogen directly from the atmosphere, which accounts for their high protein content. (Nitrogen is crucial to all plant growth, but most plants, including vegetable and fruit crops, get it from the soil.) This ability also means that legumes can grow happily in nitrogen-poor soil, where other crops would require heavy-duty fertilizer. In fact, beans actually enrich the soil in which they grow.

WHAT THE EXPERTS GOT RIGHT

Beans pack a lot of nutrients, including potassium, zinc, iron, magnesium, folate, and vitamin B_6, among others. They deliver as much as one-quarter of their weight in protein, and contain a healthy dose of fiber, which is good for gut bacteria and keeps us regular. Plus, they're cheap. And, as noted, they're easier on the environment than other crops. All true. In addition, the PURE study of more than 135,000 people in eighteen countries over ten years found that consumption of fruits, veggies, and beans (not grains) was associated with less heart disease and risk of death.[1] It's an observational study so can't prove cause and effect, but certainly they are not harmful for most people.

WHAT THEY GOT WRONG

Beans contain a lot of carbs — up to three-quarters by weight. And most of those carbs are starch, meaning chains of sugar, the same as in grains. The starches are different from those found in grains in an important way, which we'll explain in a bit. But still, carbs are... well, by now you know the story with carbs. They can be a disaster if you have pre-diabetes or type 2 diabetes, which, taken together, affect more than half of all Americans. If you are not pre-diabetic or type 2 diabetic, beans can be part of healthy diet. As carbs go, beans, aside from nonstarchy veggies, are best.

But legumes also contain substances called lectins and phytates, which actually prevent our bodies from accessing all the nutrients we eat. Lectins are beneficial for plants and not so good for humans. They act as natural pesticides that ward off predators. But when you eat and absorb them, they can wreak havoc in the body. In fact, lectins are most abundant in many common allergens, including peanuts, wheat, grains, and shellfish. They have been shown to stick to red blood cells, promoting blood clots and inflammation.[2] And they may be linked to leaky gut[3] and autoimmune disease.[4]

Cooking beans is not much help. In the case of kidney beans, it can make the lectins *more* potent. But fermentation is a great way to reduce the harmful effects of lectin. During the process, bacteria break down and digest the lectins, making them less likely to cause harm. This is one reason I advise people to stick with fermented bean foods like nattō, miso, and tempeh. Pressure cooking can also reduce lectins.

Strike two against beans is that the quality of their protein is not as useful as animal protein, as you saw in the nutritional quiz at the top of this chapter. As we age, the quality of the protein we eat matters. We need more of it to help build new muscle and maintain the aging muscle that we already have.[5] Aging muscle needs more of the amino acid leucine to build new muscle. Beans have very little; animal protein has a lot more. And it appears that the plant proteins in beans are not as effective as animal proteins when it comes to maintaining muscle.

Finally, beans can promote the overgrowth of bad bacteria in the gut, which can create gas and systemic inflammation in some people. So, when you balance out their nutritional benefits and disadvantages, our blind faith in beans may have been misplaced. And the advice to eat them freely may be misguided. They can be part of a healthy diet, but not a staple.

WHAT WE STILL DON'T KNOW FOR SURE

While the data is not all in on how beans (and the lectins, phytates, and starch they contain) affect everyone, it is clear that for many people, especially those with autoimmune disease, pre-diabetes, and type 2 diabetes, they are problematic and worth avoiding. Even type 1 diabetics may benefit from a very-low-carbohydrate diet, which is hard to achieve if you eat beans.[6]

And it depends on your overall health and whether or not you have diabetes or autoimmune disease. I have many vegan or vegetarian Indian patients. For most of my patients it is fairly simple to control their blood sugars and get them off medications and even insulin. But it is very hard for those vegan or vegetarian patients to reverse type 2 diabetes. Some are successful with vegan ketogenic diets, which are hard to do.

NINE THINGS YOU NEED TO KNOW ABOUT BEANS

1. Beans Are Not a Great Source of Protein (Sorry, Vegans)

Don't vegans have to get their protein somewhere? Yes. But as they age, it's hard to get all the protein they need from beans.

As we grow older, we lose muscle — it just disappears. (The scientific term is "sarcopenia.") It happens because our bodies produce less testosterone and growth hormone, and higher levels of cortisol (the stress hormone) and more insulin. On top of that, we don't utilize the protein we eat as well as we once did.

So we need to eat a little more than we did when we were kids. It's no surprise that people who consume animal foods—meat, fish, eggs, dairy—have an advantage here, since these foods are richest in protein. But if your diet doesn't include those foods, you need to get it somewhere else, and while most plant foods contain some protein, legumes are the best candidates.

Beans have protein for sure—and without all the baggage that comes with meat. But bean protein is not enough to provide all we require. It's low in an important amino acid, leucine, which is necessary for building and maintaining skeletal muscle. In addition, the proteins in beans aren't as plentiful or as bioavailable as those in animal-based foods. The recommended dietary allowance, or RDA, for dietary protein for a sedentary American is 0.36 grams per pound of body weight; that's about 53 grams of protein for a fifty-year-old woman who weighs 140 pounds. What most people don't realize is that this is the *minimum* necessary to prevent protein deficiency, not the *optimal amount* needed for robust health or building muscle—one of the most important organs in your body. A group of forty scientific protein experts gathered at a "Protein Summit" and published a report called "Introduction to Protein Summit 2.0: Continued Exploration of the Impact of High-Quality Protein on Optimal Health" in the *American Journal of Clinical Nutrition* in 2015.[7] The experts agreed that most

Americans are not getting enough protein (the average American gets about 16 percent of their calories from protein) and that an active adult may need twice the RDA recommendation. Following the RDA guidelines for protein would provide you with about 10 percent of your calories from protein, whereas most of us need from 15 to 30 percent of our calories from protein. We need more if we are physically active and as we get older to maintain muscle mass. It is best to eat protein spread evenly throughout the day at each meal.

You can get protein from plants, but they contain less leucine and come with lots of carbs. To get the same protein you would get from a 6-ounce piece of salmon (0 carbs) you would need about 3 cups of beans (123 grams of carbs). You can do the math yourself [8]:

	Amount	Calories	Protein (grams)	Carbs (grams)
Salmon	3 ounces	184	23	0
Ground beef	3 ounces	218	22	0
Black beans	1 cup	227	15	41
Kidney beans	1 cup	225	15	37
Lima beans	1 cup	216	15	39
Almonds	1 ounce	164	6	6
Couscous	1 cup	176	6	36
Special K cereal	1 cup	115	6	22
Large egg	1 egg	75	6	1

2. Beans Contain a Special Starch and a Lot of Fiber

For years scientists wondered how our bodies handled the high levels of carbs found in beans. The mystery was cleared up in the 1980s by two scientists who came up with the term "resistant starch" to describe what's found in beans—an unusual form of starch that largely bypasses our blood and goes straight to our intestines. It "resists" digestion, in a sense. That's significant because it means those starches don't get metabolized and stored as fat, as sugar and other starches would. Rather, resistant starches act more like fiber, feeding our gut bacteria, which in turn create short-chain fatty acids that keep our colons healthy.[9] One of these fatty acids in particular, butyrate, can speed up your metabolism and help prevent cancer.[10] Compared to grains, legumes have a less dramatic impact on your blood sugar, thanks to their resistant starch.

A study published in the *Archives of Internal Medicine* compared the effects of high-glycemic plant foods like grains (which sharply raise blood sugar) and low-glycemic plant foods like legumes (which don't hike your blood sugar or insulin as much) on subjects with type 2 diabetes. The group that was assigned a diet with plenty of low-glycemic foods—or what I call "slow carbs"—were instructed to eat at least 1 cup of lentils, garbanzo beans, or other legumes daily. The other group was put on a "high wheat" diet and told to eat a variety of grains. After three months, the diabetics in the beans group had greater reductions in blood pressure and other heart disease risk factors compared to the grains group. They also had lower hemoglobin A1c levels, which is a measure of how high a person's blood sugar has been over the previous six weeks.[11] Remember, eating beans is better than eating grains, especially for type 2 diabetes, but not better than animal protein or fat for type 2 diabetes.

As you can see, beans are a better source of carbs than grains. And some beans, like lentils and garbanzos, are better than others. But as with potatoes and rice — both of which are also starchy — if you cook beans, then let them cool before you eat them, you raise the resistant starch content.[12] Nonetheless, the fact remains that legumes contain a hefty dose of carbs, and for that reason I recommend you steer clear if you're insulin resistant, diabetic, or overweight or have an autoimmune disease like Hashimoto's thyroiditis.

3. Beans Are Not Great for Your Gut (If You Have Gut Issues)

In three studies of beans and nutrition, participants were fed pinto beans and black-eyed peas and then asked whether they farted more than usual. According to the research, "Less than 50 percent reported increased flatulence from eating pinto or baked beans during the first week of each trial, but only 19 percent had a flatulence increase with black-eyed peas."[13] Interestingly, "a small percentage (3–11 percent) reported increased flatulence across the three studies even on control diets without flatulence-producing components." The researchers concluded, "People's concerns about excessive flatulence from eating beans may be exaggerated."

But this really depends on what's happening in your gut. Up to 15 percent of adults have irritable bowel syndrome,[14] and up to 20 percent have reflux.[15] This is often caused by overgrowth of bad bugs in the small intestine or colon. Little-known fact: Humans don't produce gas. Bugs eating your food and fermenting it create it. And these bad bugs go crazy for the starch in beans. So, if you have tummy troubles, it's best to stay away from beans and get help fixing your inner garden with a good functional medicine doctor (you can search for a practitioner at the Institute for Functional Medicine: www.functionalmedicine.org).

4. Beans Contain Substances that May Cause Disease

Because a tree can't run from its predators, all fruits and vegetables naturally contain toxic or otherwise irritating substances—chemicals that protect the plant by making life uncomfortable for the creatures (us included) that would eat them. Legumes contain lectins and phytates. Lectins, as we saw earlier, are inflammatory proteins that may damage and penetrate the lining of the small intestine, leading to leaky gut syndrome. This can trigger inflammation throughout the body, which has been linked to everything from obesity and type 2 diabetes to autoimmune diseases, depression, and even neurodegenerative diseases. The other anti-nutrient, phytates, also known as phytic acid, is actually a form of phosphorus, one that we humans can't digest. But lectins and phytates are a double-edged sword, in that they may also be beneficial to our health. Research suggests they have anti-cancer, antidiabetic, anti-obesity, and anti–heart disease properties. Phytates are not exclusive to beans: Other vegetables such as spinach and chard contain them in significantly higher quantities. And I don't advise people to avoid those, because their nutrient density and low caloric content balance out a little plant toxin.

Another little-known fact: There is a group of humans, mostly from the Mediterranean, who have a gene that makes eating fava beans toxic. People with this rare disorder, called favism, can develop a sudden fever and racing heart rate and fall into a coma and die just hours after eating fava beans.[16]

5. Canned Beans Are Convenient but Not Risk-Free

They usually come with ungodly levels of sodium: You'll get one-fifth of your recommended daily allotment from ½ cup of typical canned black beans. (Though, in fairness, you'd also get one-quarter of the dietary fiber advised.) There's also the matter of cans lined with BPA, or bisphenol A, which is an epoxy resin also found in plastic bottles. It's a hormone disrupter that damages the brains and prostate glands of fetuses, infants, and children, so pregnant women and kids should steer clear. It's also been linked to obesity, type 2 diabetes,[17] male sexual dysfunction, and hypertension.

The FDA says the levels of BPA found in food sold in cans are too low to be worrisome, but why take chances? It's the same FDA that said trans fats were fine. One clinical trial published in the journal *Hypertension* found that when people drank a beverage from a can, the levels of BPA in their urine spiked within two hours—and so did their blood pressure. But when they drank the same beverage from a glass bottle, there was no increase in their BPA levels and no troubling changes in their blood pressure.[18]

Nowadays many canned foods and beverages carry a "BPA-free" claim on their labels. But that doesn't mean you're in the clear. Studies show that packages advertised as BPA-free often contain other hormone disrupters, like BPS and BPF, that are even more potent and potentially harmful than BPA.[19] If you insist on eating beans, then look for organic, low-sodium varieties in a jar or sold fresh at the supermarket, or buy them dried and soak them before using.

6. Green Peas and Green Beans Are More Like Veggies than Beans

Technically speaking, green peas are beans, though they're more vegetable-like. Their sweet taste is your first clue that they have more sugar than, say, kale. But they have less starch than most beans, and similar amounts of protein, and 1 cup provides 40 percent of the vitamin K and 35 percent of the manganese we're supposed to eat daily. So, they're actually healthier than most legumes, on balance. And that goes for green beans too. Plus, who doesn't like fresh green peas or beans? Enjoy. Low starch, lots of crunch, full of vitamins and minerals — what's not to love?

7. Peanuts Are Legumes Too, but Not So Good for You

That's right, the "nut" is a misnomer, and so is the "pea," for that matter. Peanuts have the same advantages as most legumes. They are rich in monounsaturated fats (but they also have a lot of inflammatory omega-6 fats). Peanut oil is a problem, but a handful of peanuts is not. They have more antioxidants than apples, plus folate and vitamin E, not to mention bean levels of protein. But today, peanut allergies and sensitivities have become ubiquitous. Even more serious is the fungus aflatoxin, which is both a toxin and a carcinogen, and which grows on peanuts when they're improperly stored.

While I'm a big fan of including plenty of natural fats in your diet, raw peanuts and even peanut butter should not be staples, which may come as puzzling news to those of us who grew up on them. Just read the label on most peanut butters to see all the bad fats, sugars, and chemical additives you'll be sparing

yourself if you abstain. Most common brands of peanut butter are full of added trans fats (hydrogenated
soybean oil) and high-fructose corn syrup. Even a
national brand's "natural" variety that boasts no trans
fats and "no preservatives, artificial flavors, or colors"
on the label may include plenty of sugar and salt.

Peanut oil is highly processed and contains high
levels of omega-6 fats. It's fine to have the occasional
handful of fresh peanuts, or additive-free peanut butters on occasion, but you should keep it to a minimum.
Try almond, cashew, or macadamia nut butter instead.
(See the chapter on nuts and seeds for more information.)

8. Soybeans Can Be Good for Us

Soy is practically synonymous with health food, but
this may have more to do with good PR and wishful
thinking than anything else. There is only *some* truth
in its reputation.

Edamame—whole soybeans—are usually purchased frozen, then steamed, salted, and served warm
or cold. As legumes go, they're on the starchy side, and
they contain high levels of enzyme inhibitors that
prevent us from absorbing the very nutrients they contain. Fermenting them solves this problem, something
we have known for millennia, since people first began
consuming soybeans in China. The four fermented
soybean products—tempeh, natto, miso, and soy
sauce (gluten-free)—are the healthiest ways of eating

the bean. Tempeh is soybeans that have been cooked and fermented; miso is a fermented paste used in soup and sauces; authentic soy sauce is brewed and fermented from whole beans (the American knockoff uses extracts and a bunch of artificial additives); and don't ask about natto—it's so weird and stinky you'll never eat it, although if you can get used to its smell and gooey texture, you can take advantage of its anti-inflammatory and blood-thinning properties. Fermentation neutralizes the toxins and enzyme inhibitors and leaves the nutrients and protein intact. Tempeh and tofu are very protein-rich, low-carb vegetable foods.

Tofu came along later—it's not fermented, but instead cooked to yield the soft, smooth curds. But even this health food store staple comes with the same toxins, irritants, and other issues associated with unfermented soy. And remember that around 95 percent of soy grown in the United States is genetically modified[20] and doused with pesticides. Buying organic solves those concerns.

9. And This Soy Product Is Pure Health Hazard

Soybean oil is one of those products that nobody uses and everybody eats. It's the oil of choice for most processed, packaged foods. It is produced using highly industrialized methods, which strip the bean of whatever nutrition it once had. And most of the soybean oil used in food manufacturing shows up as hydrogenated fat, or trans fat. Remember that soybean oil is the primary source of omega-6 fatty acids in our diet, the type of fat that makes our tissues inflamed and increases our risk of heart disease, cancer, dementia, and even depression, homicide, violence, and suicide.[21]

Once the oil has been extracted from soybeans, what's left is also put to use. Today, soy protein isolates can be found everywhere from livestock feed to meat substitutes sold as though they are healthy alternatives to the real thing. But the way soy protein is processed causes its chemical nature to change for the worse. It has been shown to cause cancer. All those soy shakes, soy protein bars, soy hot dogs, and fake meats are bad news! Turkey is better for you than Tofurky any day. Soy protein is found in bread and some soy milk. It's even in baby formula, which is scary.

And then there's soy milk, a weird drink that humans never consumed until recently. Though it's considered a health food by many, I have seen men and little girls grow breasts from chugging it. Use it in your coffee as a creamer, but stay away from soy lattes and soy milk in everything else. Try almond or coconut milk instead.

GEEK ALERT: A LITTLE MORE SCIENCE ABOUT BEANS

Advocates of the Paleo diet, which is based on the foods we ate when we were cavemen and -women, advise us to avoid legumes altogether, since they, like grains, are pretty much a product of the agricultural revolution. This is mostly true. Our hunter-gather ancestors did not consume beans as a staple in their diet. However, researchers have found plaque deposits on the teeth of Neanderthals, evidence that they ate wild peas and beans.[22] And there are contemporary hunter-gatherer societies today that eat throwback legume varieties. The !Kung San, who inhabit the Kalahari Desert, for instance, are fond of the tsin bean (though chances are you won't find it at your local Whole Foods).

SUMMING IT UP

Beans have some good stuff going on. Resistant starch may be their best quality. But they don't offer us anything that we can't get from other sources, like vegetables (for fiber and minerals) or animal foods (for protein and other nutrients), without all the issues associated with beans (starches, overall digestive difficulties, leaky gut). So beans are absolutely *not* a necessity. Based on the research and my experiences using food to treat tens of thousands of patients, I can say that beans are not always man's best friend either.

Large population studies do in fact show that people who eat beans regularly tend to be in good health, but this is not proof that beans are healthy. Like all observational studies, it could just be that people with good habits—eating responsibly, avoiding cigarettes, getting plenty of exercise and sleep—are also the type to eat legumes, among many other healthy foods. Nobody can say for sure. But no one thing creates a good life, not even beans. And many of us who suffer from common ailments like digestive disorders, food sensitivities, difficulty with weight control, insulin insensitivity, and so on might see improvements if only we avoided beans and processed soy-based foods.

Though I generally advise against eating too many beans, that does not mean they're off-limits for everyone. If you're healthy and have a varied diet, beans can be a great addition. How do you know if beans are right for you?

If you're a vegan: You need to get your protein somewhere, and you're probably accustomed to spending a lot of time and effort on food prep, so the soaking won't seem like a big inconvenience. But you shouldn't kid yourself into thinking you're getting all the protein your body needs, because you're probably not. In fact, the quality of protein matters even more as you age, and maintaining muscle mass is not very easy on beans or vegetable protein in general.

If they're organic: This means they're also non-GMO.

If you really just love them: Look, there are worse things you could be eating. But you should probably limit your bean intake to once or twice a week—not the daily cup or so that some experts advise, which could have a big impact on your blood sugar levels. And stick with the beans and bean products in the following "Beans: What the Heck Should I Eat?" list.

How Much Should I Eat?

The maximum serving is ½ cup once a day. If you are a big guy you can double it. If you are very active you may be able to tolerate more beans.

And How Should I Prepare Them?

- Soak them overnight, then throw out the water.
- Cook them with kombu to make them more digestible.
- Use organic, BPA-free canned beans for convenience.

Avoid Beans If:

- You are insulin resistant or have type 2 diabetes.
- You're prone to food allergies or sensitivities.
- Weight control is an issue for you or if you have a lot of belly fat.
- You have irritable bowel syndrome or any other digestive difficulties.
- You have any autoimmune diseases, such as rheumatoid arthritis, psoriasis, lupus, or any of the rest.
- You're a man trying to father a child, since there's research showing that even half a serving a day of soy-based foods or milk can lower sperm count significantly.

- You have breast cancer. But traditional soy foods (not processed-soy meat alternatives) in moderate amounts (a few times a week) may be protective.

BEANS: WHAT THE HECK SHOULD I EAT?

- Non-GMO, organic, traditional soybean-based foods such as tofu, tempeh, natto, and miso, and gluten-free organic soy sauce or tamari
- Lower-starch varieties like peas and lentils (especially red ones, though French and traditional are also fine)
- Black beans, garbanzo beans, and adzuki beans
- Organic green beans and snow peas
- Black-eyed peas, asparagus beans, and other members of the cowpea family
- Whole soybeans, aka edamame, but don't overdo it
- Mung beans

BEANS: WHAT THE HECK SHOULD I AVOID?

- Lima beans (high in starch)
- Kidney beans (ditto)
- Baked beans (high in sugar)
- Peanuts, for the most part (due to toxins)
- Any beans in a can lined with BPA

GRAINS

NUTRITION IQ QUIZ

True or False?

1. Whole wheat bread is a great way to get your whole grains.
2. Oatmeal is the most nutritious thing you can eat for breakfast.
3. Corn is starchy and not nutritious.
4. You should eat at least two to three servings of grains each day.
5. Gluten-free foods are part of a fad that you shouldn't buy into.
6. Of all the grains you can eat, rice is the most nutritious.
7. Grains contain good fiber that helps keep you regular.

Answers

1. False: Whole wheat bread usually contains very few whole grains. In fact, the number one ingredient is

usually "wheat flour," which kind of sounds like something healthy. It's not. It's white flour with a few whole-grain flakes in it—and usually a lot of sugar or even high-fructose corn syrup. Can you really believe that whole-grain Cookie Crisp cereal is healthy? Hardly. It has almost 6 teaspoons of sugar in one serving. Don't be fooled by the whole-grain label. It's also finely ground, which makes it act like sugar, whole wheat or not.

2. False: While it's a better breakfast than sugary cereal, oatmeal has a high glycemic index, which means having some for breakfast virtually guarantees that you'll spend the rest of the day overeating. Steel-cut oats are not much better. Protein and fat are the best things to eat for breakfast.

3. True and false: Corn is starchy but contains fiber and antioxidants, which give it its bright yellow color.

4. False: You don't *need* grains at all. You can get the nutrients they contain from other less problematic foods. In fact, you have no biological need for carbohydrates. And a high-grain, high-carb diet is the last thing you need if you want to lose weight.

5. False: It turns out that we'd all probably be better off without gluten. Dr. Alessio Fasano of Harvard, the world's leading expert on gluten, says that non-celiac gluten sensitivity is a real ailment[1] and that anyone who eats gluten is doing small

amounts of damage to their intestinal lining, creating leaky gut and inflammation. Even if you're not celiac, gluten isn't something you should eat regularly.

6. Mostly false: Some rice varieties are healthier than others, but there are more nutritious grains with fewer carbohydrates—black rice, quinoa, and buckwheat, for example.

7. True: Whole grains contain fiber that helps keep your bowels healthy, but so do other plant-based foods.

Get a new food fact and weekly recipe directly from my kitchen. Sign up for free at www .foodthebook.com.

As good PR goes, this is hard to beat:

O beautiful for spacious skies, for amber waves of grain...

See what I mean? It comes right after the sky and even before purple mountain majesties, which says a lot about the place grains occupy in the American psyche, not to mention our diet. Bread is the "staff of life." As much as anything else, grains made America. The evidence is in the sheer acreage of farmland we devote to wheat, corn, barley, and sorghum and the tonnage of grain we consume and export to the rest of the world. Grain-based foods are by far the number one source of calories in the American diet.[2] Among adults, the number one source of calories is baked desserts, followed by yeast breads. And among adolescents and teenagers, the number two source of calories is pizza—in other words, flour and cheese. The grains that go into those foods—mainly wheat, corn, rice, and sorghum—are among the crops that receive billions in federal farm subsidies annually, so even our tax dollars are devoted to keeping grain-based foods like bread, pasta, rice, cereals, cookies, cake, pizza, oatmeal, and crackers on top. And it doesn't stop there. Most of these federally subsidized crops are fed to livestock, which means that Americans are also getting grains indirectly, too, from all the grain-fed beef, chicken, and dairy we consume. The average American consumes 133 pounds of flour a year in their food (down from 146.8 pounds in 1995); that's more than a third of a pound per person per day, and some of us consume much more. And that doesn't include all the other grains and potatoes. We were never designed to handle this much starch. It's a toxic drug dose that leads to obesity,[3] heart disease,[4] type 2 diabetes, dementia,[5] and even cancer.[6]

So, let's dig into the science of grains and what we should and shouldn't do.

THE SCIENCE OF GRAINS

Grains are the seeds of the grass family. They've always existed in the wild, of course, but became edible after humans invented farming about 10,000 years ago. Thanks to our new ability to cultivate food, we no longer had to forage. That was the good news of the Neolithic era. But there was some bad news, too. The state of our physical being took a downturn—our skeletons actually shrank in response to our dependence on this new source of nutrition, a sign of grain's influence on our health.[7] The trade-off was that grains gave us a reliable source of sustenance.

WHAT THE EXPERTS GOT RIGHT

Each part of the whole grain has its benefits. The fiber in bran (which is composed of a grain's outer layers) passes through our intestines undigested but drags everything in its path along with it, thereby promoting regular bowel movements, eliminating toxins, and maintaining colon health. Bran also helps keep your blood sugar on an even keel by slowing digestion. In theory at least, this means a reduced risk of diabetes. Eating bran has also been associated with healthy cholesterol numbers,[8] normal blood pressure,[9] and even the prevention of heart disease and cancer.[10] Best of all, fiber is the favored food of the trillions of beneficial bacteria that live inside the gut.

The germ (the reproductive part of a grain that grows into a new plant) contains virtually all of a grain's nutrients, such as B vitamins, vitamin E, and tocopherols, plus minerals like magnesium and potassium, proteins, and even some fats. So far, so good.

The third component of grain, the endosperm, or the energy stores of the plant, is all starch. Since a grain is a seed, this part is necessary for the growth of the new plant. For animals who eat the grain—us included—it performs the same function: It breaks down into glucose, which spikes the hormone insulin, the body's fat fertilizer or fat-storage hormone. High levels of insulin induced by starch and sugar are the driving force behind our obesity and chronic disease epidemics. They are linked to heart disease, type 2 diabetes, cancer, and even dementia.

This could be trouble.

WHAT THEY GOT WRONG

The nutrition community has been guilty of disseminating a lot of bad information over the years. It suggested that we could all lose weight just by cutting calories. That was a major blunder because only certain types of calories cause weight gain (carbs) — others cause weight loss (fats). It advised us to cut back on cholesterol and avoid egg yolks — another disaster. But its erroneous insistence that carbs are better for you than fats will probably go down in history as the most catastrophic nutritional screw-up of the twentieth century. It has literally killed millions of people. First, the medical community urged us to improve our heart health by cutting back on fats and replacing them with grains. (Wrong.) Then the federal government got into the business of issuing dietary guidelines and created the fabled food pyramid in 1992, which placed grains at the foundation of a healthy diet. (Wrong.) We were told to eat six to eleven servings of bread, rice, cereal, or pasta a day. Really? *Eleven servings of bread every day?*

In hindsight, it clearly wasn't the soundest nutrition advice. In fact, it was atrocious. But we all bought it — the public, doctors, dietitians, the entire public health community. As a result, we all got fatter and sicker. It turns out that the starches and carb-laden foods the experts urged us to devour contributed mightily to our current epidemic of diabesity (which is the spectrum of pre-diabetes to full-blown type 2 diabetes that now affects one out of two Americans and one in four children) and heart disease. The carbs, sugars, and starches in our diet have been tied to cancer[11] and even mental illness.[12] Dementia, for example, is now also called type 3 diabetes. Nearly all the grains we consume today have been processed to death, so the good stuff they once contained is lost.[13] Yet grain's halo stubbornly persists. A recent survey found that 70 percent of Americans think granola bars are healthy, even though they're really just cookies with a wholesome-sounding name. The scariest part of that survey? The fact that 28 percent of nutritionists said that granola bars are good for us.[14]

The truth is that only by cutting way back on grain-based foods could we ever hope to reverse the trend of metabolic diseases that they cause. If you are diabetic, you shouldn't eat more than 25 to 50 grams of carbs a day (less than two slices of bread). If we limited ourselves to moderate amounts of whole grains—*certain* whole grains, I should say—we might be okay. But most whole grains aren't much fun to eat, at least not compared to the foods we make by refining and processing them until they are deliciously unrecognizable, which of course is when all the trouble begins. They cease to become food and enter the realm of food-like substances. Edible, but not entirely qualified to join the ranks of real whole foods.

TEN THINGS YOU NEED TO KNOW ABOUT GRAINS

1. You Don't Have to Eat Them — At All!

Don't get me wrong. There are plenty of vitamins, minerals, nutrients, and fatty acids contained in whole grains. But you can easily get all those beneficial substances from other sources — vegetables, fruit, nuts, seeds, and other foods that don't have the baggage that comes with grains. The same is true of the fiber contained in whole grains. It's absolutely vital to healthy living but easily available in other plant-based foods. For us to live, our bodies need the amino acids contained in protein and the fatty acids contained in fats. Believe it or not, we don't need to eat carbs. At all! For nearly all of our history, humans consumed no grains, and our bodies are designed to work very well without them. Our hunter-gatherer ancestors occasionally binged on buffalo and antelope meat, but never on a sheet cake!

2. Flour = Sugar

When we talk about grains, we use the word starch. (We use it for some vegetables, too, as we've seen.) But we don't all realize that starch is just sugar with a slightly more complex molecular structure. This is important: Starch and sugar are essentially the same thing. The whole complex vs. simple carb idea has retired to the dustbin of history. What matters is how much a particular carb raises your blood sugar. Bread is a complex carb, sugar a simple carb. But eating two slices of whole wheat bread raises your blood sugar more than eating 2 tablespoons of table sugar does! So whenever you eat something containing wheat flour, you might as well be mainlining sugar. On the glycemic index, which measures the amount that any given food raises your blood sugar, white bread is a 75, while sucrose (table sugar) comes in at 65 (and chocolate at 45).[15] This rapid rise in blood sugar brought on by consuming starchy carbs and all forms of sugar is essentially the metabolic mechanism single-handedly responsible for today's global epidemics of diabetes, heart disease, and obesity (and it contributes to dementia and cancer as well). Eating refined grains prompts your body to release insulin, which ushers the glucose from your bloodstream into your fat cells, making them bigger and plumper. Then, before you know it, you're hungry again for more carbs. In the meantime, the insulin acts like a lock that prevents fat from being mobilized from your fat cells. If you consume more than minimal amounts of sugar and starch, the calories will be stored in your fat cells but won't be able to get out. Which is why we always feel hungry and keep getting fatter!

My friend David Ludwig, the Harvard professor and obesity expert, often says that below the neck, your body can't tell the difference between a bowl of cornflakes without the sugar and a bowl of sugar without the cornflakes. That's how bad flour is.

Today, grain-wary people who bake at home use flours made from almonds, coconuts, or some other substitute. And that's generally a good idea. But in commercial food products, we're getting grains. And when we get grains, we almost always get one or more sweeteners—sugar, high-fructose corn syrup, molasses, honey, dextrose, maltodextrin, maltose. Look at the label on any loaf of bread next time you go shopping. There may be five or six different kinds of flour and sugar in there. That's a lot of ways to inflame your body in addition to whatever damage the flour itself is doing.

3. Your Body Doesn't Know What to Do with Gluten

Vegetarian Buddhists in China began eating gluten, a protein found in wheat, rye, barley, and a few other grains, back in the sixth century. Under its Japanese name, seitan, it's long been a staple in health food stores as a substitute for meat. Gluten is what makes dough doughy and bread airy (it shares the same root as the word "glue"). Normally, getting some of your protein from plants is a good thing. Except when it comes to gluten. Celiac disease, an autoimmune condition just like rheumatoid arthritis, multiple sclerosis, or lupus, causes confusion in your immune system. Here's what happens: Your body mistakenly reacts to gluten as if it were an external threat, and that prompts your immune system to attack your own tissues. Celiac is a root cause of at least fifty different diseases, including cancer, lymphoma, osteoporosis, kidney disease, irritable bowel syndrome, autoimmune diseases such as colitis or rheumatoid arthritis, anemia, and psychiatric and neurological diseases like anxiety, depression, schizophrenia, dementia, migraines, epilepsy, and autism.[16] Quite a list. But only an estimated 1 percent of the population has been diagnosed with celiac. That's terrible for them, but why should it matter to you and me?

Many more of us are afflicted with NCGS—nonceliac gluten sensitivity—which is essentially an extreme inflammatory reaction to the same protein. Even those of us without celiac may damage the cells of our intestinal lining when we eat gluten.[17] Today, the most advanced research on the subject has concluded that nobody—not one of us—can properly process gluten. But because we may not show any obvious symptoms, we could all be doing harm to our bodies without knowing it.

We've only recently learned how exactly gluten affects us. Scientists from the University of Maryland discovered the existence of a protein called zonulin, which is produced by our bodies whenever we eat gluten. Zonulin creates a leaky gut by opening up the tight junctions between intestinal cells that are normally stuck together like Lego pieces so that food and microbes can't "leak" into the spaces between cells of the small intestine's lining. Normally food and particles get filtered through the cells and don't go between them. That's important because 60 percent of our immune system is right under the one-cell-thick lining of our intestine. If those foreign food and microbe particles leak through our protective gut lining, they activate our gut immune system. That's when inflammation and disease happen. When those tight junctions become loose, we suffer what's become known as leaky gut syndrome, which allows microbes and even microscopic particles of food to escape into our bloodstream, where they don't belong.[18] Recent evidence has found that anyone who consumes gluten may have a mild form of leaky gut. Over the past 50 years there's been an almost unbelievable 400 percent rise in the number of Americans suffering with celiac.[19] We're still figuring out why that might be so, but it may be because wheat itself changed during that period. Or because our environment, habits, and medications — a rise in Cesarean sections, lack of breastfeeding, overuse of antibiotics, and use of acid-blocking medications, anti-inflammatory medications, and more — have created a bad situation for our guts. Which brings us to our next topic...

4. The Grains We Eat Aren't the Grains Our Grandparents Ate

New hybrids have been developed, most notably dwarf wheat, which is heartier than its predecessors but contains a "superstarch" called amylopectin A that has a greater impact on our blood sugar than the traditional kinds of starch—it actually promotes insulin resistance.[20] The new varieties also have more gluten, which is not doing us any favors. And while most wheat isn't genetically modified, it *is* dosed with a chemical herbicide called glyphosate just before harvest, which increases its yield. The trade name for this nasty stuff is Roundup, made by Monsanto, and although it didn't exist until 1974, it's now the most heavily used weed killer in global agriculture. (It's also the second-most popular herbicide for home use.) The EPA says it's safe for us, but there's evidence suggesting it may have something to do with the rise in celiac disease and other gluten sensitivities. Glyphosate exposure has been associated with increased risk of cancer, kidney disease, lymphoma, reproductive difficulties, and damage to our gut bacteria.[21] GMO products containing glyphosate are banned in Europe.

5. This Is Not to Say Gluten-Free Is Always Good for You

You might remember in years past when foods suddenly began proclaiming themselves "free"—as in sugar-free cookies or fat-free yogurt. More often than not, those were marketing ploys designed to cash in on our (sometimes justified) fear of certain ingredients. But the word "free" doesn't necessarily mean good for you. "Gluten-free" doesn't just mean the protein has been removed. Often it means the gluten has been replaced with something else harmful, like refined vegetable oils, artificial additives, a ton of sugar, or higher-glycemic flours. Remember: A gluten-free cookie is still a cookie! So, beware of "freedom," at least when it comes to food. Because it usually means increased processing, which in turn means less healthy and more expensive. If you want to go gluten-free, you should stop eating foods that contain gluten, period. Apples and almonds are gluten free—stick with whole foods.

6. You Should Be a Cereal Killer

Breakfast cereal should be called breakfast candy. When you eat it, your body immediately begins breaking down all those refined grains, starches, and added sugars into an avalanche of glucose. Most breakfast cereals are 75 percent sugar. But if you walk down any supermarket cereal aisle, you'll see misleading food labeling at its most creative. Today, virtually every cereal box makes some bogus health claim related to the theoretical benefits of eating whole grains. But those cereal grains are highly processed, even when technically "whole," and the added sugar content and chemical additives more than nullify any nutrition the stuff contains.

For all this we can thank John Harvey Kellogg, the nineteenth-century physician and Seventh-Day Adventist who ran a health spa in Battle Creek, Michigan. He (with his brother Will) created a vegetarian, non-protein alternative to the standard heartburn-inducing breakfast foods of his time (flapjacks and sausages). Kellogg's invention, flakes made of toasted corn, immediately caught on. His name endures thanks to the cereal giant he inspired, but his invention's connection to good health is long gone. I wonder how he would feel knowing that a cereal that bears his name — Kellogg's Honey Smacks — contains an insane 55.6 percent sugar by weight.[22] Breakfast cereal today is just a sugar-delivery system. Some are healthier than others, of course, but even the "healthy" cereals, the ones that look and taste like they were made from wood chips, should be avoided. We've somehow gotten the impression that granola is a better choice, but often the opposite is true — there are brands that contain more sugar than Cocoa Puffs. And the bad news just gets worse: When you start your day with sugar, you kick off an addictive cycle of sugar and carb cravings that will last all day long.

7. Oatmeal Is Not a Health Food

Can a food as boring as oatmeal really be unhealthy? Many Americans eat it religiously, as though it's a

miracle breakfast. It's not. It may lower your cholesterol,[23] but that isn't the lifesaving change you might
have thought it was. In fact, a large, eye-opening study
published in *BMJ Open* in 2016 found that people
above the age of sixty with low cholesterol levels have
higher mortality rates than people older than sixty
with high cholesterol.[24] And regardless, it's not the
oatmeal that lowers cholesterol; it is the oat bran.

The major problem with oatmeal is the same problem with every other grain: It spikes your blood sugar
and makes you hungrier. In one oft-quoted study,
overweight children were fed one of three breakfasts:
instant oatmeal, steel-cut oats, or omelets, all of which
had the same number of calories. The kids who had
the instant oatmeal ate 81 percent more food in the
afternoon than the omelet eaters. The kids who ate the
steel-cut oats did a little better, but still consumed 51
percent more than the children who ate eggs. That
wasn't the only difference: Compared to the omelet
group, the kids who ate the oatmeal had higher levels
of insulin, sugar, adrenaline, and cortisol (which suggests that the body perceives oatmeal as a stressor).[25]
The lesson? Even "healthy" cereal will increase your
food cravings more than protein and fats. And if you're
eating instant or microwavable oatmeal, you're getting
a cereal grain refined to the point that its nutritional
value has been compromised. I still talk to plenty of
people who believe that oatmeal is a healthy way to
start the day. It is—compared to Froot Loops! One

more thing to keep in mind: Although oats don't contain gluten, they can be contaminated with it when processed in factories where wheat is present. So, add oats to your list of gluten-containing foods to avoid. Even gluten-free oats can be a problem for those who are sensitive.

8. Your Corn Has Been Abused

Corn's an unusual case. It's a grain many of us believe isn't particularly healthy, mostly due to its high starch content. But we're at least partly wrong. Corn itself—fresh corn, also known as sweet corn—contains both soluble and insoluble fiber, which our gut bacteria turns into short-chain fatty acids that lower our risk of intestinal ailments, including colon cancer. Each variety of fresh corn—yellow, white, red, blue, purple—contains vitamins and minerals such as potassium and magnesium, and antioxidant phytonutrients, especially carotenoids like lutein and zeaxanthin, which are good for eye health.[26] However, corn these days does contain lots of starch, thanks to the newer hybrids that emphasize its sweetness. This means it's not ideal for those of us struggling with weight or blood sugar control. Still, we can eat it in its natural, whole, fresh state, as long as it's organic and non-GMO—and on the cob.

That said, nearly 90 percent of corn grown in the United States is GMO.[27] And GMO corn in some form or another shows up in an estimated 70 percent of processed foods — either as a sweetener (the notorious high-fructose corn syrup) or in other additives with long, unrecognizable names. GMO corn is also routinely grown using the pesticide atrazine, which is banned in Europe because it is a proven endocrine disrupter. (Researchers say that exposure turns male frogs into females![28]) Among humans there's a possible connection between a mother's exposure to atrazine and newborn male genital malformation.[29] So if you're going to eat corn, be sure to shop with care.

9. And Your Rice Isn't So Nice Either!

We've always thought of rice as a health food, but that's not really the case. All rice is starchy, and white rice is so refined that the fiber's all gone. It's associated with an increased risk of type 2 diabetes; the opposite is true of unrefined brown rice.[30] Brown rice contains more vitamins, minerals, and phytonutrients than white rice, which is so devoid of anything good that the government requires producers to supplement it with B vitamins and iron.

But why stop at brown? We can go all the way to red, purple, and my personal favorite, black rice (also known as emperor's or forbidden rice), which may sound scary but tastes great. (Give it a try; you won't be disappointed.) These colorful varieties have even more fiber than brown rice, and more beneficial substances, too, including anthocyanins, the flavonoids that make blueberries blue and cabbage red.

Traditionally, pigmented rice was eaten in Asia for its medicinal properties—it provides antioxidant, antitumor, hypoglycemic, and antiallergic protection.[31]

So, all rice is starchy, but the colored varieties less so than the white. However, there's another, potentially more serious issue: arsenic. Rice contains both the harmless organic kind as well as the inorganic type, which may cause cancer.[32] It ends up in the soil, thanks to pesticides and poultry farming, where it's absorbed by rice plants. (It may also be naturally present in the soil.) California white basmati rice has the least arsenic and brown rice has the most. I am not saying you should avoid eating rice altogether, but you should probably limit yourself to no more than one serving a week.

10. Some Grains Are Always Okay to Eat

Lest you get the impression that no grain belongs in a healthy diet, let me suggest a type we can all eat safely: weird grains. By that I mean the whole grains that contain no gluten, have not been turned into highly refined, industrialized products, and will never be found in Twinkies, cookies, or pizza crust—grains like quinoa and amaranth. These are nutritious as well as delicious, but most important, they won't send your blood sugar soaring. If the word *weird* makes you uneasy, feel free to think of them as exotic instead, which is accurate since these are more commonly eaten in Africa, Asia, and Latin America than they are in the

United States. There are many more weird grains just as beneficial, and they're listed at the end of this chapter. You might see some of these varieties referred to as "ancient grains," a name that reflects the fact that they have not been bastardized or genetically engineered.

GEEK ALERT: A LITTLE MORE SCIENCE ABOUT GRAINS

When we eat food with labels touting "whole-grain flour," we automatically assume that we're eating whole grains. We're not. The labeling rulebook says that as long as all three parts of the kernel are present in the flour in their original proportions, then the resulting product can be called "whole," like "whole wheat bread."[33] Except that the whole grain has been processed into flour, which is *not* the same thing as whole kernel. A whole kernel is just that — intact. Once a grain has been milled into flour, it may be called "whole grain," but it's no longer *whole*. If the label on a loaf of bread says it contains whole grains, it just means it contains some whole-grain flour. And as you know, flour acts more like sugar in your body than a whole unprocessed grain.

I've seen bread from a major commercial bakery boasting not one, but several "ancient healthful grains," like amaranth. But when you read the ingredients (in small print on the back), you see that these grains are way down at the end of the list, meaning they are the smallest part of the mix. Chances are, you're not going to get a whole lot of unrefined grain nutrition in that loaf.

Ideally you want to eat nongluten whole grains, not grains made into flour. Even worse, bread can be mostly white flour, deceptively described as "wheat flour," and be labeled whole wheat bread as long as it contains a tiny bit of whole wheat flour. If that wasn't bad enough, a serving of even two slices of completely whole wheat bread raises your blood sugar more than 2 tablespoons of table sugar. Hardly a health food.

THE DOWNSIDE OF MONOCULTURE

Crops like wheat, rice, and corn are typically grown as monocultures, meaning that a single crop is planted repeatedly on the same land, season after season. Monocultures deplete the soil of its nutrients, and as a result they require huge amounts of chemical fertilizers and pesticides. Damaged soil leads to erosion and runoff, which contaminates the water supply with pesticides and fertilizers. The USDA has found residues from fifteen toxic pesticides on corn.[34] About 95 percent of cornfields in America contain seeds coated with neonicotinoids, an insecticide known to kill bees, which are a crucial part of our entire system of agriculture.[35] Most of the grains grown in monocultures are used to feed livestock, so buying organic meat (as well as organic grains) helps to reduce the negative effects of industrial agriculture.

Here are some resources that can help you purchase the right grains—the ones that are most nutritious, not bastardized, and best for the environment and the planet.

- **Bluebird Grain Farms:** Bluebird sells plow-to-package whole grains that are organically grown, harvested, and milled on their certified organic farm: http://www.bluebirdgrainfarms.com/.
- **Agrilicious:** This website is a great way to search for sellers of fresh, locally farmed foods. You can use it to locate farms in your area that sell ancient and organic whole grains: http://www.agrilicious.org/.
- **Bob's Red Mill:** This is one of the leading brands of natural, certified organic, and gluten-free grain products in the United States: http://www.bobs redmill.com/.
- **The Teff Company:** Based in Idaho, this is one of the leading brands of teff, an African grain, in the United States. Their teff is grown in Idaho and sold throughout the country: https://teffco.com/.
- **Thrive Market:** You can find all sorts of cool and weird grains and rice varieties on Thrive Market's website. Examples include organic heirloom quinoa, amaranth, wild rice, sprouted brown rice, and even organic sprouted coconut rice: https://thrive market.com/.

SUMMING IT UP

Grains can be a great source of vitamins, minerals, and fiber. And let's face it: They taste pretty good too. That's one reason Americans have been binging on them for decades. But grains are not for everyone. There are many people who should absolutely avoid them for health reasons, which we'll get to in a bit. But even if you are among the people who can safely include some grains in your diet, you should still keep your grain intake to a minimum. Cutting down on your consumption of ubiquitous starches like rice and corn protects your health and improves your microbiome, plus it lessens the environmental impact of industrial agriculture. Corn, rice, and wheat are the most popular grains in the world, but growing them consumes a lot of resources, including water, fossil fuels, and fertilizer. If you have any doubts, keep this in mind: A study in the *Journal of the American Medical Association* found that people on government-subsidized food or food programs (56 percent of the population) have the worst health, including higher risk for diabetes, obesity, inflammation, and bad cholesterol. Government subsides support corn (high-fructose corn syrup), wheat, rice, and soy, mostly turned into processed foods.

In general, we need to recognize grains for what they are—treats. I think of most grains like I think of alcohol. I love wine, and I'm partial to tequila. But I make them both a "sometimes" pleasure. I don't partake every day, or even every week. It's the same with most grains. I see them as an occasional indulgence, not an everyday thing. Although I'm not a fan of most grains, it's fine to include small amounts in your diet. But you should eat them only if...

They are whole grains: If you're going to eat grains, they should be in their natural, whole, fresh state. Once they're pulverized and turned into flour — including whole wheat flour or brown rice flour — they act a lot like candy in your body, ramping up your blood sugar and insulin levels.

They're organic: Organically grown crops prevent water, soil, and air contamination. And they provide a safe space for honeybees and other wildlife. They're grown without pesticides like Roundup, which pollute the environment, harm wildlife, and leave behind toxic residues on your food. Look for organic, non-GMO grains and corn.

They're weird: Experimenting with millet, buckwheat, amaranth, quinoa, and black rice and other "weird" grains, and cutting down on corn (except organic corn on the cob), white rice, and wheat, is a step in the right direction. It's better for the environment and better for your health.

They're gluten-free: Our bodies don't know what to do with gluten. So, when you consume it, it can confuse your immune system, setting off a cascade of health issues. Even if you don't have celiac disease, it's best to avoid gluten as much as possible. Stick with gluten-free grains and pseudo-grains like quinoa, teff, and amaranth instead.

Grains Are Entirely Off-Limits If:

- You have type 2 diabetes or high blood glucose.
- You have issues with weight control or cravings.
- You suffer from any food sensitivities, since many of them can be traced back to gluten or other substances found in grains.
- You have any digestive issues, including irritable bowel syndrome or acid reflux.
- You have any autoimmune disease.
- You feel bloated after eating.
- Blood testing shows that your inflammation markers are high.

Do We Really Have to Give Up Bread?

Not entirely. There are health food brands that make bread with whole kernels of grains (not just the flour) and seeds, like spelt or dark German rye (both of which contain gluten), or sunflower seeds, and no added sugar. And usually the slices are thin, an added plus. They're a good choice. There are also great recipes for making bread using nut, seed, and coconut flours. Experiment. I made great pancakes the other day from coconut flour, almond meal, eggs, and macadamia milk. They were awesome and you can find the recipe on my website www.foodthebook.com.

Other than that, I'll repeat my best advice: Eat weird grains. No wheat, rye, barley, kamut, couscous, or oats.

How Often Should I Eat Grains?

Once a day. Tops.

How Much Should I Eat?

A ½ cup serving, max.

What to Do if You Think You Might Be Gluten-Sensitive

In this chapter, I've talked a lot about gluten and why you should avoid it. Some people need to avoid it more than others, particularly those who are gluten-sensitive or intolerant. So how do you find out if you fall into that category?

First, eliminate from your diet all grains and anything else that might contain gluten, including prepared foods and anything from a restaurant, for three weeks. Then reintroduce the foods one by one and track your reactions, if any.

If that doesn't tell you what you want to know, ask your doctor to order:

- Cyrex 3 testing (for reaction to twenty different gluten and wheat proteins)
- Conventional lab blood testing for celiac:
  - Anti-gliadin antibodies IgG and IgA

- TTG (tissue transglutaminase IgG and IgA)
- HLA DQ2 and DQ8 testing (genetics)

GRAINS: WHAT THE HECK SHOULD I EAT?

If you've never heard of a grain before, try it. The following grains can be served as side dishes, cooked in water or broth, and flavored with whatever vegetables, herbs, and spices you prefer.

- Buckwheat, from which pancakes, soba noodles, and kasha are made (it's a cousin of rhubarb, not wheat at all, despite the name)
- Whole-kernel rye (if you're not gluten-sensitive)
- Amaranth
- Millet
- Teff
- Sorghum
- Black rice
- Brown rice
- Red rice
- Wild rice (actually a seed)
- And the current champion weird grain: quinoa, also a non-grain; it's technically a pseudo-grain, related to beetroots and tumbleweeds, but it cooks like a grain, looks like a grain, and is supernutritious
- Non-GMO whole corn

What About White Rice?

White rice is not always bad. New research has found that when white rice and white potatoes are cooked and then allowed to cool, they develop something called resistant starch, which resists digestion, a good thing. It also provides fuel for healthy bacteria in your gut and helps improve metabolism. Cook. Cool. Warm gently. Enjoy.

GRAINS: WHAT THE HECK SHOULD I AVOID, IF I'M GLUTEN-SENSITIVE?

- Wheat (try einkorn or ancient wheat)
- Barley
- Rye
- Spelt
- Kamut
- Farro
- GMO wheat
- Bulgur
- Oats
- Semolina
- Couscous
- Any refined grains

NUTS AND SEEDS

NUTRITION IQ QUIZ

True or False?

1. Nuts are fattening, so you should limit your intake to avoid weight gain.
2. Peanut butter is a good source of protein.
3. Pistachios can help with erectile dysfunction.
4. Women who eat tree nuts like walnuts and almonds have a lower risk of breast cancer.
5. Almond milk is a great source of protein and fiber.
6. You should eat nuts two or three times a week for maximum benefit.

Answers

1. False: Studies show that eating nuts can actually help with weight loss because the fat and protein help cut appetite, speed metabolism, and prevent type 2 diabetes.
2. False: Peanuts aren't nuts; they're legumes. And most peanut butter contains high-fructose corn

syrup and industrial hydrogenated oils. Peanuts also contain aflatoxins (a kind of mold that causes cancer).

3. True: Pistachios improve arterial health and blood flow. They've been proven to help combat erectile dysfunction.

4. True: Fiber, which is contained in tree nuts, improves the health of the gut microbiome, helping to prevent cancer. Tree nuts also prevent diabetes and insulin resistance, which also causes cancer. Furthermore, adolescent girls who eat tree nuts have been shown to have a reduced risk of breast cancer when they're adults.[1]

5. False: There is hardly any protein in most brands of almond milk, and almond milk often contains lots of sugar and thickeners that can harm your gut. Whole almonds are a good source of fiber, protein, and good fats, but not almond milk— unless you make it yourself.

6. False: You should eat nuts every day because they help fight weight gain, type 2 diabetes, and heart disease! Don't go crazy, but a few handfuls a day is healthy.

Get a new food fact and weekly recipe directly from my kitchen. Sign up for free at www .foodthebook.com.

"On paper, nuts don't have much going for them," writes an Australian wellness blogger. He's right—on paper. Of all whole foods, nuts and seeds are the most energy-dense, which means we can get all the nutrients they offer from foods that are lower in calories. Americans have never really considered nuts a health food. Tree-nut consumption in the United States lags behind that in countries in Europe and the Mediterranean. The reality is that we've never expected much from nuts—we tend to eat them from bowls while sitting around a bar drinking beers, or maybe roasted over an open fire once a year during the holidays. Even at the supermarket, jars of nuts and seeds are found in the snack aisle, by the microwavable popcorn and the bags of Doritos—as if they were just another junk food.

The bad rap on nuts began in the 1980s, when the country was awash in the low-fat diet advice that convinced us all to think of high-fat foods as calorie bombs that would blow up our waistlines. Then the government's misguided 1992 Food Guide Pyramid told us to limit fat as much as possible. At the top of the pyramid, making up a small sliver that may as well have had a skull and crossbones on it, were the things we were told to eat "only sparingly": fats, oils, nuts, meats, poultry, dairy, and eggs.

Of course, as soon as the government steered us down this path of fat phobia, the food industry was all too happy to jump on the bandwagon, pumping out an avalanche of sugar-laden, fat-free junk foods marketed as healthy. (Remember SnackWell's? Yikes.) But before the ink on the government's food pyramid had time to dry, experts were already pointing out its major flaws. How could the government discourage people from eating nuts, eggs, avocados, olive oil, and other whole foods that have been dietary staples for thousands of years, even in countries where obesity and heart disease are scarce?

Some, like Walter Willett, the chair of Harvard's nutrition department, were so outraged that they campaigned against the Department of Agriculture's pyramid, pointing out that it was not based on rigorous science.[2] Willett and his colleagues even created an alternate food pyramid with no limits on nuts and other healthy oils and fats. Today we know that the government's dietary recommendations were wrong in many ways. But its advice to cut back on nuts due to their fat and calorie content will likely be remembered as some of the worst dietary advice we ever received.

When it comes to choosing what to eat, you should always look for foods that won't spike your blood sugar. That's why protein and fat should be your dietary staples. Nuts, it turns out, are an excellent source of both. They also contain plenty of fiber, minerals, and other healing nutrients. Best of all, as you're about to see, you need only a handful a day to make a powerful impact on your health.

THE SCIENCE OF NUTS AND SEEDS

Basically, a nut is an edible fruit seed contained in a hard shell. There are lots of similarities between nuts and other seeds, the main one being that both are full of energy—specifically polyunsaturated, monounsaturated, saturated, and omega-3 fats—which are necessary for the growth of a new fruit. That has always been held against them. But the calories or fat in nuts don't contribute to obesity, diabetes, or poor health like those in sugars do. They don't even make us fatter—in fact, studies show the opposite is true.[3] Nuts are good sources of healthy, anti-inflammatory polyunsaturated fats. Furthermore, nuts and seeds contain antioxidants and minerals like zinc and magnesium in abundance. They're good for weight loss (especially dangerous belly fat),[4] they're good for arterial health and blood pressure,[5] they lower the risk of heart disease and cancer,[6] they prevent type 2 diabetes,[7] and they may even keep you alive longer.[8]

WHAT THE EXPERTS GOT RIGHT

Recently, nuts and seeds have had a revival. New research points to their power for weight loss and for preventing heart disease, type 2 diabetes, and more. It's an about-face from the "nuts are fattening" days.

WHAT THEY GOT WRONG

Until recently, everything. If you followed the most popular dietary advice in the eighties and nineties, it's likely you seldom ate nuts. Their benefits were ignored, and they were treated like high-calorie junk food. This isn't that surprising if you look at the way we've traditionally served them — highly salted, encased in chocolate, or turned into butters and mixed with sugars, industrial oils, artificial colorings, chemical additives, and preservatives.

SEVEN THINGS YOU NEED TO KNOW ABOUT NUTS AND SEEDS

1. Nuts Look Like a Miracle Food

In February 2013, one of the largest dietary clinical trials ever published showed that eating fat could protect you from heart attacks and strokes. How did the researchers find this out? By making people add nuts and olive oil to their diets.

The randomized controlled trial, published in the *New England Journal of Medicine*, was called PRE-DIMED (for Prevención con Dieta Mediterránea), and it was one of the biggest and most rigorous nutrition studies ever conducted.[9] In the study, researchers from Spain assigned nearly 8,000 overweight and diabetic (or otherwise at risk for heart disease) people to follow a

Mediterranean diet supplemented with either nuts or olive oil. A third group, the control group, followed a low-fat diet. Those in the nut group were told to eat a large handful of walnuts, almonds, and hazelnuts daily, in addition to the standard Mediterranean diet. The other Mediterranean group was instructed to consume a liter of olive oil each week. The trial was designed to run for many years, but it was stopped early, after just five years, because the benefits of eating nuts and olive oil became so clearly enormous it would have been unethical to force the control group to stay on the low-fat diet!

Those who ate nuts every day reduced their risk of having a heart attack by 30 percent. Any drug that could produce that effect would be a blockbuster. In fact, eating nuts slashed the risk of a heart attack as much as taking a statin — but without any of the side effects (or expense). In later studies that further analyzed the PREDIMED data, scientists found that compared to the low-fat diet group, the subjects who ate nuts lost more belly fat[10] and had greater reductions in blood pressure,[11] LDL cholesterol, and inflammation.[12]

Another clinical trial published in the journal *BMJ Open* in 2014 compared people assigned to eat a low-fat vegan diet with a group of people who were instructed to eat a high-fat vegan diet that included nuts, avocados, and olive oil.[13] The group that consumed more nuts and other high-fat foods lost more weight and saw greater improvements in their cholesterol and other heart disease risk factors.

In 2016 a team of researchers published a meta-analysis of twenty-nine of the most rigorous studies of nut consumption in *BMC Medicine*. When evidence from all of those studies was combined, the researchers concluded that eating a handful of nuts each day reduced coronary heart disease risk by 30 percent, cancer risk by 15 percent, and diabetes risk by 40 percent. It also protected against kidney and neurodegenerative disease and lowered overall mortality. Extrapolate those findings to other countries and the impact of increased nut consumption would be enormous. The researchers estimated that just one serving of nuts per day could prevent 4.4 million premature deaths annually in the United States, Europe, Southeast Asia, and the Western Pacific.[14]

2. Nuts Can Help You Lose Weight

Nuts are a good lesson on how all calories are not the same. An Oreo has around 50 calories, about the same as three or four macadamia nuts. So what's the difference?

Quite a bit, it turns out. For starters, the ample dose of sugar in that Oreo will raise your triglycerides, lower your good cholesterol, contribute to a fatty liver, and increase your stress hormones. It will also spike your blood sugar and insulin, which will cause your body to store fat and make you hungrier. In fact, that one cookie could punch your ticket for a roller-coaster ride of blood sugar spikes and crashes, cravings, and binges, which will ultimately lead to weight gain. The macadamia nuts, however, have the opposite effect. They are high in protein, fiber, vitamins, and minerals. They are packed with satiating, healthy fats that improve your cholesterol profile and make you less hungry, not more. They won't spike and crash your blood sugar or insulin levels.[15] In fact, they'll keep them steady. Nuts are the perfect antidote to hunger pangs, which is why research shows that people who regularly eat them gain less weight than those who don't.

A study published in the journal *Obesity* followed 8,865 men and women in Spain and found that over a twenty-eight-month period, those who ate nuts two or more times per week were 30 percent less likely to gain weight than those who seldom or never ate nuts.[16]

The results of a review of the evidence of the relationship between body weight and consumption of nuts and other foods were published in the *American Journal of Clinical Nutrition*. In this review, the researchers examined three large prospective epidemiological studies— the Nurses' Health Study, the Health Professionals Follow-Up Study, and the Nurses' Health Study II. When the data were combined, the researchers found that people who replaced carbohydrates with nuts, poultry, seafood, and other low-glycemic foods had greater weight loss over a four-year period.[17]

The evidence is clear that eating nuts, for many reasons, won't make you fat. But it will improve your heart health and protect you against chronic disease. So, should you include them in your diet? Absolutely. But do so within reason. Avocados are fantastic. But you shouldn't eat ten in one day. The same goes for nuts. Enjoy them. But don't go *too* nuts. The research shows that all you need is one or two handfuls a day. Now let's look at their individual benefits.

3. Nuts Are Antioxidant Powerhouses

All nuts contain antioxidants, which are great for preventing cancer. But which have the most? In order:

- Pecans
- Walnuts
- Hazelnuts
- Pistachios
- Almonds[18]

4. Which Nuts Should I Eat for What?

Every nut is nutritious, but researchers have singled out some for their specific nutritional powers.

Almonds	Almonds lower bad cholesterol and the risk of heart disease; the magnesium they contain lessens the chance of sudden heart attack; they help prevent diabetes by stabilizing blood sugar, and they deliver minerals like copper and manganese, along with antioxidants such as vitamin E.

Walnuts	Walnuts are good for everything from bone health to cancer prevention to blood sugar control, but the main benefit is to our arterial function.[19] They also contain a good dose of omega-3 fats (ALA, or alpha-linoleic acid).
Pecans	Pecans are high in minerals (especially manganese and copper) and are as powerful as walnuts when it comes to cancer-fighting antioxidants.[20] They've also been associated with favorable cholesterol and triglyceride levels.[21]
Brazil nuts	Brazil nuts are valued mostly for their high levels of selenium, a mineral that's important for our metabolism, digestive health, thyroid function, detoxification, and protection against arthritis.[22] Just two Brazil nuts a day is all it takes, and they're proven to improve cholesterol and cardiovascular health, too.[23]
Hazelnuts	Like walnuts, hazelnuts are good for endothelial function and keep bad cholesterol from oxidizing. Their total antioxidant capacity is more than double that of almonds.[24]
Pistachios	Arginine is an amino acid found in meat, fish, shellfish, seeds, and abundantly in pistachios. It produces nitric oxide in the body, which improves arterial function and blood flow. In fact, men who ate three to four handfuls a day for three weeks had better penile blood flow and harder erections — a side effect no one complains about.[25]
Macadamias	Unlike most nuts, macadamias contain the same monounsaturated fats as olive oil and can improve overall cholesterol.[26]

5. Be Sure to Leave the Skin On

That's because it contains extremely high levels of polyphenols, micronutrients that help prevent cancer and heart disease.[27] In fact, hazelnut skin alone has more polyphenols than whole almonds. Skins of walnuts and almonds are also nutrient-rich and should be eaten along with the nut.

6. Don't Forget About Seeds!

Like nuts, each variety of seed has its own distinctive nutritional profile of fats, minerals, antioxidants, proteins, and fiber. The omega-3 fatty acids in flaxseeds reduce inflammation and help prevent heart disease and rheumatoid arthritis. And they're great for relieving and preventing constipation. Flaxseeds are one of my favorites (the whole seeds, not the oil) because they contain special compounds called lignans, which are protective against hormone-related cancers of the breast and prostate.[28] While many plants contain these compounds, flaxseeds have more than seventy-five times the amount found in fruits, vegetables, beans, and other seeds.[29] They also have high levels of plant-based omega-3 fats, or ALA.

You can't go wrong adding a variety of different seeds to your diet: Pumpkin seeds, hemp seeds, sesame seeds, and chia seeds are some that you should try to include often. You can throw hemp and chia seeds into your favorite salads, shakes, and smoothies. Sesame seeds are great in savory dishes like veggie stir-fries or sesame-crusted wild salmon. Tahini, made from ground sesame seeds, is one of the best sources of calcium and makes great creamy salad dressings. Pumpkin seeds are a great source of zinc. You can toast them in the oven and eat them as a snack (go easy on the salt), or add them to salads for crunch and flavor. One of my favorite lunches is what I call a "fat salad." I throw together a bunch of greens, crunchy veggies, olives, avocado, and a can of wild salmon, and then I top it all off with some fresh toasted pumpkin seeds. You can add seeds to all sorts of foods and dishes. Just try not to eat the extracted oils. Think of seeds like fruit: They're fine for most people when consumed whole. But you run into problems when you refine them and highly concentrate their individual components. Small amounts of walnut, macadamia, almond, flax, or hemp oil are fine.

7. Nut Butters, Flours, and Milks Can Be Healthy — but Only Certain Ones

Nut butters are becoming more popular because they make a great, quick snack (except peanut butter, which is discussed in the beans chapter). When I travel, I always throw a couple of packets of almond and cashew butter in my suitcase to keep me from having to rely on airport food or vending machine snacks. The brand I like is Artisana.

One reason most people don't succeed in eating

well is that they don't plan their food day. They plan their vacations, they plan their kitchen redesigns, but they don't think ahead about what they'll eat — and that's a recipe for nutritional disaster. So, I always know where I'm going to get my food every day of every week. And I carry with me a set of snacks so that I'm never in a food emergency. I have to protect myself from myself because I'll eat all the wrong foods if I'm hungry in an airport lined with fast-food options. That's why I always have packets of nut butter, a Primal Kitchen bar, a Tanka bar, or a Bulletproof bar when I'm on the road. I carry fat and protein as my snacks, and I keep enough food in my bag to last an entire day. I recommend you do the same. You can purchase little packets of nut and cashew butters at many grocery stores or at Thrive Market (an online grocery store where you can get healthy products at 25 to 50 percent off).

But be judicious with nut butters. Eat them in moderation, and choose the kinds that don't have added oils, sugars, or anything else — the nutrition label should mention just one ingredient. Look for a store that grinds the nuts into butter, so they're not subjected to industrial processing, which can damage the fragile fatty acids. A final consideration: Buy it in small quantities so the oils don't go rancid. You should keep your nuts and nut butters in the fridge or freezer.

I recommend flours made from almonds, cashews, hazelnuts, coconut, and hemp seeds, all of which are healthier than any grain-based flour. But remember that no flour is a whole food. When almonds or any other nuts are milled, it changes the way our bodies digest them. Nut flours are never a license to go crazy. A cookie made from almond flour is still a cookie.

Nut milks don't come with the same baggage as dairy—meaning no hormones (which even organic milk contains). But they contain additives like xanthan gum and carrageenan, both of which can alter the gut flora and create a leaky gut. And you have to read the labels carefully, because even organic nut milk can contain sugar and other additives. Barley malt, which is a sweetener used in some nut milk, contains gluten, too. Look for brands without those ingredients.

GEEK ALERT: A LITTLE MORE SCIENCE ABOUT NUTS AND SEEDS

Lectins are proteins present in all plants. They keep them healthy and protect them from predators.[30] But when you eat them in high amounts, they can damage the lining of your intestine and even contribute to leaky gut.[31] The phytates in nuts and seeds may be beneficial, but they have also been shown to disrupt the body's ability to absorb the iron (and potentially other nutrients) in food.[32] Thankfully this is a problem that can be fairly easily overcome. Soaking and cooking reduce the concentrations of these compounds substantially. So, I recommend soaking your raw nuts or seeds in a bowl of warm water overnight. Problem solved. You can also buy sprouted nuts. And in the context of the overall benefits of nuts and seeds, the lectins are a minor issue that I wouldn't worry about.

ARE NUTS AND SEEDS BAD FOR THE ENVIRONMENT?

A few years ago, my inbox was flooded with articles that had headlines like this: "Your Almond Milk Obsession Is Destroying the Environment." As I am a seed and nut lover, my friends and family turned to me for reassurance. "Should we be eating nuts and seeds? We know they're good for us, but are they bad for the environment?"

Almonds are now the most popular nut consumed in the United States, and California is the only state in the country that produces them commercially. In fact, if you eat an almond anywhere in the world, there's a good chance it came from California, since the state produces almost 85 percent of the global supply.[33]

Unfortunately, California is prone to severe droughts, and high demand for almonds is using up a lot of the water available to farmers. The king salmon population in Northern California is threatened, because already low river water is being diverted for use in almond farming.[34] But the truth is that almonds aren't the only food or crop that uses a lot of water. Everything grown—including meat, dairy, vegetables, fruit—requires extensive irrigation. We aren't going to stop eating, so what can we do? We can stop wasting. When we buy food and don't eat it, we squander water, fertilizer, pesticides, and animal lives, too. Another thing we can do is realize that almond milk isn't really as nutritious as we've been led to think; it's usually loaded with other ingredients and not so many actual almonds. (See the chapter on beverages for details.) You can use other kinds of milk, such as hemp, cashew, or macadamia.

The key to making the best nut and seed purchases is to buy organic. Nuts and seeds are fatty and oily, so they absorb pesticides easily. A lot of the chemicals used on nuts and seeds are potentially carcinogenic and have been shown to cause harm to human beings and surrounding wildlife. Your local health food store should have great options for organic nuts and seeds, but here are some other options as well.

- My favorite place to buy organic nuts and seeds is Thrive Market: https://thrivemarket.com/nuts-seeds -trail-mixes. Everything is 25 to 50 percent off, making eating healthy more affordable.
- Agrilicious is a website that you can use to find organic nuts for sale in your local area. Just go to this web page and type in your zip code to find the nearest vendor: http://www.agrilicious.org/local/nuts.

- Tierra Farm is a great website that sells raw, certified organic nuts and seeds in bulk. They source their products responsibly too: http://www.tierra farm.com/rawseedsandnuts.aspx.
- When you buy organic nuts and seeds, look for those that are certified Fair Trade so you can support the ethical treatment of workers. You can learn about the Fair Trade certification program here: https://fairtradeusa.org.

SUMMING IT UP

It's hard to go wrong with most nuts and seeds, as long as you're eating them raw and organic when possible. But you should always make sure they're not adulterated with additives like sugar, refined oil, artificial flavors and colorings, or excessive amounts of salt. Buy nuts and seeds in small quantities so the fats don't go rancid, or store them in the freezer. Soak them overnight and then keep them around as daily snacks. Don't eat more than a couple of handfuls a day, and go easy on nut butters and flours.

NUTS AND SEEDS: WHAT THE HECK SHOULD I EAT?

- Almonds
- Walnuts
- Pecans

- Hazelnuts (filberts)
- Brazil nuts
- Pistachios
- Macadamia nuts
- Cashews
- Pumpkin seeds

The following seeds aren't really convenient for eating whole, but you should have these as well, either in smoothies or mixed into other dishes:

- Chia seeds
- Ground flaxseeds
- Hemp seeds
- Sesame seeds

NUTS AND SEEDS: WHAT THE HECK SHOULD I AVOID?

- Nuts enrobed in sugar, chocolate, or any form of candy
- Nut butters with added oil, salt, or sugar (which often contain toxic trans fat and high-fructose corn syrup)
- Peanuts, except in small amounts (and they're not nuts anyway)

SUGAR AND SWEETENERS

NUTRITION IQ QUIZ

True or False?

1. The main problem with sugar is that it's just empty calories.
2. Agave syrup is a healthy alternative to high-fructose corn syrup and sugar.
3. Saturated fat from butter or meat causes heart disease, not carbs or sugar.
4. Sugar may be more addictive than cocaine.
5. One of the benefits of eating sugar is that it provides fuel to your brain.
6. High-fructose corn syrup is sugar with a different name.
7. If you want to lose weight, replace sugary drinks with diet soda.

Answers

1. **False:** Sugar isn't mere empty calories. It causes heart disease, diabetes, cancer, and more. It doesn't just make you fat; it makes you sick, even if you don't gain weight.

2. **False:** It may sound healthy, but it's pure fructose, which causes fatty liver, diabetes, and inflammation, and it creates dangerous types of cholesterol. Plus, it is processed with toxic chemicals.[1]

3. **False:** That was the lie we were told. Now we know that sugar[2] in all its forms, not fat, is the leading cause of heart disease.[3]

4. **True:** Eating sugar has a potent impact on the same parts of the brain that are stimulated by addictive drugs like cocaine or heroin.[4] In animal studies, rats will work eight times harder to get sugar than cocaine. If they are already cocaine addicted, they will switch to sugar as their preferred drug when given the chance.[5]

5. **False:** You get all the sugar you need from eating fruits and other whole foods, and your brain can get energy from fats, too. In fact, it runs better on fats such as MCT oil (from coconut).

6. **False:** High-fructose corn syrup is an industrial product that's metabolized differently than sugar and does even more harm, including damage to the gut and liver. It may also contain mercury as a by-product of how it's produced.

7. False: The artificial sweeteners in soda and other junk foods make you eat more than you would if you just consumed sugar instead. And they can alter your gut flora to promote obesity[6] and type 2 diabetes.[7] Don't drink soda—diet or otherwise.

> Get a new food fact and weekly recipe directly from my kitchen. Sign up for free at www .foodthebook.com.

If it weren't for the fact that we eat so much of it, sugar might not even deserve its own chapter in this book. It's not something you need, and I hesitate to call it food. If it were a brand-new product, the government would treat it like a dangerous substance to be controlled and regulated, not something that should be given to babies and added to 74 percent of all packaged foods in supermarkets.[8] In fact it would not be approved as a food additive because it is so toxic when consumed in anything but small amounts. When you look at the damage caused by sugar—obesity, diabetes, heart disease,[9] cancer, dementia, stroke, depression[10]—you have to wonder why we continue to eat it as we do, and, even worse, why we spoon-feed sugary junk foods to our children. Once, when I worked in an urgent care center, a woman came in with her seven-month-old infant. He was drinking a brown liquid out of his baby bottle. I asked what it was. She said, "Coke." I asked her why she was giving him Coke. She said, "Because he likes it." Of course he likes it—our brains are programmed to love sugar. Sweet things in nature are always safe to eat and they are a quick source of energy that helps us store fat for times of scarcity. But sugar has become such a pervasive part of our food landscape that we're chronically overdosing on it. Almost 20 percent of our daily calories come from sugary beverages like soda, sports drinks, juice, and sweetened coffees and teas.[11] Some estimates from US government surveys say that the average American consumes 152 pounds of sugar and about 133 pounds (down from 146.8 pounds in 1995) of flour annually.[12] Combined, that's more than three-quarters of a pound of sugar and flour every day for every man, woman, and child in America. That's a pharmacologic dose our bodies were not designed to handle.[13]

Our obsession with sugar stems partly from the fact that for the past 50 years, we've been brainwashed into thinking that dietary fat causes heart attacks and obesity and that sugar is nothing more than harmless empty calories. The federal government's dietary guidelines convinced us to replace our scrambled eggs and butter with low-fat strawberry yogurt (which has about the same amount of sugar as a can of soda) and orange juice. Many of us followed those recommendations dutifully, swapping saturated fat for sugar. But instead of getting slimmer and healthier, we got fatter and sicker. That's because sugar is more than empty calories: It spurs inflammation, accelerates weight gain[14] (especially belly fat), sets the stage for heart attacks and strokes, and contributes to cancer and Alzheimer's disease. The government was dead wrong. That misguided advice—which was embraced and echoed by governments around the world—has likely killed millions and millions of people. A study in the journal *Circulation* attributed 184,000 deaths around the world each year to sugar-sweetened beverage consumption.[15] Just imagine the toll from candy, cookies, cakes, pies, breakfast cereals, chocolate milk, fruit yogurt, and all the other commonplace foods that are loaded with sugar.

The World Health Organization, the American Heart Association, and nearly every other major health organization now warn people to limit their added sugar intake to 10 percent of their daily calories or less.[16] Yet most people consume far more than that. The average American child eats triple that amount,[17] and studies show that many adults have no idea how much sugar they're eating and, when asked, drastically underestimate the actual amount.[18]

That's because the food industry adds sugar to seemingly everything. It's not only in the obvious places, like drinks and snacks, but in surprising places, like chicken soup, spaghetti sauce, multigrain crackers, bacon, smoked salmon, even most salad dressings. Why do we need sugar on our lettuce? Nearly all our added sweeteners come from processed foods purchased in grocery stores and meals from fast-food joints and restaurants, rather than the foods we cook for ourselves from scratch.[19] It's not the sugar you add to your food, but the sugar added by corporations. Far too many of us have allowed the food industry to hijack our kitchens, and in return the food industry has poisoned us for profit.

The key to ridding yourself of this problem is recognizing the special harm that sugar represents, knowing where to look for it, and eliminating it completely for a few weeks (try the Blood Sugar Solution 10-Day Detox Diet or just use the 10-Day Detox Plan in Part IV of this book). Then eat only the sweeteners that you personally add to your food. When you cut out sugar, you'll experience fewer cravings and a lower tolerance for overly sweet foods. And best of all, as you're about to see, your health will drastically improve.

Still want that cookie?

THE SCIENCE OF SUGAR

There's a good reason why we crave sweet foods. In the pre-agriculture era — that is, for most of human existence — sugar was a rare substance, a concentrated form of quick energy found mainly in wild fruit and honey. Bears binge on fatty wild salmon but don't gain weight; when they gorge themselves on berries they gain 500 pounds by the end of the summer. Then they hibernate and lose the weight while we just keep eating all winter! Our food environment has changed a lot since the Stone Age, but the news hasn't reached the reward centers of our brains, which have always been worried about nutritional scarcity. Evolution has wired our brains to desire the easy access to energy that glucose provides. Our brains may be smart, but they still don't understand that all this sugar is killing us.

It's easy to see how our excessive consumption of sugar is causing the diabetes pandemic: In 2014, the World Health Organization estimated that 422 million adults had type 2 diabetes, up from 108 million in 1980; that's a 400 percent increase.[20] And remember, 1980 was the dawn of the low-fat, high-carb era of dietary recommendations. Even though it has less than half the calories of fats, sugar sets off a spike and then a plunge in insulin production, which inspires more cravings for sugar and starches. Before long, our cells no longer respond to insulin, and trouble sets in — diabetes, which ravages the entire body. And that's not all. Sugar causes high blood pressure, high cholesterol, high triglyceride levels, and heart disease.[21] It promotes cancer and can increase recurrence and mortality rates in cancer patients.[22] It speeds up the aging process in cells,[23] including the neurons in your brain, leading to an increased risk of dementia.[24] It damages the liver exactly like alcohol does.[25] In fact, fatty liver from sugar consumption has now become the number one cause of liver disease. And if you think the best alternative to sugar is using artificial sweeteners, well, think again. Artificial sweeteners may be even worse for your brain and metabolic health.[26] Rather than satisfying cravings, they'll push you to binge on more sugar and junk food, creating a vicious cycle that leads to obesity and diabetes.

WHAT THE EXPERTS GOT RIGHT

For decades, there has been evidence of the dangers sugar and processed carbs pose, especially where diabetes is concerned. Type 2 diabetes was called "sugar diabetes" long ago because doctors would taste their patients' urine for the telltale sweetness that indicated the disease. William Banting, a British undertaker, documented the link between sugar and obesity as far back as 1863 and urged the public to adopt low-carbohydrate diets.[27]

WHAT THEY GOT WRONG

The first federal dietary guidelines in 1980 warned against fat and cholesterol but barely mentioned sugar at all. There was a recommendation to eat less sugar because of tooth decay, but the guidelines incorrectly declared that sugar has nothing to do with type 2 diabetes or heart disease.[28] Wrong.[29] We were told it was better to eat sugar than fat because sugar contained fewer calories. But now we know that was wrong. By misplacing the blame for obesity and related health problems on fat, the government gave the food industry a license to pour unlimited amounts of sugar into the food supply. Americans gave up fat and got hooked on sugar—and we know how well that turned out.

SEVEN THINGS YOU NEED TO KNOW ABOUT SUGAR

1. It Was Sugar All Along

You can thank one man for launching the anti-fat crusade that spawned the explosion of sugary foods in America. That man was Ancel Keys, the University of Minnesota physiologist whose research in the 1950s and '60s shaped the government's dietary guidelines that convinced the world to look away from the toxic nature of sugar. Keys, a hugely influential scientist, worked closely with the federal government and the American Heart Association and was even featured on the cover of *Time* magazine for an article advocating low-fat diets. As we saw in the chapter on meat, Keys convinced the world that saturated fat was the world's biggest dietary villain. But he made a crucial error: Although he had access to data on fat and heart disease from twenty-two different countries, he cherry-picked the six countries that most helped his argument and ignored the sixteen countries that did not.[30]

When other nutrition experts included the data from all twenty-two countries, they saw a very different picture from the one Keys painted. A paper published in 1957 that analyzed all the countries together found that there was *zero* association between fat intake and heart disease.[31] At around the same time, John Yudkin, a British physician and founding professor of the Department of Nutrition at Queen Elizabeth College in London, argued that Keys and his colleagues were overlooking all the evidence that clearly implicated sugar. Yudkin carried out numerous studies on the physiological effects of sugar. He found that it increased triglycerides, insulin, and weight and stress hormones,[32] while lowering HDL cholesterol and causing blood to thicken—a deadly combination that makes heart attacks and diabetes more likely.[33] Yudkin published an acclaimed book, *Pure, White, and Deadly*, which sounded the alarm on sugar and urged the public to adopt low-carb diets. But Keys' vision had taken hold, and Yudkin was shamed and ignored.

"If only a small fraction of what is already known about the effects of sugar were revealed in relation to any other material used as a food additive," Yudkin wrote, "that material would promptly be banned."[34]

Keys was not alone in scapegoating fat and ignoring sugar. In the 1950s and '60s, the sugar industry was gravely concerned by the research that Yudkin and other sugar critics were publishing. One leading sugar industry executive, John Hickson, wrote a letter to a pair of scientists at Harvard—Fred Stare and Mark Hegsted—asking them to write a review that would downplay the research on sugar and shift the nutrition community's focus to saturated fat. The two Harvard scientists obliged. In 1967, they published a review paper in the prestigious *New England Journal of*

Medicine that dismissed the link between sugar and heart disease and shifted the blame to saturated fat. For their work, the sugar industry paid Hegsted and Stare the equivalent of $50,000 in today's dollars—a fact they failed to disclose in their paper. It was only in 2016 that Hegsted and Stare's ties to Big Sugar came to light, after researchers uncovered thousands of internal sugar industry documents and published an exposé in *JAMA Internal Medicine*.[35] Today that 1967 paper would never have been published due to rules about conflicts of interest. But it set the stage for nearly 50 years of failed nutrition policy.

The 1967 review paper was enormously influential. It all but declared the debate over sugar dead, forcing other researchers to turn their attention to saturated fat. And its authors went on to shape the government's official nutrition recommendations and policies. Hegsted became the head of nutrition at the USDA, where in 1977 he wrote the forerunner to the government's dietary guidelines, which convinced generations of Americans to adopt low-fat diets. His coauthor, Stare, was the chairman of Harvard's nutrition department, which also trumpeted the low-fat diet advice.

Today the sugar and junk-food industries and their scientific allies continue to mislead the public about the harms of sugar. In 2015 the world's largest producer of sugary beverages, Coca-Cola, was caught paying scientists millions of dollars to downplay the link between soda and obesity.[36] Candy companies have been exposed for paying scientists to publish studies suggesting that kids who eat candy weigh less than kids who do not.[37] And in 2016, a group of scientists funded by Coke, Pepsi, Kraft, Hershey's, Mars, and other multinational junk-food makers published a high-profile paper in the *Annals of Internal Medicine* calling recommendations to reduce sugar intake "untrustworthy" and unscientific—a tactic reminiscent of those used by the tobacco industry.[38]

Big Sugar wants to hide the truth about its product. But don't be fooled. There is overwhelming scientific consensus that sugar consumption is the driving force behind the obesity epidemic. After personally reading thousands of scientific papers and seeing more than 10,000 patients over 30 years, I'm convinced that the science could not be clearer: Sugar calories are deadly calories. Anyone who tells you otherwise is either wrong or lying to you.

2. Sugar Is Addictive

Despite the industry's best efforts, it's no longer a secret that sugar is bad for you. Yet despite its deadly reputation, millions of Americans struggle to give up their cookies, cake, ice cream, and sugary drinks. Why?

It's not just that we love sugar and sweet tastes—it's that we're hooked. The awful truth is that sugar can dramatically alter your metabolism and your brain chemistry, causing you to suffer intense cravings. In a study published in the *American Journal of Clinical Nutrition*,[39] obese men were given milk shakes that contained equal amounts of nutrients and calories. But half of the subjects got shakes containing high-glycemic corn syrup, which causes a rapid spike in blood sugar, and the other group's milk shakes contained low-glycemic cornstarch, a carb that is digested more slowly than syrup, causing just a gradual rise in blood glucose. After drinking the shakes, the corn syrup group reported feeling much hungrier than the other group and ended up eating a lot more later on. All of the subjects were given brain scans, which showed that the syrup group had increased blood flow in the nucleus accumbens, the part of the brain that regulates cravings, rewards, and addictive behaviors. This is the same part of the brain that lights up when alcoholics have a drink, when compulsive gamblers walk into a casino, or when drug addicts take a hit of cocaine. When this reward center lights up in response to stimuli like sugar, it reinforces the desire for that stimulus, which, over time, gives rise to intense cravings that play a role in addictive behavior.

A group of neuroscientists published a study in *Neuroscience and Biobehavioral Reviews* that looked at the effects of sugar on brain chemistry. They concluded that sugar produced binge-like behavior and stimulated the nucleus accumbens, "the classic effect of most substances of abuse."[40] This has huge implications for how we think of obesity. If much of the food

Americans eat is biologically addictive, then the whole concept of willpower and personal responsibility for weight loss is a fiction. It's not your fault that you're fat. Blame the conscious behavior of big corporations to create ever-more addictive foods. Michael Moss, a *New York Times* reporter, interviewed 300 business executives, employees, and scientists and wrote *Salt Sugar Fat: How the Food Giants Hooked Us*, a bruising behind-the-scenes look at how Big Food deliberately designs addictive foods.

3. Quitting Sugar Improves Your Health Rapidly

Sugar is so ubiquitous, and its effects on our brain chemistry so powerful, that breaking free of its grip can be enormously difficult. But here's some motivation: As soon as you quit sugar, your health will improve rapidly. In fact, it takes just ten days without sugar to see substantial metabolic and neurological benefits.

In a study published in the journal *Obesity* and sponsored by the National Institutes of Health, scientists recruited forty-three overweight teenagers who had at least one feature of metabolic syndrome, such as high blood sugar, hypertension, or abnormal cholesterol.[41] On average the subjects had been getting about 27 percent of their daily calories from sugar. But the researchers made one simple modification to their diets: They replaced all the sweet foods they were eating—candy, pastries, doughnuts, and chicken teriyaki (that sauce contains a lot of sugar!) — with starches. They kept the amount of calories they ate the same, so the subjects didn't lose any weight. The goal of the study was to see whether replacing sugar with slower-acting carbs could improve health even without weight loss.

After only ten days, there were marked changes. On average, the subjects' diastolic blood pressure fell 5 points. Their LDL cholesterol dropped 10 points. Their triglyceride levels plummeted 33 points. And their fasting blood sugar and insulin levels — both of which are predictors of diabetes — improved significantly. In a separate paper, the researchers dug deeper into the subjects' cardiovascular profiles.[42] They found that the ten-day break from sugar reduced their levels of APOC3 — a protein associated with heart disease — by 49 percent. It also caused their small, dense LDL particles, the most atherogenic (heart-disease-causing) cholesterol particles, to all but disappear. While too many starches can be problematic, the study demonstrated that fructose — which is found in sugar but not in starches — is a primary driver of heart disease risk through its impact on triglycerides, APOC3, small, dense LDL, and blood pressure.

Unlike glucose, which can be used by nearly every cell in the body, fructose is processed almost exclusively in the liver. When you consume regular table sugar, your body breaks it down into glucose and fructose and sends the fructose straight to your liver, where, through a process known as lipogenesis, it is converted into fats such as triglycerides and harmful forms of cholesterol. This sets off a cascade of metabolic damage. Fructose drives the development of fatty liver disease, increasing liver fat and inflammation.[43] In addition to creating visceral fat or organ fat, triglycerides, and small, dense LDL particles that cause heart disease, it wreaks havoc on your intestinal lining,[44] which leads to leaky gut and systemic inflammation. Free fructose punches little holes in your intestine. And then poop and food particles leak into your blood, activating your immune system.

Fructose, as you can see, is toxic when consumed without the fiber that accompanies it in fruit, and it is especially toxic when it comes in high-fructose corn syrup. But unfortunately, fructose is everywhere. While regular table sugar is 50 percent fructose and 50 percent glucose, other sweeteners added to processed foods are usually much worse. High-fructose corn syrup contains anywhere from 55 to 90 percent fructose. Because it's extremely cheap, food companies love it and often use it in place of regular sugar in processed foods. High-fructose corn syrup accounts for more than 40 percent of caloric sweeteners added to foods and beverages today.[45]

The best way to avoid sugar, high-fructose corn syrup, and other sweeteners is to focus on eating real, whole, unprocessed foods. All it takes is a ten-day sugar detox to see major improvements in your heart disease risk factors. I wrote *The Blood Sugar Solution 10-Day Detox Diet* to help guide people through an effective ten-day sugar detox. The health benefits were amazing. Not only did a group on our program lose weight and decrease their blood sugar and blood pressure; they also experienced a 62 percent reduction in all symptoms from all diseases in just ten days.

If you do buy packaged foods, look at the ingredients list with a close eye, and be wary of the numerous euphemisms that food manufacturers use to disguise the sweeteners in their products. There are more than 250 different names for sugar, such as maltodextrin, that you wouldn't even recognize. Even trained nutritionists and dietitians have trouble spotting all the sugars hiding in ingredients labels these days. So, here's a handy little guide...

4. There Are Many Ways to Say "Sugar"

There's an old cliché that says Eskimos have one hundred words for snow. It makes sense, then, that we Americans have so many ways of saying "added sugar." For the most part, you won't find these in your cupboard — they're nearly all ingredients used in processed foods. The *New York Times* compiled a list of ninety such terms you might find on labels, all of which are just different kinds of added sugar. Here are a few clues that an ingredient is really just sugar:

- Anything with the word "agave."
- Anything with the word "corn" (unless it's whole corn), like high-fructose corn syrup or corn sweetener.
- Any derivative of rice (unless it's vinegar), like brown rice syrup.
- Anything that begins with the word "cane," like cane juice or cane syrup. Many food manufacturers try to disguise the sugar in their products by using terms like "evaporated cane juice" in their ingredients labels. But don't be fooled. Anytime you see a fruit concentrate or juice among the ingredients, you're just seeing sugar in disguise.
- Any word with the suffix "-ose," like fructose, dextrose, maltose, sucrose, or trehalose.
- Anything with the word "malt," like malt syrup or flo-malt or maltodextrin.
- Anything that starts with the prefix "iso-," like isoglucose or isomaltulose.
- Anything with the word "syrup," like maple syrup, sorghum syrup, or corn syrup. And bear in mind the difference between maple syrup and "pancake syrup," which is usually pure fructose.
- Obviously, anything that's sweet, like molasses.
- And of course, anything with the word "sugar" in it, like date sugar, coconut sugar, brown sugar, beet sugar, and confectioners' sugar.

5. Artificial Sweeteners Are Bad for You

Here is a classic example of what happens when you try to outsmart Mother Nature. Rather than accept the fact that we're eating too much sugar and try to eat less, we look for a magic loophole—an easy way to avoid doing the smart thing. We saw it with trans fats and margarine, which were created as replacements for butter but turned out to be unsafe for human consumption. And it is happening again with artificial sweeteners. There are five that have received FDA approval—saccharin (Sweet'N Low), acesulfame (Sunett, Sweet One), aspartame (NutraSweet, Equal, and others), sucralose (Splenda), and neotame, which is used by food manufacturers only. They're all bad for you. In a study of heart disease, people who consumed diet drinks every day had a greater risk of diabetes and metabolic syndrome.[46] Artificial sweeteners have proven to be carcinogenic in animal studies.[47] They wreak havoc on your gut microbes, destroying beneficial bacteria and causing glucose intolerance.[48] They contain substances called excitotoxins, which can damage neurons and have been linked to neurologic side effects.[49]

Something that tastes sweet but contains zero calories may sound like the perfect cure for sugar addiction. But it's not, and here's why. Normally, when you eat or drink something sweet, it's accompanied by lots of calories. But not when you consume artificial sweeteners. This confuses your brain. It senses that the taste of sugar without the accompanying calories from glucose and fructose is wrong, and it tries to correct the imbalance by making you hungrier. As a result, you end up eating *more* food, not less.[50] Scientists have identified this as the mechanism responsible for the fact that cutting calories the wrong way — by using artificial sweeteners — can make you fatter, not thinner. This imbalance has also been found to cause hyperactivity, insomnia, and glucose intolerance. It has even been shown that eating yogurt flavored with saccharin or aspartame results in weight gain, not loss, compared to eating yogurt with table sugar.[51] The artificial sweeteners increased hunger, slowed metabolism, and increased body fat by 14 percent, while increasing food consumption in just two weeks. A big part of the problem is that artificial chemicals can be many thousands of times sweeter than sugar, which amps up your brain to expect more intensely sweet flavors.

A team of scientists at Imperial College London analyzed the research on artificially sweetened beverages and obesity and determined that they are just as big a problem as sugar-sweetened drinks.[52] In a paper they published in *PLOS Medicine* in 2017, they concluded that there was no good evidence that artificially sweetened beverages helped prevent weight gain and that there were major questions surrounding their long-term effects on health. They also pointed out that the vast majority of the studies (about 99 percent) that have found benefits to consuming artificial sweeteners were funded by industry. Most of these studies were small, poorly done, and riddled with flaws, the researchers found. They offered a blunt assessment of diet beverages, calling them a risk factor for chronic disease and saying, "They should not be promoted as part of a healthy diet."

6. The Bitter Truth About Sugar Alcohols

Sugar alcohols are the mystery sweeteners, with weird names and murky origins. They're derived from plants such as fruits and vegetables, and they're used mainly by food manufacturers in everything from candy and bubble gum to cough drops and chewable vitamins. Unlike artificial sweeteners, which can be thousands of times sweeter than sugar, sugar alcohols are usually less sweet. And they have calories, though many fewer than sugar, and we don't absorb them very well. They're easy to identify on food labels — their names end in the suffix "-ol," for instance, mannitol, sorbitol, xylitol, and malitol.

Some experts recommend consuming these instead of sugar or artificial sweeteners. But I suggest keeping them to a minimum. Sugar alcohols are imperfectly absorbed by your intestines, which can cause diarrhea, bloating, flatulence, and other forms of digestive distress. They also mess with your gut microbes and cause bacterial overgrowth. And worst of all, they keep you hooked on sweetness.

But as sugar alcohols go, there's one that may be better than the rest. Erythritol is virtually calorie-free (0.2 calories per gram) and about 60 percent as sweet as sugar. It's the only sugar alcohol that doesn't cause digestive distress, because your intestines absorb it rather than sending it to your colon to ferment and cause trouble. It won't raise your blood sugar or insulin levels, and to my knowledge it's the only sugar alcohol that's sold in stores for home use. There seems to be only one problem. New research links it to weight gain because it can be absorbed and metabolized.[53] Sorry, no free lunch, or free cookies, as the case may be.

7. Some Natural Sweeteners Are Better Than Others

To recap: Sugar is poison at the right dose. Don't consume more than 5 teaspoons a day (although even that may be too much for some of us). Most adults consume an average of 22 teaspoons a day, and kids consume up to 35 teaspoons. Artificial sweeteners are no better, and sugar alcohols present their own problems. Now what? Well, there are natural alternatives to refined sugar. But they're not perfect. They have as many calories as refined table sugar, and they, too, reinforce cravings for sweet tastes. However, a few also deliver beneficial substances, like antioxidants. The natural sweeteners with the lowest levels of antioxidants are agave, corn syrup, and brown rice syrup, all of which provide calories but nothing else worthwhile.

Agave nectar, which sounds like it should be good for us, is almost pure fructose, a giant metabolic red flag. Even raw cane sugar has more going for it. On the other hand, date sugar and blackstrap or dark molasses have practically the same levels of antioxidants as a serving of blueberries.[54] That should come as no surprise, since date sugar is just pulverized whole dates. Almost as good: maple syrup and raw honey. When you absolutely need to sweeten something, you should try using one of these. Remember, the biggest problem is not the sugar *you* add to your food; it is the sugar corporations add to your food. One 20-ounce soda contains 16 teaspoons of sugar. You wouldn't put that in your coffee.

SUGAR PRODUCTION IS DAMAGING TO THE ENVIRONMENT

Sugar: The production of sugar, according to the nonprofit World Wide Fund for Nature, has severe consequences for our air, soil, water, and wildlife. One of the biggest concerns is that sugar mills pollute waterways, creating toxic environments for aquatic life. An extensive report from WWF described how waste and processed by-products from sugar mills have been shown to "suffocate freshwater biodiversity, particularly in tropical rivers that are already low in oxygen." In 1995, for example, the cleaning of mills in Bolivia killed millions of fish in local rivers.[55] Additionally, conventional production of sugar cane and sugar beets requires massive amounts of pesticides, including glyphosate, which are hazardous for farmworkers, wildlife, and even consumers.

High-Fructose Corn Syrup: As you might remember from the grains chapter, growing corn depletes soil of its nutrients. Milling and chemically transforming that corn into high-fructose corn syrup is an energy-intensive process. And perhaps even worse, the production of corn requires more fertilizers and insecticides than the production of other crops. The herbicides and pesticides used in corn production pollute waterways, which can create dead zones. If that weren't bad enough, when refining high-fructose corn syrup, chlor-alkali is used—and it contains mercury.

Splenda: According to researchers at the University of North Carolina, our love of Splenda is also bad for our rivers and oceans. When you consume a food or beverage with Splenda, your body absorbs only about 10 percent of the sucralose it contains. The rest is flushed down the toilet and eventually makes its way into the waterways. Sucralose is not regulated by the Environmental Protection Agency, so we have no idea what decades' worth of sucralose buildup in our rivers, lakes, and oceans is doing to fish and other marine life. Currently the EPA lists sucralose as a contaminant of emerging concern. The researchers who study this issue at the University of North Carolina found sucralose in samples of water collected from the Cape

Fear River in North Carolina and even in water samples collected eighty miles off the Carolina coastline![56]

Honey: Commercial beekeeping often involves practices like cutting the wings off queen bees to keep them from leaving their colony. Industrial beekeeping has essentially turned into insect factory farming, with heavy pesticide use and mysterious diseases that pop up and kill massive numbers of bees, threatening the worldwide bee population. A class of pesticides called sublethal neonicotinoids has been proven to be especially harmful to bees. According to research, "Through direct consumption of contaminated nectar and pollen from treated plants, neonicotinoids can affect foraging, learning, and memory in worker bees."[57] It's probably not so good for us either. The honeybees are dying, which spells big trouble for us humans. As you might have heard, we need them in order to survive.

My advice for purchasing ethically produced sugar:

- Choose fair-trade, organic palm sugar and organic maple syrup. You can find some good options on the website of Fair Trade USA here: https://fairtradeusa.org/products-partners/sugar.
- For noncaloric natural sweeteners, use stevia, which is derived from a plant and is generally better for your health and the environment than other options. Look for products with the Rainforest Alliance Certified seal to ensure that your stevia

was grown and harvested on farms that follow sustainable practices. But stevia may have a less-than-beneficial effect on your metabolism. In fact, in a head-to-head study with sugar and artificial, or "natural non-nutritive," sweeteners, there was no difference in total calorie intake and, more important, no difference in the blood-sugar or insulin levels between sugar and stevia and other non-nutritive sweeteners.[58] So, don't think of it as a free food. Read more about the certification seal here: http://www.rainforest-alliance.org/find-certified/stevia-one.

■ If you want honey, take a look at this Ethical Consumer Guide, which shows where to find the best brands: http://www.ethicalconsumer.org/buyersguides/food/honey.aspx.

SUMMING IT UP

There's only one long-term solution to the sugar problem: We all need to wean ourselves off sweetness as much as possible. As long as we keep eating sweets, we'll keep wanting more. Learning to live without them may take some time. It requires cultivating an appreciation for all the other tastes that make food so delicious — the savory, the sour, even the bitter. But it's possible. Having said all that, we need to be realistic. We're always going to love the taste of something sweet. Even animals love it. Just ask any bear gorging on honey and wild blueberries before winter. So, we need to find a reasonable, healthy way forward.

If you have insulin resistance, diabetes, cancer, or an autoimmune disease, then you should stay away from sugar and sweeteners altogether. But for everyone else, if you're cooking at home and your recipe calls for sugar, you should use as little as possible and stick to one of the healthier choices.

One of the most important things to keep in mind is the difference between sugar and added sugar. It's the latter that's the real problem here.

SWEETENERS: WHAT THE HECK SHOULD I EAT?

- Fresh, pureed fruit or fruit juice
- Molasses
- Organic palm sugar
- Date sugar
- Coconut sugar
- Monk fruit
- Organic maple syrup
- Honey (use the Ethical Consumer Guide mentioned previously)
- Stevia, sparingly (only brands certified by the Rainforest Alliance)
- Erythritol, also sparingly, although new data suggests it causes weight gain

SWEETENERS: WHAT THE HECK SHOULD I AVOID?

- Artificial sweeteners of all kinds
- Sugary beverages
- High-fructose corn syrup or any ingredient with the word *syrup* in its name (except for pure organic maple syrup)
- Any foods with sweeteners that purport to be "all natural." The big offenders are agave syrup, corn syrup, sugarcane, evaporated cane juice, and brown rice syrup.
- Packaged foods that contain added sugar or other unnecessary sweeteners, such as yogurt, tomato sauce, bread, ketchup, candy, soups, breakfast cereals, granola, salad dressings, and countless other ultraprocessed foods. If it has a long ingredients list, or additives with the suffix "-ose," that's usually a sign there's sugar hiding in it.
- Refined white sugar
- Brown sugar
- Aspartame, also sold as NutraSweet or Equal
- Sucralose, sold as Splenda
- Saccharin, contained in Sweet'N Low
- Acesulfame potassium, contained in Equal

BEVERAGES

NUTRITION IQ QUIZ

True or False?

1. Fruit juice is healthier than soda because of the antioxidants.
2. After a workout, a sports drink is the best way to restore your electrolytes.
3. Desserts are the main source of added sugar in the American diet.
4. Coffee is the top source of antioxidants for many people.
5. Drinks made with cane sugar are better for you than those made with high-fructose corn syrup.
6. A glass or two of wine a day is good for you.
7. Bottled water is safer than tap.

Answers

1. False: Juice contains all the sugar of fruit with none of the fiber that slows its absorption in your body. You wouldn't eat five apples at once, but you

can easily drink them. Yes, juice contains antioxidants, but you should get them elsewhere — from berries or whole fruits, for instance. Naked Juice and Odwalla drinks have more sugar than a can of Coke or Pepsi. In fact, the companies that make those drinks are owned, respectively, by Pepsi and Coke! Juice boxes are not something you should give your kids.

2. False: Most people don't need to "replenish" electrolytes after a workout. Unless you are playing hard-core sports in hot conditions, neither do you. You can actually buy liquid electrolytes to put in your water, which work better and also contain none of the sugar or dyes. Why do you need a neon-blue sugar-laden sports drink?

3. False: Sugar-sweetened beverages are the main source of added sugar in the American diet. Those who consume the most sweetened drinks have the highest rates of obesity, heart disease, diabetes, and cancer.

4. Unbelievable but true: It's not that coffee is so great, but most Americans eat a processed diet with almost no antioxidants.

5. False: Drinks made with cane sugar have about the same effect on blood sugar and insulin as drinks made with high-fructose corn syrup. But high-fructose corn syrup can also cause leaky gut and may contain mercury, and the free fructose in high-fructose corn syrup is linked to fatty liver.[1]

6. True. But if you are a woman you may increase your risk of breast cancer by 40 percent if you have one drink a day.[2] Alcohol increases your estrogen, which is why men with beer bellies grow breasts and lose their body hair.

7. Depends: Sometimes bottled water *is* tap. But neither is as healthy as filtered water.

Get a new food fact and weekly recipe directly from my kitchen. Sign up for free at www .foodthebook.com.

This ought to be a short and simple chapter, since you need to drink one thing and one thing only to be healthy: plain water. But human ingenuity hates to leave well enough alone. We have a near-infinite selection of new and interesting things to drink. But most of them are not very good for us—in fact, many of them are fueling the diabetes and chronic disease epidemic that's spreading across the planet. I'm talking about drinks containing sugar, artificial sweeteners, alcohol, chemical additives, and other things you should never be chugging. And this doesn't include all the contaminants and other garbage that have turned the one and only thing we *do* need to drink into a health hazard itself. There are good nonwater drinks on the market, but you have to be a smart shopper and read the labels carefully. In this chapter, I'll show you how you can sidestep these problems if you approach your beverages carefully.

THE SCIENCE OF BEVERAGES

As every kid who pays attention in school knows, humans are roughly two-thirds water. It's a part of every tissue, contained inside every cell, and in between. We're constantly losing water, through exhalation, sweat, tears, elimination, and many other physiological functions—and we need to replace it all or suffer dire consequences. It's fairly elementary biology, and yet the things we drink have become the source of a lot of confusion and controversy.

Here's one "expert" view: "In a well-balanced diet we need to drink two liters of liquids a day." Sure, it's hard to argue with that. But he continues, "Soft drinks can be a healthy part of that intake. I would reject any argument that they are in any way harmful."[3] Well, what else would you expect from the chair of the American Beverage Association, the soda industry trade group, in his testimony before Congress? Despite what he says, he's likely aware that sugary drinks cause an estimated 184,000 deaths each year globally—133,000 from diabetes, 45,000 from cardiovascular disease, and 6,450 due to cancer.[4] This is frighteningly like Orwellian doublespeak obscuring the truth.

This reflects the overwhelming problem with beverages today: We keep adding sugar to them. It's as though we think that liquids don't count, and so the harmful things they contain won't really hurt us. But they have the same effect on our health as the things we eat. If anything, the damage they wreak is worse, because at least when we chew and swallow solid food our hunger is sated. Sugary drinks, on the other hand, barely make a dent, which is why it's so easy to chug a 20-ounce bottle of Coke—with its 15 teaspoons of sugar—and still polish off a cheeseburger and fries. That's a whole lot of toxic junk for one meal.

WHAT THE EXPERTS GOT RIGHT

Drink plenty of water? Can't dispute that advice. Don't drink too much alcohol? Right again. But after that, it gets murky.

WHAT THEY GOT WRONG

Here the list grows lengthy. We've all been told that orange juice is nutritious. But now we know it's just a big, cold glass of sugar. Meanwhile, coffee was considered a health hazard, which is not entirely true. We've been sold "sports drinks" that have nothing to do with healthy athleticism and "energy drinks" that have zero to do with energy. But all you really need is water, so long as it's not filled with lead, contaminants, and other impurities. Then there are some drinks that are not necessary but provide a great jolt of powerful plant compounds. We'll get to those in a moment.

EIGHT THINGS YOU NEED TO KNOW ABOUT DRINKS

1. Soda and All Sugar-Sweetened Beverages Are as Bad as You Think

Sales of soft drinks in the United States are practically in free fall—in the United States, soda consumption is now at a 30-year low, and the biggest drop is among diet drinks, meaning that people are even wise to the hazards of no-calorie/artificially sweetened varieties. However, in Latin America and around the world, soda consumption has increased 25 percent. Given all that, do we really need to devote any more space to the argument against drinking this junk? I don't think so. Sugar-sweetened beverages are the single biggest factor contributing to obesity[5] and are also linked to type 2 diabetes,[6] fatty liver,[7] kidney failure[8] and high blood pressure,[9] heart disease,[10] and more. End of story. Full stop. Sugar-sweetened beverages are deadly.

2. Coffee Is neither Poison nor a Panacea

Not so long ago, many health-conscious Americans wondered whether they should stop drinking coffee. Now they ask if they should start.[11] In recent years coffee's reputation has gone from addictive health hazard to powerful potion that provides a long list of surprising benefits. There's evidence to suggest that regularly drinking coffee lowers the risk of heart disease, Alzheimer's disease, colon cancer, cirrhosis of the liver, depression, and even premature death.[12] That is quite a makeover.

It's not exactly clear why this bitter brew is linked to so many health benefits. But we know that coffee, both regular and decaf, contains an abundance of antioxidants — in fact, for many people it's the single largest source of antioxidants in their diets.[13] Coffee contains vitamin C, magnesium, polyphenols, catechins, flavonoids, and chlorogenic acids, to name a few.[14] Antioxidants, however, are its main selling point. Coffee provides around three-quarters of the average person's antioxidant intake, followed in descending order by fruit, tea, wine, cereals, grains, and lastly, vegetables.[15] This doesn't mean coffee is a universal health food—more than anything, it reflects the fact that the average person isn't eating enough broccoli, kale, and blueberries.

The news for coffee isn't entirely positive. It can increase insulin production in people who have type 2 diabetes, so they and anyone with pre-diabetes should probably abstain.[16] Because caffeine is a stimulant, it can also raise cortisol, the stress hormone, and adrenaline, which can lead to adrenal exhaustion.[17] But the way you respond to coffee has a lot to do with your genetics. Some people can have 1 cup and be wired all day. Others can drink 10 cups and still have trouble keeping their eyes open. Coffee can also lead to heart palpitations, and if you're a regular drinker who misses a dose, you may experience withdrawal symptoms like headaches, fatigue, and anxiety. If you're particularly sensitive to coffee's stimulant effects, it's a sign that you need to cut back. You can switch to gentler sources of caffeine, like green or black tea.

Finally, it's important to consider how we define "coffee" today. The old-school definition—meaning, a drink brewed using water and roasted coffee beans—has given way to an infinite number of "coffee drinks." Starbucks and many of its competitors sell milk shakes disguised as coffee: Their drinks are just big cups of milk, sugar, artificial flavors, and whipped cream with some coffee mixed in for a caffeine kick. One Starbucks White Chocolate Mocha has 470 calories—mostly sugar. These chain coffee shops are sugar dispensaries masquerading as coffee shops. Ultimately, coffee isn't a health hazard for most people, but keep in mind that it's never going to be a source of good nutrition or a replacement for the nutrient-dense whole foods you should be eating.

3. The Best Water Doesn't Come in a Bottle

The problem with water is that it's essential for life, and yet nearly everything we do as a society has a negative impact on our supplies, from our industries to our agricultural practices to our transportation systems. Even some of our most mundane, everyday habits—doing laundry, driving to work, cleaning the dishes—can pollute water sources. According to the Environmental Working Group, the EPA has regulations in place to restrict more than ninety water contaminants. Yet we're still drinking arsenic, lead, mercury, and chromium-6, the toxin famously uncovered by Erin Brockovich (but still widespread).[18] You might try to escape harm by switching to bottled water, but that's no guarantee: An EWG analysis found at least thirty-eight contaminants in ten popular bottled water brands. Despite their striking names and the images of majestic springs and mountains on their labels, a lot of bottled water companies get their water from municipal water supplies—not pristine springs and snow-capped mountains. A four-year study by the Natural

Resources Defense Council concluded that there was no assurance that bottled water is any cleaner or safer than tap water. An estimated 25 percent of the brands tested by the NRDC were found to be tap water in a bottle — "sometimes further treated, sometimes not."[19] Plus, bottled water is an environmental disaster — even if you recycle — because plastic is destroying our oceans. And plastic bottles contain phthalates and other harmful plastics including BPA.

If you want clean and untainted drinking water, the only surefire solution is to buy a reverse-osmosis water filter, which puts water through three different stages of filtration, including one that uses carbon. You can pay a couple of hundred bucks for a filter that fits under your sink, or less than a thousand for a whole-house system, which will guarantee that even the water you bathe in and use to brush your teeth isn't delivering poisonous chemicals. It may sound pricey, but if you can afford it, it's a relatively small investment that will pay dividends over your lifetime.

4. Soy Milk Is Not What It Used to Be

Soy milk has been a staple of East Asian cuisine for thousands of years. In its simplest form, it's made by soaking soybeans overnight, then grinding them in water. The beverage was commercially introduced to the United States in the 1970s and quickly gained traction as an alternative for the millions of Americans who cannot tolerate dairy. Soy milk's popularity eventually opened the door to similar "milk" concoctions made from nuts, seeds, beans, and rice. These drinks, in their homemade form, are reasonably nutritious. But it's another story when you pick up a carton of almond or soy milk at the local market and read the label.

In many cases the store-bought versions of these drinks are loaded with sugar and artificial flavoring. Even the organic, unsweetened versions contain weird additives that are there to make nut and rice water look and taste like cows' milk. One of these additives is carrageenan, a thickening agent that's used in ice cream, yogurt, cottage cheese, and other dairy products. It's derived from seaweed, but it's no innocent sea vegetable. It's an irritant that causes cancer in lab rats.[20] In humans, carrageenan has been associated with ulcers, leaky gut, and inflammation.[21] It has no nutritional value, and yet the FDA approves its use in baby formula. But you should avoid it as best as you can, just as you should steer clear of drinks that contain other thickeners, like the gums—xanthan gum, guar gum, locust bean gum— and anything else that sounds like it was made in a lab.

You're not losing much by skipping these mass-produced drinks. In fact, many milk alternatives are so bereft of nutrients that they have to be supplemented with added vitamins and minerals to appear even slightly beneficial. Only soy milk has a meaningful amount of protein. But soy milk comes with its own problems, like a hefty amount of phytoestrogens, which mimic estrogen in the body. Even worse, many varieties of soy milk are made with potent and hyperprocessed soy protein isolates instead of the whole beans. If you want the nutrition contained in almonds, soybeans, hazelnuts, hemp, or cashews, it's better to just eat the whole food.

If you really need something besides water to replace dairy, I recommend a few options. First, try making your own milk substitutes. It's easy—just soak a bag of almonds, hazelnuts, or cashews in a bowl overnight to soften them up, and then blend them with water and a little vanilla extract. Soaking them also unlocks their nutrients, which makes them easier for your body to absorb. But make small batches; the milk could turn rancid if it lingers too long. If you want detailed recipes for almond and other nut milks, you can look them up in my book *Eat Fat, Get Thin.*

Another great option is coconut milk. It's rich and creamy and full of medium-chain triglycerides, a special type of fat that's unique to coconuts. MCTs are superfats that increase your metabolism and fat-burning mechanisms.[22] Studies show that they help with weight loss because your body uses them more efficiently than it does other fats.[23]

One of my favorite times to use coconut milk is at breakfast. I'll throw a bunch of walnuts, pecans, pumpkin seeds, chia seeds, and hemp seeds into a Vitamix blender with some berries, almond butter, and coconut milk and blend it all together. I call it my Fat Shake. It's full of high-quality fats, protein, fiber, and antioxidants. It keeps me feeling energized all morning. You can pick up some coconut milk at your local health food store or supermarket. Just make sure it doesn't have any thickening agents or weird additives. Trader Joe's carries an organic brand that has no additives. You can also make your own coconut milk at home. All you need to do is puree some organic coconut chips in a blender with hot water, and then squeeze the mixture through a piece of cheesecloth to extract the milk. The resulting drink is thick, creamy, and delicious—and much more nutritious than any milk you can find at the store.

5. Juicing May Be Beneficial, Depending on What You Juice

There's been an explosion of interest in juicing lately. From juice bars to cleanses to cold-pressed juices sold in supermarkets, juicing has become a $2-billion-a-year industry—and for good reason. I'm a huge fan of green juices made without sugar, fruit, or other non-plant substances. Many "green juices" with added fruit contain more sugar than a can of soda. If they are pure green juices (added lemon and ginger are fine), they are a great way to include lots of vitamins, minerals, detoxifying nutrients, and cancer-fighting compounds in your diet. But you have to be careful. Fruit juice can get you into trouble. After all, sugar is still sugar, whether it comes from orange juice or orange soda. To get an 8-ounce glass of orange juice, you'd have to squeeze four to five oranges, which would provide about 21 grams of sugar. That's almost as much as you'd find in an equivalent amount of Coca-Cola! Juicing fruit removes its fiber, which, as we saw in the fruit chapter, negatively affects the way your body digests and absorbs its sugar.

But if you juice mostly vegetables instead, you'll get a potent dose of phytochemicals and disease-fighting compounds without all the sugar. I recommend juicing organic veggies like kale, spinach, broccoli, Swiss chard, and celery. Beets, carrots, cucumbers, and radishes are great as well. But you have to limit the beets and carrots—they turn into sugar when you juice them. To really liven up your fresh juice, you should add lemon and a bunch of spices and plants that you might not otherwise eat, such as cilantro, parsley, and gingerroot, which provide a little kick. Use organic produce whenever possible. And if you're going to add fruit, stick with lower-sugar varieties like blueberries, raspberries, and strawberries and avoid the more sugary fruits like grapes and pineapples. A little apple is okay.

It's true that by juicing vegetables you miss out on all the fiber that the plants contain. But keep in mind that fiber isn't the only beneficial part of the veggie. The phytonutrients are important too. I'm not saying you should replace every meal with green juice. But if you can get a cupful of phytonutrients without a bunch of sugar, that's a good thing. And you don't necessarily have to throw all the leftover pulp away. You can use it to make muffins, frozen ice pops, quiches, and even casseroles. Juicing is a good way to be resourceful. If you have a bunch of veggies sitting around that might otherwise go to waste, put them to good use by tossing them in your juicer. The more plants and veggies you consume, the better. One of my favorite juice combinations is kale, apples, cucumbers, celery, lemon, parsley, gingerroot, and daikon radish. It's delicious, refreshing, and full of plant chemicals that boost your body's capacity to heal, rejuvenate, and repair. Even better, blend them into a smoothie and keep the fiber.

6. The Bottom Line on Wine

By now the research on alcohol and its health benefits—while not definitive—is starting to look pretty solid. There's no shortage of large studies showing that people who consume small doses of alcohol, especially wine, are slightly less prone to disease. They also have longer life expectancies than teetotalers (maybe it's because they have more fun). A large meta-analysis published in the *Archives of Internal Medicine* combined thirty-four prospective studies on men and women around the world and found that those who consumed roughly one or two drinks per day lived slightly longer than people who did not drink at all.[24] However, these are correlation studies, so they don't prove cause and effect. But alcohol is a double-edged sword: As the number of drinks you consume surpasses one or two daily, so, too, does your risk of mortality. People who drink the most have shorter life expectancies than those who abstain. In other words, a little bit of alcohol is generally better than none, but beyond that there are no health benefits—only downsides.

The same law of diminishing returns applies to alcohol and chronic diseases. A large meta-analysis published in the *Journal of the American College of Cardiology* found that "light to moderate" alcohol consumption protects against heart attacks.[25] Another study in the *Annals of Oncology* found that light drinking lowers the risk of some forms of cancer in men.[26] But the risk of both heart disease and cancer is higher among people who consume more than roughly one drink a day.

These studies come with the usual caveats about large epidemiological studies. They can't prove cause and effect. There could be other factors at play that protect people who imbibe from time to time. It's possible they consume more nutritious diets or exercise more often. But there is evidence from more rigorous studies that suggest these findings are not a fluke. In a randomized controlled trial published in the *Annals of Internal Medicine*, researchers recruited 224 nondrinking adults with type 2 diabetes.[27] Then they assigned them to have one of three beverages each night with dinner over a two-year period: a small glass of red wine, white wine, or mineral water. The study found that the people in both wine groups had improved blood sugar control, while the group that drank only water did not. But the red wine group did the best. They experienced reductions in their cardiovascular risk factors. Their protective HDL cholesterol increased as a result of the red wine, and their overall cholesterol and lipid profile improved.

Taken as a whole, the research suggests that alcohol

in small amounts can be good for you. That's especially the case for red wine. It contains antioxidants and flavonoids such as resveratrol and quercetin, which improve arterial health, reduce inflammation, and protect mitochondria, the factories in our cells that convert the food we eat and the oxygen we breathe into energy.[28] However, the studies that demonstrated the benefits of resveratrol found that rats had to consume an amount equivalent to what would be in 1,500 bottles of red wine to reap the benefits. Therapeutic doses are available in pill form, but wine isn't really a reliable source of resveratrol. The key—and this cannot be emphasized enough—is moderation. Limit yourself to no more than one glass of wine at night or 1 ounce of hard liquor. A study published in the *American Journal of Clinical Nutrition* found that people who consumed just two alcoholic beverages in one sitting experienced a significant decrease in fat burning two hours later.[29] While wine and hard liquor are okay in small amounts, beer is off-limits. It's loaded with carbs (one can of beer has about the same amount as a slice of white bread) and gluten. Sugary cocktails are also out of the question, and beer alternatives such as hard cider are not any better than beer.[30]

7. Toss Sports and Energy Drinks in the Trash

These are useless modern concoctions, so let's deal with them all at once. "Sports" drinks like Gatorade and its imitators were invented to replenish the sodium and potassium lost under a hot sun. And while it's true that intense exercise in the hot sun can deplete those minerals, athletes certainly don't need to consume the insane, soda-rivaling levels of sugar packed into a bottle of sports drink. Most of us probably don't need to drink anything besides water when we exercise, but if you do work out so intensely that you need fluid replenishment, you can buy electrolytes in powdered or liquid form and add them to plain water for the same result without all the calories. You can also drink coconut water or watermelon water for better, healthier hydration.

"Energy" drinks like Red Bull contain massive amounts of caffeine, sugar, artificial flavors, colorings, stimulants, and a host of other chemicals. They can lead to high blood pressure, cardiac arrhythmia, and even death.[31] The aptly named Monster brand, the leader in this industry, now sells a 20-ounce drink called Mutant—with 72 grams of sugar (almost twice as much as a can of Coke) and 115 milligrams of caffeine (more than coffee) all in one big, lethal beverage. It's a heart attack in a can. Avoid these like the plague.

8. Green Tea Helps You Burn Fat Without Breaking a Sweat

And at last we come to the beverage with a well-deserved halo—a green halo. Green tea contains catechins such as EGCG (epigallocatechin gallate) and flavonoids, which are cancer-fighting phytonutrients and detoxifiers.[32] It helps protect against heart disease, high blood pressure, liver disease, high cholesterol, and inflammation, and it strengthens the immune system.[33] Drinking green tea is also one of the easiest ways to burn fat. That's because it contains an abundance of catechins, which increase thermogenesis (calorie burning) and prevent the damaging effects of free radicals on your metabolism. A study in the *American Journal of Clinical Nutrition* found that people who consumed 690 milligrams of catechins from green tea each day for three months lost more weight and body fat than a control group—and that was without changing what they ate or reducing the amount of food they consumed.[34] Green tea becomes even more beneficial in matcha form—powdered tea leaves that you can mix with water or add to smoothies, which is one of my favorite ways to consume it.

Another great choice is hibiscus, which has been used in Chinese folk medicine to treat high blood pressure and inflammation for centuries. But at the end of the day, you really can't go wrong with any commercially available organic tea—green, white, or black. One caveat is licorice tea. A little is good; a lot causes high blood pressure. According to the National Cancer Institute, herbal teas contain disease-fighting polyphenols that rid our bodies of free radicals and may even prevent cancer.[35]

THE ENVIRONMENTAL IMPACT OF YOUR FAVORITE BEVERAGES

Coffee: In exchange for doing a grueling and often demanding job, many coffee farmers receive as little as 10 percent of the retail price of their product. High demand for coffee has also led to the destruction of rain forests and animal habitats. According to the World Wildlife Fund, more than 2 million acres of forests have been cleared in Central America alone for coffee farming. Additionally, industrial coffee farming requires a massive amount of chemicals and fertilizers that pollute our environment.

Tea: Most tea is grown as a monoculture, which dramatically decreases biodiversity through habitat destruction. According to the Ethical Consumer's guide on tea, "Monocultures provide the perfect environment for pests, resulting in an increased use of toxic pesticides. Pesticides have a lasting effect upon soil quality, as well as devastating impacts on local wildlife and the workers applying the pesticides." The amount of chemicals used on tea plantations is destroying local wildlife, including elephants that are grazing on pastures treated with pesticides.

Orange juice: PepsiCo, the food giant that owns Tropicana, decided to do some research on the carbon footprint of its conventionally produced orange juice. The company discovered that 60 percent of Tropicana's carbon emissions come from fruit growing: irrigation, fertilizers, and pesticides, plus maintaining the orange groves and processing fruits into juice.[36] The remaining 40 percent of emissions come from transportation, packaging, and other aspects of the process. This ties into what we've discovered about conventionally grown, mass-produced *anything*: It uses a lot of natural resources and a massive amount of toxic pesticides. Organic juices are definitely a better choice, but my recommendation is to avoid commercial juices altogether. If the occasion really calls for it, squeeze your own!

Soft drinks: Do we need any more reasons to stop drinking soda? Well, here are a few. The waste from sugar production finds its way into oceans and waterways, killing aquatic life. It contaminates our drinking water, too. About 132 gallons of water are needed to produce 2 liters of soda. In 2009, a Coca-Cola plant in India was accused of overextracting groundwater, leaving local farmers high and dry and prompting many people to protest.[37] The sad fact is that wherever soft drinks become a part of the diet, obesity and environmental destruction follow.

All drinks come with potential social or environmental costs. So how can you drink responsibly?

When it comes to tea, coffee, and juices, my advice is to stick to organic. For tea and coffee, I recommend buying Fair Trade Certified, which ensures that farmers and workers are getting a fair price for their products. You can also look for the Rainforest Alliance Certified logo, which ensures that the coffee farms provide habitats for birds and that they protect their workers.

Here are some useful guides that can also be helpful:

- The Fair Trade USA guide to coffee and tea, which can help you find one of the 500 certified brands in North America: https://fairtradeusa.org/shopping -guide.
- The Ethical Consumer's guide for purchasing the most environmentally friendly teas: http://www .ethicalconsumer.org/buyersguides/drink/tea.aspx.
- The Mother Jones' guide to which liquor and alcohol are best for the planet: www.motherjones.com/ environment/2010/11/carbon-footprint-beer -whiskey-tequila.
- Dry Farm Wines, which is a wine club that delivers only additive-free organic wines: www.dryfarm wines.com.
- Alissa Hamilton's acclaimed book *Squeezed*, which provides an inside look at some of the sordid aspects of the juice industry.
- My website www.foodthebook.com for a list of my top five shake recipes.

BEVERAGES: WHAT THE HECK SHOULD I DRINK?

There's nothing you absolutely need to drink to be healthy other than clean, pure water. But many beverages can be okay if they're not loaded with sugar, stimulants, thickening agents, and other artificial or harmful ingredients.

- Water, as pure as possible — ideally, filtered
- Tea, especially green tea, brewed at home
- Coffee, as long as you don't overdo it
- Wine in moderation (1 glass a day, 5 ounces)
- Spirits in moderation (1 drink a day, 1 ounce)
- Homemade green juices, shakes, and smoothies, as long as you don't include high-sugar fruits
- Coconut water and watermelon water (look for WTRMLN WTR brand), which are low-sugar good choices for sports or rehydration

BEVERAGES: WHAT THE HECK SHOULD I AVOID?

- Bottled water (also because of the harm to the environment of waste plastic)
- Vitamin water or other "enhanced" waters
- Waters containing flavoring, coloring, or sweetening
- Any fruit juice you didn't squeeze yourself (and even then in moderation)
- Any fruit or vegetable smoothie or shake you didn't make yourself (because it's probably loaded with sweeteners and other junk)
- Sugary or artificially sweetened coffee drinks
- Sweetened or flavored iced teas
- Milk
- Beer (gluten plus a ton of calories)
- Did I mention that soda and sugar-sweetened beverages are bad for you?

PART III

WHAT ELSE YOU NEED TO KNOW ABOUT FOOD

Now that we've gone over the main food groups, you should be completely equipped to eat and drink properly and live a long, healthy life, correct? That *would* be true, except eating isn't as simple as that. There are plenty of things we eat that have the power to do us harm, and this is especially true of the substances—everything from pesticides to artificial ingredients—that are in our food supply without our knowledge. Even the containers that hold the things we eat can be bad for us. There's also the question of processed foods to consider—contrary to the current wisdom, they're not *all* toxic, but most are, and we need to distinguish the good from the bad. On the positive side, there are plenty of small touches we can add to our meals that bring more flavor and excitement. Our impulse to improve healthy food to better suit our tastes can be a force for good and healing, as long as we choose our spices, condiments, dressings, and seasonings wisely. In this section, we'll address all those subjects and more, plus how to purge your kitchen of everything unwholesome and replace it all in a way that will support good eating as well as good health.

THINGS TO KEEP OUT OF YOUR FOOD

The list of potentially dangerous substances is long. But these items are easy to steer clear of, once we know what to look for.

Unhealthy Processed Foods

People have been processing food virtually from day one. Until refrigeration, it was the only way we had of preserving perishables to eat later. Cooking is a form of processing. So are curing, drying, smoking, fermenting—the list goes on and on. Whole foods processed using traditional methods and ingredients are *not* something we need to avoid. Some processing actually improves food by making its nutrients more available or potent. We just have to understand which processed foods we can safely eat—we'll go over those later—and which ones *are*, in fact, to be avoided, such as foods with these ingredients:

- Anything with ingredients that are difficult to pronounce. These products surely contain substances that belong in a chemistry set, not in your body.
- Anything that didn't exist in your grandmother's day—maybe even your great-grandmother's day, depending on how old you are.

- Anything containing soybean oil.
- Anything containing high-fructose corn syrup.
- Anything with the word "hydrogenated" in its name.
- Anything advertised on TV. Have you seen a commercial for broccoli or sardines during the Super Bowl? The worst foods get the most airtime on television.
- Anything with a cute name. Froot Loops are not a good source of fruit.
- Anything you can buy at a drive-through window.
- Anything with monosodium glutamate (otherwise known as MSG), even though the FDA says it is safe. It's an excitotoxin—a neurotransmitter that is known to kill brain cells.[1] We associate it with Chinese cuisine but food companies use it in many items without our knowledge. They even try to hide its presence, calling it "hydrolyzed vegetable protein," "vegetable protein," "natural flavorings," and even simply "spices." Spices? Tricky, right? And the worst news—it induces hunger and carb cravings, so you'll eat more of it. It's what they give to lab rats in experiments to fatten them up!
- Any food in an aerosol can.
- Anything called "cheese food" (which is neither *cheese* nor *food*).
- Anything with artificial sweeteners.
- Anything with any type of additives, preservatives, or dyes (of which we eat about 2½ pounds per person per year).

- Any food with more than five ingredients on the label unless they are all things you recognize, such as tomatoes, water, basil, oregano, salt.

Pesticides and Herbicides

Conventionally grown produce is treated with toxic chemicals designed to kill insects and other pests. Should we be surprised to learn that these substances may not be completely harmless where our own health is concerned? There's no question that residues of these chemicals remain on the fruit and vegetables we eat, and then make their way inside our bodies. Once inside, these chemicals have been linked to cancers, Parkinson's disease, autism, and many other ailments. They also hurt us indirectly by contaminating our soil and water. Even nitrogen-based chemical fertilizers damage the environment. We have a dead zone the size of New Jersey in the Gulf of Mexico because fertilizer runoff has led to an overgrowth of algae that monopolizes the water's dissolved oxygen supply.[2]

Organic agriculture offers a safer alternative, but not one that's always easily available (or affordable). If our only choice is nonorganic produce or no produce at all, we should choose the former. But I believe we can do better than that. First, most of us can grow at least some of our food. That's healthy, safe, and economical. Second, we can choose the vegetables and fruit that are proven to have the least amount of pesticide residue. There really is no need to buy *everything* organic. If we buy in-season produce at farmers' markets from small local growers, we probably also wind up eating healthier food. The food stamp program, or SNAP, provides double bucks if you shop at farmers' markets. Finally, we can use the research done by the Environmental Working Group to guide us. Following you'll find their list of forty-nine foods ranked according to their pesticide risk, number one being the most toxic. I would focus on the bottom thirty if you can't afford organic. If you want to eat any of the foods listed in the top twenty, choose organic.

1. Strawberries
2. Apples
3. Nectarines
4. Peaches
5. Celery
6. Grapes
7. Cherries
8. Spinach
9. Tomatoes
10. Sweet bell peppers
11. Cherry tomatoes
12. Cucumbers
13. Imported snap peas
14. Domestic blueberries
15. Potatoes
16. Hot peppers
17. Lettuce

18. Kale/collard greens
19. Imported blueberries
20. Plums
21. Pears
22. Raspberries
23. Carrots
24. Winter squash
25. Tangerines
26. Summer squash
27. Domestic snap peas
28. Green onions
29. Bananas
30. Oranges
31. Watermelon
32. Broccoli
33. Sweet potatoes
34. Mushrooms
35. Cauliflower
36. Cantaloupe
37. Grapefruit
38. Honeydew
39. Eggplant
40. Kiwi
41. Papaya
42. Mangoes
43. Asparagus
44. Onions
45. Frozen sweet peas
46. Cabbage

47. Pineapples
48. Sweet corn
49. Avocados

Additives

How much of what we eat doesn't even qualify as food? More than is good for us. The average American child has consumed 7½ pounds of chemicals by the age of five. There are more than 15,000 chemicals in our food supply. Many don't have to be listed on ingredients labels, and many have never been tested for safety.

It's a scary thought: By the time we're adults, our bodies have been infiltrated by thousands of non-food substances, things never consumed before by human beings. Pounds and pounds of them. Chemical formulations with dubious scientific backing. Newly invented substances that make food easier to process, or that keep it fresher for longer, or that give it a color or taste or consistency that the manufacturer believes we want. Who knows what the long-term effects will be?

The Food and Drug Administration's job is to protect us, but that doesn't always work so well. Scientists began questioning the safety of trans fats a good 50 years before they were declared not safe to eat by the FDA—a half century's worth of damage done to those of us who unknowingly ate them. Even the containers that hold our food pose a danger, because they contain phthalates and bisphenol A (BPA), which we only recently learned are dangerous.

So, what's the solution? Eat food, not food-like substances. It may not always be possible, but you need to be sure to avoid the really bad ones. The roster of food additives allowed by the government is *long*; it reads like a phone book.[3] It's an eye-opener, and for most of us, completely impossible to navigate. Luckily, we have organizations looking out for us.

The Environmental Working Group (EWG) has compiled a detailed report on food additives, including a Dirty Dozen list that calls out those that pose the greatest danger to our health:[4]

1. Nitrates and nitrites (which turn into carcinogenic nitrosamines when heated at high temperatures): Used to color, preserve, and flavor processed meats like bacon, hot dogs, and salami; a "probable" carcinogen according to the World Health Organization.
2. Potassium bromate: Found in bread and other baked goods; linked to various cancers; not allowed in food in Canada, the United Kingdom, or the European Union.
3. Propylparaben: Used in baked goods; believed to be an endocrine disruptor; also may be carcinogenic.
4. Butylated hydroxytoluene (BHT): Used as a preservative in cereal and other foods; caused cancer in animal tests.
5. Butylated hydroxyanisole (BHA): Similar to BHT; listed by California as a carcinogen.

6. Propyl gallate: Used in food with animal fats, like lard and sausage; may be carcinogenic.

7. Theobromine: Used in chocolate, bread, and sports drinks; in animal testing it had possible effects on reproduction and development.

8. Flavorings, natural or artificial: Even when these say "natural," they may be extracted using other chemicals that aren't listed. Any time you see a word like "flavors" or "spices," it's cause for concern. Natural vanilla flavor comes from beavers' anal glands. Look it up if you don't believe me.

9. Artificial colorings: Associated with everything from cancer to hyperactivity in children.

10. Diacetyl: Flavoring, like the "butter" taste in microwave popcorn; has been deemed hazardous for the workers in the factories where it's used.

11. Phosphates: In thousands of foods; linked to risk of cardiovascular disease and osteoporosis.

12. Aluminum additives: Such as sodium aluminum phosphate and sodium aluminum sulfate; used as stabilizers; linked to neurotoxicity.

13. Calcium proprionate: A preservative used in flour that affects your gut flora and produces neurotoxins that cause ADHD and autism.

Another watchdog organization, the Center for Science in the Public Interest (CSPI), also compiles a list of additives, which it categorizes variously as "safe," "cut back," "caution," "certain people should avoid," or "avoid."[5] For the full list, visit https://cspinet.org/eating -healthy/chemical-cuisine. For simplicity, here's their list of what to *avoid*:

- Potassium bromate
- Artificial colorings
- Aspartame (aka NutraSweet)
- Azodicarbonamide (a yoga mat ingredient used in Subway's sandwich bread)
- Brominated vegetable oil (BVO)
- Butylated hydroxyanisole (BHA)
- Caramel coloring
- Mycoprotein (a meat substitute made from fungus, which has reportedly caused extreme allergic reactions in some people)
- Quorn (brand name of foods that use mycoprotein)
- Olestra (Olean)
- Potassium iodate
- Propyl gallate
- Saccharin
- Sodium nitrate
- Sodium nitrite
- Sucralose
- Tertiary butylhydroquinone (TBHQ)
- Artificial sweeteners

There are many more compounds that are concerning. Almost all commercial bread products contain the additive calcium propionate. This has been shown to cause autistic behavior in rats and in kids.[6] It's enough to make you wonder if there's a link between the 133 pounds of flour consumed by each American each year and the rising rate of brain disorders such as ADHD, autism, depression, and more.

Now, not every additive is equally harmful. There's a long list of them rated by the FDA as GRAS—generally recognized as safe: https://www.fda.gov/food/ingredientspackaginglabeling/gras/. But notice the wiggle room in that term. It doesn't state categorically that these substances are harmless. It just means that as of right now the consensus is that they're okay. But that can always change, so why take unnecessary risks? If you don't know whether you should eat something, you probably shouldn't.

Genetically Modified Organisms

There's conflicting evidence on this one. Some scientists say GMOs are safe and a necessity if we're going to feed all the world's inhabitants and protect the environment. But that propaganda may not be true.

When first invented, GMOs held lots of promise—they would produce high yields and be insect resistant, thereby decreasing our dependence on toxic pesticides. It hasn't worked out that way. Twenty years ago, Europe banned GMO foods while the United States went full steam ahead, especially with soybeans and corn. What happened? The yields were not better for GMO crops, and the United States increased its chemical and pesticide use by 21 percent, whereas Europe saw a 65 percent reduction.[7] Putting the safety issues aside, GMO agriculture has simply failed to fulfill its promise.

There has been a nationwide push to require producers to label all foods containing GMOs. Monsanto, the world's largest seed company, and other food corporations fought these efforts, which only reinforced the suspicion that they had something to hide. Nonetheless, the consumers persisted, and the federal government now requires labeling on all genetically modified food. However, as with most federal regulations, there is a lot of gray area. And as we've seen, the food industry is quite good at wiggling out of their legal obligations. It is best to avoid industrial food and eat organic as often as possible. That is better for your health and solves the GMO problem.

Should we be eating GMOs at all? In Europe, they're still banned. That's unlikely to ever happen in the United States. But in my opinion, until the science becomes more definitive, we should avoid genetically modified foods when we can.

Antibiotics

A reported 24 million pounds of antibiotics are used every year in the United States—most of it for farm animals, partly to prevent infections but mainly as a way to fatten livestock and poultry faster. One estimate says that 70 percent of antibiotics given to animals is purely to stimulate growth. By now we know the effects of excessive antibiotics use: It disrupts the microbiome of man and beast, causing inflammation, weight gain, and illness.[8]

Antibiotics also promote the growth of superbugs: dangerous, drug-resistant microbes that make us sick and can even kill us because we can't kill them. They are resistant to all current antibiotics. These germs make their way into produce when animal manure is used as fertilizer.

Nonmedical use of antibiotics should be banned, and only the political power of Big Agriculture prevents this from happening. The FDA merely "recommends" that their use as a growth factor be curtailed, leaving it up to the big animal factory farms to decide whether or not to use them.

So far, the food industry has been lousy at policing itself. So, we need to take matters into our own hands and buy the meat only of animals that haven't been treated with these drugs. Go with grass-fed and organic to guarantee antibiotics-free meat, although some nonorganically grown meat is grown without the use of antibiotics and is labeled that way.

Hormones

Cows and sheep, when treated with estrogens and other growth hormones, grow bigger faster, making them more profitable to the grower. This is why the use of these natural and synthetic substances is so widespread. But is there a downside? Yes.

There's some evidence that consuming the meat of animals treated with hormones is associated with higher levels of IGF-1, a growth factor in humans that's been linked with increased risk of cancer.[9] Steers raised on feedlots have DES pellets placed in their ears to fatten them up. That's the same hormone that caused major birth deformities and cancer when it was given to pregnant women in the 1960s.[10]

Dairy cows are treated with something called recombinant bovine growth hormone (rBGH), which is associated with early-onset puberty in girls as well as increased levels of IGF-1. The FDA currently allows six hormones in the food supply, including estradiol, estriol, testosterone, and progesterone—the sex hormones that can accelerate the age at which puberty occurs. Other contributors to early puberty include our high-sugar diet, caffeine, artificial sweeteners, and "xenoestrogens"—estrogen-like compounds found in plastics and petrochemical pollutants including BPA (bisphenol A).

What do we do? As with antibiotics, injecting animals with hormones does not do us any good, so why take the chance? Better to eat and drink organic and consume food made without hormones and antibiotics. It will serve you well in the long run.

Emulsifiers and Gums

Emulsifiers and thickeners are used to "improve" the texture and consistency of a wide range of processed foods. Look for these to avoid:

- Carrageenan is an additive that is commonly found in long ingredients lists. It's derived from seaweed, which makes it sound healthy. But it's not. It has been linked to colitis and other digestive tract ailments.[11]
- Xanthan gum is also extracted from plant sources, and it is also widely used to thicken packaged foods and beverages. It, too, is associated with digestive problems and may also cause extreme allergic reactions and autoimmune disease.[12]

Both these additives, of course, are approved by the FDA and considered to be safe.

There are many other thickeners that can also cause problems. Take microbial transglutaminase, for instance. It is a form of hidden gluten that is manufactured from bacteria and then put into many processed foods to make them stick together. It doesn't have to be listed on any label. So, as you can see, it is best (yet again) to stay away from processed foods and eat real food as often as possible.

Chemicals in Containers

BPA or Bisphenol A

BPA is used in plastic containers and to line metal cans, theoretically to protect us from aluminum that might otherwise leech into our food. According to the FDA, BPA is safe—or, at least no one has so far proven otherwise.[13] But there is evidence that it may mimic estrogen, meaning it might disrupt our endocrine system and could be linked to infertility and miscarriages. BPA may also increase our output of insulin, the fat storage hormone, promoting obesity and diabetes.[14] It's banned for use in baby bottles in Europe, but it is still in use in water bottles and other containers in the United States.

Phthalates

These are also used to harden plastic containers. Studies have shown that they affect the reproductive system,[15] the brain,[16] and more. Still, they're not banned. But remember trans fats? It took the FDA about five decades to listen to the science and put an end to their use. Avoid phthalates by choosing packaged foods stored in glass containers. Or, better yet, avoid packaged foods altogether.

Phony Fats and Fake Butter

We've discussed these throughout the book, so there's no need to go into detail again. In 2013, the Food and Drug Administration finally acknowledged that hydrogenated and partially hydrogenated trans fats are unsafe for human consumption and ordered them removed from our food by 2018.[17] Thanks, FDA. And even if you "can't believe it's not butter," trust me, your body can.

Refined Oils High in Omega-6 Fatty Acids

Refined oils are deceptive because they come from legitimate plant sources—like corn, soybeans, rapeseed (the source of canola oil), sunflower seeds, and safflower seeds. Still, they're anything but beneficial. Not because they're inherently unhealthy—they're not. The problem is twofold.

First, these oils are all highly processed and refined in high-heat processes that use solvents, deodorizers, and other chemicals, which the government doesn't require manufacturers to list among the ingredients on the label.

Second, they're high in omega-6 fatty acids. As we discussed in the chapter on fats and oils, the standard American diet, rich in processed foods, is also abundant in those omega-6s, which may cause chronic inflammation and all the ills that typically follow. Get your omega-6s from real food such as nuts and seeds.

THINGS YOU CAN ADD TO YOUR DIET

There are plenty of little touches we can add to our food to make it more delicious, and if we choose right they can also make meals more nutritious.

Spices, Herbs, and Other Condiments: The Powerful Medicine in Our Food

Prized for centuries, and the inspiration for trade routes established as far back as 3000 BC, spices and herbs are celebrated not only for their flavors but also for their medicinal powers. Some, like turmeric and ginger, are anti-inflammatory. Others, like oregano, are antibacterial and antifungal. These and many more were eaten daily before the invention of pharmaceuticals. And many are still revered and regularly consumed by people in places where costly drugs are out of reach. In fact, many drugs are derived directly from spices and herbs.

Dried, their potency often increases. Infused in oil and used in cooking, they retain their powers. They're easy to grow at home in tiny spaces, and although we eat just a little, herbs and spices pack a big nutritional punch. Most of us don't use nearly enough of them.

Because I love using spices and herbs when I cook, my pantry is always filled with my favorites. Here's a partial list of the ones we should keep handy in the kitchen, ready for every meal:

- Basil: good for the heart, antioxidant, antibacterial
- Black pepper: helps the absorption of nutrients
- Cayenne and all hot peppers: boosts metabolism, increases circulation
- Cinnamon: improves circulation, antimicrobial

- Cloves: protection from environmental toxins, anticancer properties
- Coriander and cilantro (the leaves of the coriander plant): lowers blood sugar, good for detoxification
- Cumin: helps immune system, anticancer
- Ginger: helps digestion, anti-inflammatory
- Oregano: antimicrobial, antioxidant
- Parsley: promotes good breath, contains antioxidants and antitumor agents
- Rosemary: stimulates immune system, improves digestion
- Sage: good for the brain, anti-inflammatory, antioxidant
- Thyme: good for lung function, antioxidant, antibacterial
- Turmeric: good for the heart, anti-inflammatory, anticancer properties

Salt

Salt is an extremely important part of history. It's prominent in the Bible. It's the root of the word "salary" and the origin of the saying that something is "not worth its weight in salt." Once, it was a rare, highly prized substance. Today it's everywhere. That's where the problem begins.

Salt, or sodium, as we all know, has been linked to hypertension, the precursor to death due to heart disease and stroke, but only in a subset of people who are genetically salt-sensitive. Sodium is important for overall health, but our sodium levels needs to be in proportion to our levels of other important minerals—mainly potassium. When the ratio of sodium to potassium in our bodies gets out of whack, high blood pressure follows. So, we need optimal amounts of both to stay healthy. The best source of potassium is whole, unprocessed, plant-based foods like cooked spinach, broccoli, squash, avocados, papayas, and bananas (though we shouldn't overeat the latter two).

If you're diagnosed with high blood pressure and hypertension, you'll be instructed to eliminate sodium from your diet as much as possible. But this isn't great advice. In fact, patients with heart failure who ate a salt-restricted diet were 85 percent more likely to die or be hospitalized than patients who didn't limit their salt intake.[18] There are some people with high blood pressure who *are* salt-sensitive. But even then, the research doesn't show much benefit to restricting salt. The trick, as we've seen time and time again, is to avoid the refined salts ubiquitous in processed foods. We'll get to that in a minute, but first let's talk about sodium in general.

Sodium is naturally found in whole foods, and, as with any other food or mineral, it's best in its purest form. Look for these foods that are rich in natural sodium to get your recommended daily allowance of about 2,300 milligrams:

- Meat
- Beets

- Carrots
- Celery
- Chard
- Seaweed
- Beans

When it comes to seasoning, be sure to choose unrefined varieties of salt. I prefer Himalayan pink salt, which is as beautiful as it sounds, as well as kosher and sea salt in moderation. We can safely add these to our food, as long as our diet is also rich in potassium. And here's a tip: If you use all the amazing, potent spices and herbs we just discussed, you really won't need to add much salt to make your meals taste great. Also, if you add salt to your dishes after you've finished cooking them, flavor-wise you'll get more bang for your buck.

Now, none of this means you can eat as much salty food as you want. You absolutely *can* be harmed by too much sodium. Although we have an unfairly negative view of salt as bad, emerging science has disproven the "salt is bad for you" mantra. The highly refined salt that food manufacturers add to processed and packaged foods is killing us. Again, it is not the salt you add to your food, but the salt added by food corporations. Refined salt has been stripped of any beneficial trace minerals (found in sea salt or other forms of salt such as Himalayan salt) and is there purely to mask the unpleasant tastes of the processed food and nasty ingredients. You should also watch for refined salt that's been "iodized," or supplemented with iodine. Iodized salt was introduced in the mid-1920s to supplement iodine-poor diets that were causing goiters. But today, if you are eating enough real food that is rich in iodine—like fish, shellfish, and seaweed—then you really don't need to get iodine from salt. Not enough iodine can cause thyroid dysfunction, but so can too much. So, I recommend staying away from iodized salt when possible. Morton's iodized salt also contains sugar in the form of dextrose.

So, as is often the case, the first thing we need to do is stop eating so much processed food that's high in sodium. Go through the supermarket shelves and look for it on the labels—it's everywhere, including many places it doesn't need to be. And use salt in its most natural form. It's that simple. If you want to learn more about how we have unfairly maligned salt and its health benefits, read *The Salt Fix* by James DiNicolantonio.

Condiments, Dressings, Vinegars, and Sauces

There are literally thousands of items that fall into this category, and if you read the ingredients you'll see that most brands contain ingredients we should be avoiding—unhealthy oils, added sugars, additives, preservatives, and weird chemicals with long names that are added to flavor or color or thicken. But condiments are meant to enhance our favorite foods. We should be able to use them freely—just be sure to use the right ones.

- Salad dressing: It's nutritionally crazy, not to mention a waste of money, to buy premade dressing when you can do so much better at home. Most store-bought dressings are full of high-fructose corn syrup, corn thickeners, and refined oils, even many of the "healthy" ones. Try this instead: Add some of the best, tastiest extra virgin olive oil you can find, ideally organic, to a jar. (I know, good olive oil is expensive, but you're worth it, aren't you?) Mix in oil from another healthy source, like walnuts or avocado, if you like the taste. Add vinegar of any kind—balsamic if you want, or wine vinegar, rice vinegar for an Asian kick, or apple cider vinegar. Next, add a little mustard, some dried or fresh herbs and spices, and a little salt and pepper. Shake it up and you're done. Now you've got a dressing that's delicious on salads and vegetables. Don't be afraid of the oil, which helps you absorb the fat-soluble vitamins in your food. If you want to make it even healthier, add a little raw garlic (½ or 1 clove) and liquefy it all in the blender. Some people also add tahini, the paste from ground sesame seeds, for a creamier dressing.
- Ketchup: Buy organic, with as little sugar as possible. And no high-fructose corn syrup.

- Mustard: It's healthy, as long as it contains just mustard seed, water, vinegar, and spices; stay away from those that contain soybean oil and additives.

- Mayo: Fine as long as it's made the traditional way, with eggs and oil, and ideally not with nonorganic canola or soybean oil. You can find it made with olive or avocado oil—my favorite kind.

- Vinegars: Take your pick—apple cider, wine, balsamic, rice—they are all delicious and add a pleasant zing to a dish.

- Fish sauce: Again, as long as you can pronounce all of the ingredients, this is a great addition to your condiments inventory for Asian cooking.

- Soy sauce and tamari: Look for brands that are brewed in the traditional way, with no sulfites, coloring, sweeteners, or, ideally, gluten.

- Worcestershire: Usually contains some form of sugar, vinegar, anchovies, and other ingredients for flavor. Any other weird stuff has no place in it.

- Chili sauce and hot spice sauces: Again, make sure there are no added chemicals such as sulfites, which can cause allergic reactions and make you feel bad. Otherwise, these make a great addition to your homemade sauces.

- Miso: Help yourself. It's a healthy fermented food you can use in soup or salad dressing. And there are many gluten-free options.

- Tahini: You can make it at home, or buy it as long as there are no extra ingredients—just ground hulled sesame seeds. It's healthy and delicious, and you can mix it with miso, rice wine vinegar, tamari, and a little water to make a great sauce for salmon or veggies.

- Barbecue sauce: Make your own. It's easy, cheap, and the only way to avoid the excess sugar and additives contained in commercial varieties.
- Cocktail sauce: Ditto—if you've got ketchup, lemon juice, and horseradish, you've got a delicious sauce for your shrimp!

You can find great versions of all these condiments at Thrive Market online (www.thrivemarket.com/foodbook), usually at 25 to 50 percent off the retail prices you would find at Whole Foods or other upscale health food stores.

Healthy Processed Foods

As we've said before, there are many unhealthy processed things to eat out there, but there are also examples made with whole food and using traditional methods. These are the ones we can safely enjoy.

- Tofu, as long as it's organic and, if you can find it, made from sprouted soybeans. Be careful with tofu that's been smoked, baked, or otherwise processed. Sometimes, a lot of sodium and flavorings are added to tofu.
- Tempeh, if it's organic.

- Yogurt, as long as there's no sugar, fruit, or flavoring added. You can make your own additions if necessary once you get it home. Be sure it's made from organic, whole (full-fat), grass-fed milk, or better yet goats' or sheep's milk if you have trouble digesting cows' milk. They are healthier options for you.

- Kefir, as long as you follow the same rules as yogurt.

- Cheese, which we've been eating since before recorded history, is made from milk, bacteria, rennet, and salt. Sometimes herbs, spices, and even fruit may be added. But that's it — any variety that contains anything that doesn't sound like food should be avoided. American cheese cannot legally be called cheese because it is mostly a "cheese-like substance" containing very little actual cheese. They are typically called American "slices" or "singles." I encourage you to stick to organic sheep's or goats' cheese.

- Chocolate, as long as it's organic and dark (not milk), at least 70 percent cacao. In moderation, naturally.

- Kimchi, a Korean spicy cabbage condiment, is a great source of probiotics due to natural fermentation.

- Sauerkraut, as long as it was fermented naturally, meaning without the use of vinegar.

- Jerky made of meat, poultry, or fish, as long as there's no sugar or other weird and unnecessary ingredients or preservatives. Watch out for gluten and MSG.

- Hummus is a great food if it's organic and chemical-free. It's easy to make at home in a food processor by combining chickpeas, tahini, cumin, olive oil, garlic, and lemon.
- Nut butters, as long as there's no sugar or palm oil added. Nuts contain a lot of fat, so there's no need to add any more. Most peanut butter contains high-fructose corn syrup and emulsifiers. Read ingredients lists, not just the nutrition facts.

GOOD HEALTH STARTS IN THE KITCHEN

It's no coincidence that as the percentage of meals Americans prepare and eat at home has dwindled, our rates of obesity and type 2 diabetes have skyrocketed. In 1900, 2 percent of all meals were eaten away from home; now it is 50 percent. But we can completely overhaul our lives as eaters by performing a kitchen purge and restocking. Cooking is the best thing you can do for your health and your budget, and it's fun! It begins with a very large trash bag (or, even better, a recycling bin). We'll spend the first half hour finding and throwing away the bad stuff that's damaging us every day. Then we'll head over to the supermarket to replace it all with foods that will restore our good health.

Toss These

- Sugar in all its forms (except a little honey or maple syrup)
- Artificial sweeteners
- All-purpose, refined white flour
- Any packaged food made with high-fructose corn syrup
- Anything with sugar among the first five ingredients on the label (ingredients must be listed in order of prominence in the food)
- Anything with ingredients that don't sound like food (Maltodextrin, anyone?)
- Anything made with refined white flour, including pasta, bread, bagels, pretzels, muffins, and so on
- Anything made with soybean oil, vegetable oil, or hydrogenated oils
- Soft drinks or any sugar-sweetened beverages including energy drinks, sports drinks, sweetened teas or coffees, and so on
- Anything made from refined grains, like hot cereal (even unsweetened), instant or microwavable oatmeal, or anything else not made with whole grains
- Powdered flavored drinks
- Breakfast cereals, sweetened or not
- Any food with MSG
- Any food with soy-based protein
- Anything deep-fried like potato chips or other kinds (baked vegetable chips are fine)

- Anything that includes preservatives, flavorings, colorings, or thickeners
- Any butter or fat replacements
- Any yogurt containing sugars or fake sweeteners
- Any frozen dish containing non-food ingredients (check the list on page 375)
- Anything white — rice, bread, potatoes (except onions, cauliflower, daikon radish, or white fish)
- Skim milk or any non-grass-fed or nonorganic dairy

Keep or Purchase These

- Canned wild-caught salmon, mackerel, sardines, and anchovies
- Nuts (almonds, Brazil nuts, walnuts, pecans, macadamias, cashews, pine nuts, hazelnuts; all raw and unsalted)
- Nut butters (no added sugar, salt, or oil)
- Extra virgin olive oil
- Virgin organic coconut oil
- Seeds (pumpkin, ground flax, hemp, and chia seeds)
- Vinegar (balsamic, apple cider, wine, rice)
- Unsulfured molasses or raw honey
- Whole grains (quinoa, millet, teff, amaranth, black rice, brown rice)
- Beans (smaller beans such as lentil, adzuki, and navy beans)
- Green tea or hibiscus tea
- Herbs and spices
- Healthy condiments (see the list on page 396)

Perishables

- Fresh, organic, seasonal, nonstarchy vegetables
- Fresh, starchy vegetables such as sweet potatoes and winter squash
- Fresh, organic, seasonal, low-glycemic fruit
- Fresh or frozen organic or wild berries
- Grass-fed beef and lamb
- Pasture-raised pork and poultry
- Pasture-raised eggs
- Wild-caught salmon, mackerel, and others from the low-mercury list, which is in the chapter "Fish and Seafood."
- Any kind of shellfish (keep lobster to a minimum because of high mercury levels)
- Grass-fed butter or ghee
- Whole-milk, grass-fed, unsweetened, organic yogurt or kefir, ideally goats' or sheep's
- Whole-milk cheese made from grass-fed animal milks without preservatives or chemicals

IS FOOD ENOUGH, OR DO WE REQUIRE MORE?

Do we really need to take nutritional supplements? No, not as long as we follow a traditional hunter-gatherer lifestyle, eating only wild plants, game, and fish; live where the air, water, and soil are pure and untouched by pollution; get lots of physical exercise and direct sunlight; sleep soundly nine hours a night;

and stay untroubled by the stresses and anxieties of modern living. If that describes your life, feel free to skip this section.

Up to 90 percent of Americans aren't getting enough of the nutrients that are critical for healthy functioning.[19] We're functionally deficient in vitamins, minerals, micronutrients, and fatty acids. We don't suffer noticeably in the short term from scurvy or rickets. But these insufficiencies damage us decades down the line. We get too little folic acid today and suffer cancer in the future. Or we get too little vitamin D and wind up with osteoporosis someday. These are called long-latency deficiency diseases. You won't get rickets, but you can get cancer and die early and will be more susceptible to infections, depression, fatigue, and muscle weakness if you are insufficient in vitamin D for a long time.[20]

The vegetables and fruits we eat may look healthy, but they have been compromised. Thanks to modern agricultural practices, the soil where they grow has been depleted of nutrients, so strong chemical fertilizers are used instead of the gentler natural kind. Pesticides and herbicides take their toll on the entire ecosystem, us included. Plus, in order for produce to reach us and still be edible, it must be harvested prematurely, before the nutrients have had a chance to fully develop. Then it's shipped long distances and stored in warehouses, further diminishing its benefits. The average apple you buy at a supermarket is stored for about a year. Organic is better because it has no agricultural chemicals, is more nutrient-dense, and contains more phytonutrients. But even organic produce is picked early, shipped long distances, and stored for ages. Try organic broccoli from the store, then grow some and eat it right out of the garden. You will taste the difference immediately. So, if you can't get all the nutrients you need from your produce, how can you get them?

This brings us back to the importance of supplementation. Most people I talk to are confused about supplements. Even doctors, nutritionists, and other health experts are uncertain of how to advise their patients. Why? Because there's so much conflicting information out there. One day we're told that extra vitamin E is necessary; the next, we hear that too much may cause cancer. We're informed that taking folate is healthy; before long, the headlines say it's harmful. We all need to take a multivitamin; no, now we all need to stop. First we're told that supplements are an important part of a healthy lifestyle; then we read that we're wasting our money on worthless junk that may not even contain what it says on the label. Or our doctors tell us that vitamins are just excreted, so all we really get from them is expensive urine. Your body uses what it needs and gets rid of the rest (except for fat-soluble vitamins such as A, D, E, and K).

Let's start with a little background. Every one of the thousands upon thousands of chemical reactions that take place inside our bodies every second is made possible by the work of enzymes and coenzymes. Nearly all coenzymes are vitamins and minerals. Magnesium and zinc, for example, are each responsible for activating more than 200 enzymes. Folic acid is critical for creating neurotransmitters, regulating our DNA, and determining which of our genes are turned on and off. That plays a crucial role in preventing (or allowing) cancer, heart disease, and dementia. Most of us don't eat enough leafy greens and other vegetables to maintain proper levels of these nutrients. That's why we need to supplement.

Because so many of us work indoors all day, more than 80 percent of the US population has insufficient levels of vitamin D, which our bodies synthesize from sunlight. Another reason to take supplements. Omega-3 fatty acids are critical for supporting brain function and mood, regulating metabolism, and preventing diabetes and inflammation. The modern diet, rich in processed oils and fats, doesn't include enough omega-3s from healthy sources like fish and nuts. Most of us need more than our food delivers.

A final piece of advice: Be very picky about which brands of supplements you take. The federal government doesn't evaluate or regulate them the way it does prescription drugs or food, even though many supplements are as potent as any medicine. As a result, the nutritional supplement industry is as lawless as the Wild West. Dosages may not match what's on the label. The capsules may be filled with additives, colorings, flavorings, or allergens. The supplement's formulation may not be optimized for absorption by your body. There have even been instances where capsules contained virtually none of the contents advertised. So, how can you know you're getting pure, properly manufactured supplements? Do some research about the brands before you buy, and take the advice of experts you trust.

Supplements are a healing cornerstone of my practice, so I have investigated manufacturers, toured factories, and studied independent analyses of their products. I have learned that there are a few companies I can rely on. You can learn more about these companies in our online resource section at www .foodthebook.com/resources.

Now we are going to put everything we've learned into practice. In Part IV, we will talk about how to use a combination of supplementation and food as medicine to heal your body and achieve overall well-being.

PART IV

THE PEGAN DIET AND HOW TO EAT FOR LIFE

By now, we've discussed pretty much everything there is to eat and drink. It's time to put all that knowledge to work. You may be ready to plunge right in with a healthy nutritional plan. But chances are you may have some dietary damage you need to undo. All those years, or even decades, of eating poorly definitely take their toll. If you've become a sugar junkie, you'll have to get that monkey off your back. Same if you're hooked on grain-based carbs, which are sugar in disguise. If you've been eating things that promote inflammation, you need to give your body a break and allow it to reset. Everybody is different, and so we each need to discover what we as individuals can tolerate and what does us harm. That's the first part of the plan—the detox. After that comes the regimen you can adopt for the rest of your life—what I call the Pegan Diet, a sensible, inclusive way of eating that integrates all the current science while poking fun at the extremes of vegan and Paleo diets. Once I explain the details, I'll provide you with meal plans and recipes—everything you'll need to bring yourself and your family to optimal health.

BEFORE THE DIET, THE DETOX

Until the twentieth century, the chronic ailments that beset us today—cancer, heart disease, diabetes, Alzheimer's, autoimmune diseases, allergies, and digestive diseases—were uncommon. Environmental toxins, lack of physical activity, and chronic stress have all played a part in their rise, but the most important factor has been diet. I realize this isn't exactly news. And yet we go on eating refined and processed foods that contain sugars, starchy carbs, unhealthy fats, and chemical additives. It turns out that food is medicine. What you put on your fork is truly more powerful than anything you will find in a prescription bottle. It works faster, is cheaper, and has only good side effects, including tastiness. Most people know that eating healthy is good for them. But most don't understand the scope of food's medicinal power when it comes to preventing, treating, and even reversing disease.

Eating a highly processed diet low in nutrients will always catch up to you in some way or another. It might make you sluggish. It might make you feel groggy. It can give you irritable bowel syndrome, acne, autoimmune disorders, or worse. This is when therapeutic diets can help.

In 2014, I published *The Blood Sugar Solution 10-Day Detox Diet* to address the epidemic of sugar addiction, obesity, and diabetes in the United States and all over the world. The goal of the 10-Day Detox is to reverse processed food and sugar addictions, which come from years of eating industrial-made, drug-like foods that hook our taste buds with every bite, hijack our brain chemistry and metabolism, and give rise to everything from heart disease to cancer, dementia, diabetes, depression, and much more. Although I created the 10-Day Detox with the intention of helping people who are overweight, sugar addicted, diabetic, or suffering with autoimmune disease or chronic disease, it turned out to be a great plan for nearly anyone who wanted to reboot their biology and see how good they can feel. In our study of the program, our subjects saw a 62 percent reduction in all symptoms from all diseases in that group in just ten days! There is no drug on the planet that can do that.

We could all use a reboot once in a while. I revisit the 10-Day Detox whenever I return from a long period of traveling or even when I've just had a particularly exhausting few months at work. Therapeutic diets like the 10-Day Detox are the building blocks for optimal health. The idea of a detox might sound extreme or trendy, but when done correctly, detoxing can be a powerful way to balance your blood sugar and hormones as well as prevent insulin spikes that are a result of eating a diet filled with processed sugars and carbohydrates. Unfortunately, many of these foods (breads, rice, potatoes, pasta) have become daily staples in the American diet. Again, it's not your fault if you are having trouble breaking away from these foods. You're not weak-willed. These foods are biologically addictive, and using willpower to drop pounds and feel good again rarely works. The good news is that there is something that does work—the 10-Day Detox Diet. This program is an important tool that you can use to reclaim your health and break away from cravings for these highly addictive and damaging foods.

You're not meant to stay on this program forever. Rather, it is designed to reset your body so that you can develop healthy eating habits for life. Not everyone needs to do a therapeutic diet, but if you're feeling sluggish, are addicted to sugar, or have brain fog, skin challenges, or chronic health issues, or if you have FLC Syndrome (that's when you Feel Like Crap), it's important to reset your body.

If this program feels like a big shift from your normal diet, I highly recommend transitioning slowly to give your body time to adjust to this new way of eating. To read more about easing your way into the 10-Day Detox Diet and how to manage detox symptoms, please visit food thebook.com/resources.

Let me break down the 10-Day Detox Diet in three easy steps that anyone can start today.

1. ELIMINATE SUGAR, PROCESSED FOOD, AND POTENTIALLY INFLAMMATORY OR TOXIC FOODS FOR 10 DAYS.

The first step is to eliminate the junk. It's simple. First, you stop eating certain addictive and inflammatory foods for ten days, and then, after ten days, you'll have the opportunity to add some of these foods back in to see how your body responds. I'll talk about how to reintroduce foods in "The Pegan Diet" chapter, but the first step is to remove the following items from your diet for ten days.

Avoid These Foods

Carbs	Gluten, all grains
	Legumes, beans
	All fruit (with the exception of berries, kiwi, lemon, lime, pomegranate seeds, watermelon)
Animal foods/ proteins	Processed meats: bacon, canned meat, hot dogs, salami, etc.
	High-mercury fish: king mackerel, tuna, swordfish, Chilean sea bass, halibut, lobster, marlin, shark, tilefish, orange roughy (avoid these for the long term)

Fats	Dairy products (except for grass-fed ghee or clarified butter, which has no dairy proteins)
	All refined vegetable oils: canola, corn, safflower, soy, sunflower, etc.
Condiments	Additives, preservatives, dyes, MSG (avoid these for the long term)
	Artificial sweeteners: Splenda, Equal, aspartame, sorbitol, xylitol and all sugar alcohols (avoid these for the long term); some stevia may be okay, but it's not a free food—the science is still coming in
	Natural sweeteners: honey, maple syrup, raw sugar, etc. (avoid these for the short term)
Drinks	Soda, diet soda, milk, fruit juices, sports drinks, energy drinks, alcohol, caffeinated beverages

2. FOCUS ON EATING REAL, WHOLE FOODS FOR TEN DAYS.

Eliminating inflammatory and toxic foods is just part of the 10-Day Detox. The other part involves adding in the good stuff—real, whole foods that nourish your body with every single bite. Like I said before, we all know that food can harm us, but we should all take advantage of the fact that food can heal us, too. For ten days focus on eating the following foods.

Eat These Foods

Carbs (raw, steamed, roasted, or sautéed; approximately 50 to 75 percent of your plate should be made up of nonstarchy veggies) (½ to 1 cup of starchy veggies up to 4 times a week at dinner: beets, celeriac, parsnips, pumpkin, sweet potatoes, winter squash [butternut, kabocha, acorn, etc.]) (4 oz of low glycemic fruit per day: blackberries, blueberries, raspberries)	Artichokes, arugula, asparagus, avocados, bean sprouts (not alfalfa sprouts, which contain natural carcinogens), beet greens, bell peppers, broccoli, Brussels sprouts, cabbage, carrots (no juicing because it turns them into pure sugar), cauliflower, celery, chives, collard greens, dandelion greens, eggplant, endive, fennel, fresh herbs, garlic, ginger, green beans, hearts of palm, jalapeños, kale, lettuce, mushrooms, mustard greens, onions, radicchio, radishes, seaweeds (kelp, wakame, arame, kombu, etc.), shallots, snap peas, snow peas, spinach, summer squash, Swiss chard, tomatoes, turnip greens, watercress, zucchini
Animal foods/ proteins (aim for 4 to 6 ounces of protein per meal)	Bison, beef, elk, lamb, ostrich, venison Pasture-raised eggs, chicken, duck, turkey Lard, tallow, duck and goose fat (free-range, pasture-raised) Non-GMO tempeh and tofu

	Fresh or canned fatty fish: black cod, herring, mackerel, perch, sardines, scallops, wild salmon, anchovies
	Shellfish: clams, crab, mussels, oysters, scallops, shrimp
	Get organic or grass-fed animal protein whenever possible
Fats (aim for 3 to 5 servings of healthy fats a day)	Nuts: hazelnuts, macadamia nuts, pecans, walnuts, almonds, cashews (except for peanuts and sunflower seeds, which may contain mold toxins); seeds: chia, flax, sesame, black sesame, hemp seeds, pumpkin seeds; and nut butters
	Nut flours: almond and coconut flour
	Nut and seed milks: macadamia, almond, Brazil, cashew, coconut, hemp (avoid ones with carrageenan and xanthan gums)
	Avocados, olives, ghee, coconut butter
	Oils (extra virgin and cold-pressed): avocado, coconut, macadamia nut, MCT, olive, walnut, sesame
Condiments	Apple cider vinegar, arrowroot, balsamic vinegar, black peppercorn, coconut flour, Dijon mustard, kelp noodles, kimchi, miso, nutritional yeast, organic vegetable and chicken stock, sea salt, spirulina, tahini, ume plum vinegar, unsweetened vanilla and chocolate (cacao) powder, wheat-free

	tamari, dried or fresh herbs and spices such as basil, cayenne pepper, chili powder, cinnamon, coriander, cardamom, ginger, cumin, onion powder, oregano, paprika, parsley, rosemary, sage, thyme, turmeric
Drinks	Water, hot lemon water, sparkling water with lemon or lime, green tea, homemade green juice (no fruit), herbal teas, bone broth

3. TAKE SUPPLEMENTS TO SUPPORT YOUR HEALTH.

Supplements can be a powerful way to get your body the nutrients it needs. I recommend taking supplements on the 10-Day Detox to support your body while it goes through this deep reset. To learn more about these supplements and purchase them in a ready-made kit, visit foodthebook.com/resources.

Take These Supplements

Supplement	Benefits	Dosage (Per Day)
High-quality multivitamin	The right multivitamin will contain all of the basic vitamins and minerals.	Take as directed on the label
Purified fish oil (EPA/DHA)	Omega-3 fats are crucial for healthy	1 to 2 grams

	cardiovascular, nervous system, and immune function; they also bolster insulin sensitivity and support healthy blood sugar balance.	
Vitamin D_3	Known for its role in healthy immune function and skeletal support, vitamin D_3 also supports healthy metabolism by influencing many genes involved in blood sugar balance and insulin sensitivity.	1,000 IU to 2,000 IU Some may need more. You need 1,000 IU to raise your vitamin D level by 10 ng/dl. Ideally your levels should be at least 50 ng/dl to 60 ng/dl.
Magnesium glycinate	Magnesium is known to support health in a number of ways since it impacts the function of more than 300 enzymes. It is known to improve metabolic function, blood sugar levels, and insulin sensitivity, and it helps with sleep and constipation.	200 to 300 mg
Chromium*	Chromium supports lipid and glucose metabolism and is	500 to 1,000 mcg

	important for fat metabolism, enzyme activation, and glucose support. It promotes healthy lipid and carbohydrate utilization.	
Alpha-lipoic acid*	Alpha-lipoic acid may be useful in supporting healthy nerve function in those with diabetes and pre-diabetes. It is also a powerful antioxidant and mitochondrial booster.	300 to 600 mg
Cinnamon*	Cinnamon is helpful in controlling blood sugar and improving insulin sensitivity.	500 to 1,000 mg
Green tea catechins*	Catechins support insulin sensitivity, healthy fat burning, and metabolism.	100 to 200 mg
Zinc*	Zinc plays a crucial role in immunity and absorption of B vitamins, among other benefits.	15 to 30 mg

* Chromium, alpha-lipoic acid, cinnamon, and green tea catechins are usually found combined in special blood sugar–balancing supplements; check your local health food store or go to www.foodthebook.com/resources to purchase the 10-Day Detox Kit.

That's it. Follow these three steps for ten days. After ten days, you have the option of staying on the 10-Day Detox if you want to lose more weight or address abnormal cholesterol, high blood pressure, pre-diabetes, or type 2 diabetes, or you can transition to the Pegan Diet.

In the next chapter, we'll talk about how to reintroduce foods after the 10-Day Detox Diet and how to transition to the Pegan Diet. To learn more about my recommendations for following the 10-Day Detox Diet and transitioning off the program, I highly recommend reading *The Blood Sugar Solution 10-Day Detox Diet*. For all of this information and my top lifestyle recommendations to enhance the 10-Day Detox Diet, visit www.foodthebook.com/resources.

After you reset your body, you can move on to a healthy way of eating *for life* or you can transition to the Pegan Diet.

ENHANCING YOUR DETOX EXPERIENCE

A well-designed detox plan starts with food, but food isn't the only mechanism that can enhance detoxification. Sleep, relaxation, and movement are also powerful ways to support the detox process and create better health.

There are plenty of tools I keep in my detox tool box, but the three most important for you to use during your program are the following:

- **Actively relax.** No, I don't mean sitting on the couch watching Netflix. I mean meditating, deep breathing, yoga, journaling, or spending quality time with friends and family.
- **Move your body.** There are so many benefits to gain from exercising. I recommend moving every single day. You don't have to work out at the gym. Find something that works for you, like bike riding, hiking, dance, or sports.
- **Prioritize sleep.** Inadequate sleep, especially while detoxing, can sabotage your efforts at getting healthy. Make time for at least eight hours of sleep every night. My biggest tip for getting better sleep is to avoid your phone and TV for an hour before bed. Stretching, meditation, journaling, or talking to a loved one are ways to actively relax and get ready for a good night's sleep.

Sometimes my patients require a special dietary program and you might too. I've put together several e-books for individuals who have specific dietary needs. We have e-books on pregnancy, thyroid, autoimmune conditions, irritable bowel and leaky gut, and more, available here: www.foodthebook.com/resources.

THE PEGAN DIET

The choice of nutritional philosophies is endless these days: We can go vegan; vegetarian; ketogenic; Paleo; flexitarian; pescatarian; Mediterranean; high-fat low-carb; high-carb, low-fat; raw; and on and on. Trying to find the best one can be overwhelming. I've spent many years studying nutrition and even I have trouble sometimes sifting through all the conflicting science and opinions. For years I tried different diets. I was a vegetarian. Then I went Paleo. But eventually, I got fed up. It seems like the world of nutrition is being divided into armed camps, each proclaiming its superiority and decrying the fatal flaws in all the others. The obvious fact is that they all have advantages and disadvantages.

The vegan diet, for example, ideally incorporates plenty of whole, plant-based foods. As a result, vegans get lots of vitamins, minerals, antioxidants, fiber, and healthy fats with none of the baggage that comes with feedlot meat. They're also making the world a more humane place for the creatures that are treated cruelly by industrial farms, along with reducing their carbon footprint. But even a perfect vegan diet won't provide enough DHA and EPA, which are important omega-3 fatty acids. Neither will it provide enough iron, zinc, copper, or vitamin D. Vegans are also unlikely to be getting the amount of quality proteins and essential amino acids they require, especially as they age. It's possible to find sufficient amounts in non-animal sources, but it is incredibly challenging. But they're definitely not getting B_{12} because it only comes from animal foods. Finally, it's entirely possible to be a vegan and still eat a poor diet filled with sugar, refined grains and flour, highly processed oils, soy-based protein substitutes, and foods loaded with chemicals and additives. You can live on Oreos, potato chips, and root beer and still call yourself a strict vegan. Even if you were to swear off wheat and gluten, a common staple in many vegan diets, the food industry is booming with "gluten-free" food items that trick us with misleading health claims on the label. Just because the gluten has been removed from something doesn't mean it's healthy; often, it means the exact opposite. If you eat a gluten-free brownie full of gluten-free refined flours and tons of sugar, you're still wreaking havoc on your blood sugar and weight.

In the last six years, the Paleo diet has become the most popular diet among health and wellness advocates. As we all know by now, this regimen is based on the idea that our bodies do best when fueled by foods that existed in the Paleolithic era, before agriculture came along

10,000 or so years ago. That means no sugars (except maybe honey and those occurring naturally in fruit), no grains, no dairy, no legumes or beans, and only nonindustrial meat, fish, whole nonstarchy vegetables, some starchy root vegetables and winter squashes, fruit (but not too much), nuts, and seeds. And that's about it. As extreme as that may sound, it can be a healthy, low-glycemic diet, especially at a time when so many people are in ill health from eating grain-based sugary foods made with overly processed fats and oils. In fact, emerging research is using this approach, and a more aggressive approach called a ketogenic diet (very-low-carbo hydrate, high-fat diet), to reverse type 2 diabetes (www .virtahealth.com).[1]

However, some use the Paleo philosophy as an excuse to eat too much meat and too few plant-based foods. As critics point out, there were many diets in the Paleo era, depending on what part of the world we're talking about. Back then, humans foraged for their food, mostly plants, and ate animals only when they could find, catch, and kill them. Meat wasn't nearly as abundant as it is now. Meanwhile, our prehistoric ancestors had a huge amount of healthy plant fiber in their diets (100 to 150 grams a day vs. 8 to 15 grams a day, which is the modern average). Our healthy plant fiber intake doesn't come anywhere close.

I've tried both of these diets (vegan and Paleo) and plenty of others, but I always wind up finding my way back to a happy medium. A few years ago I was on a panel with two other doctors; one was a Paleo advocate and the other a strict vegan cardiologist. I was sitting in the middle, and to lighten things up I joked, "Well, if you're Paleo and you're vegan, then I must be a Pegan."

All joking aside, the best versions of both diets are built on the same foundation: Eat real, whole food. Vegan and Paleo diets focus on foods that don't raise our blood sugar, plenty of fresh vegetables and fruits, healthy protein and fats, and no crap. I synthesized the best aspects of each and integrated them with the anti-inflammatory and detoxification principles of functional medicine to create a balanced, inclusive dietary plan that changed my life and my patients' lives, too. Now thousands of people all over the world are following the Pegan Diet.

This is not a quick fix that you follow for ten or thirty days and then quit. After you reset your body, I recommend eating this way *every single day*. It is inclusive, not exclusive, and based on sound nutritional science and working with patients for more than 30 years.

Let's look at the thirteen pillars of the Pegan Diet:

1. **Stay away from sugar.** That means a diet low in anything that causes a spike in our insulin production—sugar, flour, and refined carbohydrates. Think of sugar in all its various forms as an occasional treat, that is, something we eat occasionally and sparingly. I tell people to think

of it as a recreational drug. You use it for fun occasionally, but it is not a dietary staple.

2. **Eat mostly plants.** As we learned earlier, more than half your plate should be covered with veggies. The deeper the color, the better. The more variety, the healthier. Stick with mostly non-starchy veggies. Winter squashes and sweet potatoes are fine in moderation (½ cup a day). Not a ton of potatoes! French fries don't count even though they are the number one vegetable in America.

3. **Easy on fruits.** This is where there could be a little bit of confusion. Some Paleo champions recommend eating mostly low-sugar fruits like berries, while some vegan advocates recommend all fruit equally. I find that most of my patients feel better when they stick to low-glycemic fruits and enjoy the others as a treat. Stick with berries, kiwis, and watermelon, and watch the grapes, melons, and so on. Think of dried fruit as candy and keep it to a minimum.

4. **Stay away from pesticides, antibiotics, hormones, and GMO foods.** Also, no chemicals, additives, preservatives, dyes, artificial sweeteners, or other junk ingredients. If you don't have that ingredient in your kitchen for cooking, you shouldn't eat it. Polysorbate 60, red dye 40, and sodium stearoyl lactylate (also known as Twinkie ingredients), anyone?

5. **Eat foods containing healthy fats.** I'm talking about omega-3 fatty acids and other good fats like those we find in nuts, seeds, olive oil, and avocados. And yes, we can even eat saturated fat from fish, whole eggs, and grass-fed or sustainably raised meat, grass-fed butter or ghee, and organic virgin coconut oil or coconut butter.

6. **Stay away from most vegetable, nut, and seed oils,** such as canola, sunflower, corn, grapeseed, and especially soybean oil, which now accounts for about 10 percent of our calories. Small amounts of expeller or cold-pressed nut and seed oils like sesame, macadamia, and walnut oils are fine to use as condiments or for flavoring. Avocado oil is great for higher-temperature cooking.

7. **Avoid or limit dairy.** As we learned in earlier chapters, dairy doesn't work for most people, so I recommend avoiding it, except for the occasional yogurt, kefir, grass-fed butter, ghee, and even cheese if it doesn't cause any problems for you. Try goat or sheep products instead of cow dairy. And always go organic and grass-fed.

8. **Think of meat and animal products as condiments** or, as I like to call them, "condi-meat" — not a main course. Vegetables should take center stage, and meat should be the side dish. Servings should be 4 to 6 ounces, tops, per meal. I often make three or four vegetable side dishes.

9. **Eat sustainably raised or harvested low-mercury fish.** If you are eating fish, you should choose low-mercury and low-toxin varieties such as sardines, herring, anchovies, and wild-caught salmon (all of which have high omega-3 and low mercury levels). And they should be sustainably harvested or farmed. Check out www.cleanfish.com and www.foodthe book.com to learn more about your fish options.

10. **Avoid gluten.** Most gluten comes from Franken-wheat, so look for heirloom varieties of wheat like einkorn. Eat wheat only if you are not gluten-sensitive, and even then, only occasionally. Dr. Alessio Fasano of Harvard, the world's top gluten expert, has done research showing that gluten damages the gut—even in nongluten-sensitive people who show no symptoms.[2]

11. **Eat gluten-free whole grains sparingly.** They still raise blood sugar and can trigger autoimmunity. All grains can increase your blood sugar. Stick with small portions (½ cup per meal) of low-glycemic grains like black rice, quinoa, teff, buckwheat, or amaranth. For type 2 diabetics and those with auto-immune disease or digestive disorders, a grain- and bean-free diet may be key to treating and even revers-ing your illness. Stick to the 10-Day Detox Diet or even a ketogenic diet for diabetes.

12. **Eat beans only once in a while.** Lentils are best. Stay away from big starchy beans. Beans can be a

great source of fiber, protein, and minerals. But they cause digestive problems for some, and the lectins and phytates they contain may impair mineral absorption.[3] If you are diabetic, a high-bean diet can trigger spikes in your blood sugar. Again, moderate amounts (up to 1 cup a day) are okay.

13. **Get tested to personalize your approach.** What works for one person may not work for another. This is called bio-individuality and it is why I recommend that everyone eventually work with a functionally trained nutritionist to personalize their diet even further with the right tests. If you're interested in getting tested and coached by one of my nutritionists, visit www.foodthebook.com/diet for more information.

THE TWO-STEP TRANSITION TO THE PEGAN DIET

1. Follow the 10-Day Detox plan (see the previous chapter, "Before the Diet, the Detox") while slowly adding one new food group to your diet every three days, such as gluten-free grains, beans, or any other food that you'd like to experiment with, like goats' or sheep's cheese or the occasional treat. I highly recommend sticking to one new food group at a time. Here's an example: After your

detox, try eating gluten (i.e., pasta, bread) on Days 11, 12, and 13. Notice how your body responds. On Day 14, take a break and stick with approved foods from the 10-Day Detox. On Days 15, 16, and 17, try eating dairy. Notice how your body responds. Then on Day 18, go back on the 10-Day Detox approved foods. Repeat this method. This might seem tedious, but I truly feel that this is the best way to understand what works for you and what doesn't. You might discover that certain foods just don't work for you, and that's okay. If something bothers your gut, makes you foggy, achy, or congested, you might have an intolerance, sensitivity, or allergy to it. And now you know to avoid it. Eat a plethora of plant foods in addition to healthy fats and good-quality proteins. Use this combination as the basis for your meals (plant foods plus healthy fats plus protein). Then, when the occasion calls for it, you can incorporate your favorite pleasure foods. That does not mean a can of Coke and a Twinkie! They still have to be real foods that follow the Pegan principles.

2. Take the Pegan Diet supplements to support daily detoxification, reduce inflammation, and support mitochondrial function and cardiovascular health. These include CoQ10, resveratrol, milk thistle, curcumin, glutathione, lipoic acid, magnesium, and a special form of folate.

DAILY SUPPLEMENTS FOR THE PEGAN DIET

Supplement	Benefits	Dosage (per day)
High-quality multivitamin	The right multivitamin will contain all of the basic vitamins and minerals.	Continue to take as directed on label
High-quality purified fish oil (EPA/DHA)	Supports healthy cardiovascular, nervous system, and immune function; bolsters insulin sensitivity and supports healthy blood sugar balance	Continue to take 2 grams
Vitamin D_3	Supports the immune system	Continue to take 1,000 IU to 2,000 IU (total)
Magnesium glycinate	Supports healthy metabolism, blood sugar, and insulin sensitivity	Continue to take 100 to 200 mg
Chromium	Supports healthy metabolism	Continue to take 200 mcg to 500 mcg
Alpha-lipoic acid	Boosts mitochondria and cellular energy production	Continue to take 300 to 600 mg

Supplement	Benefits	Dosage (per day)
CoQ10	Provides energy for cardiovascular health and cellular energy production	25 to 50 mg
Resveratrol	Provides antioxidant and cardiovascular support	50 to 100 mg
Milk thistle	Provides liver support	50 to 100 mg
Curcumin	Supports healthy liver, colon, musculoskeletal, and cell function and is a powerful anti-inflammatory	100 to 200 mg
Glutathione	Helps protect and support cellular function and detoxification	25 to 50 mg
Folate or methyl folate	Supports DNA synthesis and repair, as well as heart and brain health	400 to 800 mcg

Many of these can be found in special combination formulas. Check with your local health food store or visit foodthebook.com/resources, where you can find my maintenance kit, which includes all of the daily supplements.

PEGAN DIET — A WAY OF LIFE

Many of us are used to thinking about diets as something we do short term without much enjoyment, but I designed the Pegan Diet not to be something we go "on" and "off" of. As I mentioned in the intro, the Pegan Diet is not a *diet*, but rather a way of life. Remember the goal is not to be perfect, but rather to have simple guiding principles that can continue to keep us healthy for years to come. The Pegan Diet is a philosophy and approach to health. It's about doing your best and letting go of food stress and anxiety.

My highest hope is that his book and the principles in it give you a sense of food peace and confidence when it comes to your overall health and wellness. Remember, true health isn't just about losing a few pounds or about the absence of chronic disease; it's about feeling good, showing up, and giving your highest gifts to the world.

MEAL PLAN AND RECIPES

I hope that by the time you start the Pegan Diet, you'll have equipped your kitchen with tons of beautiful produce and healthy ingredients. But I don't want to leave you without ways to prepare all those delicious foods. With the help of my friend Chef Frank Giglio, I've created a 7-Day Pegan Meal Plan inspired by some of my favorite dishes. You don't have to follow this meal plan exactly. Sometimes I like to double a recipe so I can have leftovers for lunch the next day. You can also interchange any breakfast, lunch, or dinner from one day to another. The key is to explore, experiment, enjoy. Eating well doesn't necessarily mean spending hours cooking. Sometimes I just throw a quick salad together. But other days, I love to spend time in the kitchen making delicious and intricate recipes. I encourage you to play in the kitchen and find what works for you.

Some recipes are labeled *10D*, which means they are compatible with both the 10-Day Detox Diet and the Pegan Diet. The rest of the recipes are designed to be enjoyed on the Pegan Diet.

If you need additional support for creating the right personalized meal plan, consider working with one of my trained functional medicine nutritionists. You can learn more about our nutritional coaching at www .foodthebook.com/diet.

A 7-DAY PEGAN MEAL PLAN

Day 1

Breakfast: Scrambled Eggs with Tomatoes, Herbs, and Goat Cheese   439

Lunch: Kale Salad with "Bacon" Vinaigrette *10D*   449

Dinner: Beef Curry *10D*   460

Dessert: Warm Spiced Apple Slices   483

Day 2

Breakfast: Savory Buckwheat Porridge   440

Lunch: Mediterranean Steamed Mussels *10D*   450

Dinner: Braised Chicken with Fennel and Endive *10D*   462

Dessert: Blueberry Soft Serve   484

BREAKFAST

SCRAMBLED EGGS WITH TOMATOES, HERBS, AND GOAT CHEESE

This makes an amazing breakfast or quick lunch that is most enjoyable when tomatoes are fresh and in season. It's incredibly versatile, protein-packed, and easy on your digestive system. And it's always a hit with kids!

Serves: 4   Prep time: 5 minutes   Cook time: 5 minutes

- 8 large eggs
- ½ teaspoon sea salt
- ¼ teaspoon freshly ground black pepper
- 2 tablespoons filtered water
- 1 tablespoon clarified butter or ghee
- 1 small tomato, roughly chopped
- 2 ounces soft goat cheese
- ¼ cup fresh herbs (chives, thyme, parsley, dill, oregano), roughly chopped

In a large bowl, whisk together the eggs, salt, pepper, and water.

In a large nonstick skillet, warm the butter over medium heat until shimmering. Add the egg mixture and stir with a wooden spoon until the eggs form soft curds, about 3 minutes.

Fold in the tomatoes and remove the pan from the stove. Gently fold in the goat cheese and herbs, divide among four serving plates, and serve immediately.

Nutritional analysis per serving: calories 250, fat 10 g, saturated fat 15 g, cholesterol 359 mg, fiber 0.3 g, protein 16 g, carbohydrate 2 g, sodium 480 mg

SAVORY BUCKWHEAT PORRIDGE

A yummy alternative to oatmeal, this porridge has a delicious nutty flavor and a slightly crunchy texture. You can easily make it sweeter by adding some honey or maple syrup, but this savory version is definitely something you'll want to try!

Serves: 4   Prep time: 5 minutes, plus overnight soaking time   Cook time: 15 minutes

- ¾ cup buckwheat groats
- 1 tablespoon apple cider vinegar
- 2½ cups bone broth or filtered water
- ¼ cup unsalted grass-fed butter
- ½ teaspoon sea salt
- ¼ teaspoon freshly ground black pepper
- 1 large sprig fresh thyme, stem removed, leaves chopped (about 1 teaspoon)

To prep the buckwheat groats, place them in a large bowl with 2½ cups of filtered water and the apple cider vinegar. Cover the bowl and let it sit at room temperature for 8 to 12 hours (or overnight), then drain and rinse well.

Place the soaked buckwheat in a 2-quart saucepan and add the bone broth. Cover the pan and turn the heat to medium-high. Bring the liquid to a simmer, then lower the heat to medium and continue to cook while stirring occasionally until the buckwheat is soft, 10 to 12 minutes.

Once the buckwheat is tender, finish by stirring in the butter, salt, pepper, and thyme. Divide between two serving bowls and enjoy. If you want, top each serving with a fried egg.

Leftover porridge can be stored in the refrigerator for 2 to 3 days. Patties can be formed with the leftovers and pan-fried in ghee or coconut oil until browned and warmed throughout.

Nutritional analysis per serving: calories 276, fat 13 g, saturated fat 8 g, cholesterol 30 mg, fiber 4 g, protein 11 g, carbohydrate 32 g, sodium 430 mg

ZUCCHINI–SWISS CHARD HASH AND FRIED EGGS

10D

Hashes are quick, easy, and endlessly adjustable. This one is potato-free but still amazingly good. The perfect way to make a meal right from the garden!

Serves: 2   Prep time: 15 minutes   Cook time: 20 minutes
- 2 tablespoons extra virgin olive oil
- 1 small onion, finely diced
- 1 large zucchini, diced into ½-inch cubes
- 1 large red bell pepper, stemmed, seeded, and diced into ½-inch pieces
- 3 to 4 large Swiss chard leaves, stems removed, cut into small pieces
- 2 tablespoons filtered water
- ½ teaspoon sea salt
- ¼ teaspoon freshly ground black pepper
- 4 large eggs

In a large sauté pan, heat 1 tablespoon of the olive oil over medium-high heat. When the oil is shimmering, add the onion and zucchini, and toss gently to combine them. After 5 minutes, add the red pepper. Stir to combine and cook for an additional 3 to 4 minutes.

Add the Swiss chard and water. Cover the pan immediately and allow the ingredients to steam for 1 to 2 minutes. Turn off the heat, remove the cover and sprinkle with the salt and pepper.

While the hash rests, warm the remaining 1 tablespoon olive oil over medium heat in an 8-inch skillet. Carefully crack the eggs into the pan and cook until the egg whites are fully set but the yolks are still runny, 3 to 4 minutes. (For over-easy eggs, use a spatula to gently flip each egg and cook for 1 additional minute.)

Divide the hash between two serving plates and top with two eggs. Serve immediately.

Nutritional analysis per serving: calories 160, fat 12 g, saturated fat 2 g, cholesterol 146 mg, fiber 2 g, protein 8 g, carbohydrate 8 g, sodium 382 mg

Pesto Frittata

10D

You won't even miss the cheese in this dairy-free version of traditional pesto. Eggs and pesto are a perfect match, and you can enjoy this dish warm or cold. Feel free to adjust the garlic and nutritional yeast content to your taste.

Serves: 4   Prep time: 15 minutes   Cook time: 30 minutes
- 1 cup packed basil leaves
- ¼ cup pine nuts
- 2 garlic cloves
- 2 tablespoons nutritional yeast
- 1 teaspoon sea salt
- ¼ cup plus 1 teaspoon extra virgin olive oil
- ¼ teaspoon freshly ground black pepper
- 6 large eggs
- ½ cup unsweetened almond milk

Preheat the oven to 350°F.

Combine the basil, pine nuts, and garlic in a food processor. Pulse until the mixture is finely chopped, 4 or 5 pulses. Scrape down the sides of the bowl, and then add the nutritional yeast, black pepper, and ½ teaspoon of the sea salt and begin processing. Drizzle ¼ cup of the olive oil slowly into the processor until well incorporated, about 30 seconds.

In a medium bowl, whisk together the eggs, almond milk, and the remaining ½ teaspoon sea salt. Stir in the pesto, reserving 2 tablespoons for garnish, and whisk to combine. Brush an 8-inch seasoned cast-iron pan with the remaining 1 teaspoon olive oil, pour in the egg-pesto mixture, and place in the oven.

Bake until fully set, about 20 minutes. Carefully remove the pan from the oven and spread the reserved pesto over the top. Cut into four wedges and serve.

Refrigerate any leftovers in an airtight container for 3 to 4 days.

Nutritional analysis per serving: calories 273, fat 26 g, saturated fat 4 g, cholesterol 246 mg, fiber 1 g, protein 11 g, carbohydrate 3 g, sodium 583 mg

GRASS-FED BEEF BREAKFAST PATTIES

10D

Flavorful and packed with iron, a mineral we often don't get enough of, these patties are the perfect way to start your morning. They couldn't be easier to make, and they're great any time of day, especially since the crumbled-up leftovers make a great taco or frittata filling!

Serves: 4   Prep time: 10 minutes   Cook time: 5 minutes
- 1 pound grass-fed beef
- 2 teaspoons onion powder
- 2 teaspoons dried sage
- 1 teaspoon ground fennel seed
- 1 teaspoon garlic powder
- pinch of sea salt
- ½ teaspoon freshly ground black pepper
- 1 tablespoon extra virgin olive oil

Place the beef in a bowl and add in the seasonings. Mix thoroughly and then divide evenly into 8 portions.

Flatten the portions into thin patties.

To cook, heat the olive oil in a medium sauté pan over medium-high heat. Add the patties and cook for 2 to 3 minutes. Carefully flip the patties and cook for an additional 1 to 2 minutes. Serve alongside fried, poached, or scrambled eggs.

Store the meat, cooked or uncooked, in an airtight container in the refrigerator and use within 3 to 4 days.

Nutritional analysis per serving: calories 186, fat 9.5 g, saturated fat 3.5 g, cholesterol 70 mg, fiber 0.1 g, protein 24 g, carbohydrate 1.5 g, sodium 365 mg

RICH AND CREAMY BLUEBERRY SMOOTHIE

Adult- and kid-friendly, this is a yummy way to get greens into your daily routine disguised as a sweet treat! Don't be afraid of the saturated fat in the coconut milk. It's the best possible fuel for your body, especially when combined with the protein from the almond butter.

Serves: 2   Prep time: 5 minutes
- 1 (12.5-ounce) can (or homemade) full-fat unsweetened coconut milk
- ½ cup frozen blueberries
- optional: 2 Medjool dates, pitted
- 1 heaping tablespoon almond butter
- ½ teaspoon alcohol-free, gluten-free pure vanilla extract
- 2 cups baby spinach
- 2 large ice cubes

Place all the ingredients into a blender and blend on high speed until smooth and creamy, about 45 seconds. Drink immediately.

Nutritional analysis per serving with dates: calories 421, fat 36 g, saturated fat 27 g, cholesterol 0 mg, fiber 4 g, protein 6 g, carbohydrate 21 g, sodium 81 mg

TROPICAL CHIA PORRIDGE WITH KIWI AND COCONUT

This breakfast bowl will really start your day off right. Protein and saturated fat keep your brain focused, energy levels high, and blood sugar stable. No energy crashes after this breakfast of champions!

Serves: 2   Prep time: 10 minutes, plus 30 minutes to 12 hours chilling time

- 2½ cups unsweetened almond milk
- ½ cup chia seeds
- optional: 2 tablespoons maple syrup
- 1 teaspoon alcohol-free, gluten-free pure vanilla extract
- ½ teaspoon ground cardamom
- 3 ripe kiwis, peeled and diced into small pieces
- 1 tablespoon unsweetened large coconut flakes
- 2 tablespoons full-fat unsweetened coconut milk

Combine the almond milk, chia seeds, maple syrup (if using), vanilla, and cardamom in a quart-size mason jar. Cover tightly and shake well to incorporate all the ingredients.

Place the jar in the refrigerator for at least 30 minutes and up to 12 hours, to allow the mixture to thicken as the chia seeds soak up the liquid.

When ready to serve, divide the chia mixture between two serving bowls and top with kiwi and coconut flakes. Drizzle the coconut milk over the top and serve.

Leftover porridge can be stored in an airtight glass container in the refrigerator for up to 3 days.

Nutritional analysis per serving: calories 254, fat 12 g, saturated fat 5 g, cholesterol 0 mg, fiber 0.3 g, protein 5 g, carbohydrate 37 g, sodium 233 mg

LUNCH

KALE SALAD WITH "BACON" VINAIGRETTE

10D

This antioxidant-rich combination is the perfect mix of crunchy, salty, and just a hint of sweetness to balance out the fresh greens. You'll make this again and again and feel amazing when it's part of your weekly routine.

Serves: 4   Prep time: 15 minutes   Cook time: 20 minutes
- 2 tablespoons plus 2 teaspoons extra virgin olive oil
- 4 strips turkey or regular bacon
- 2 tablespoons apple cider vinegar
- 2 teaspoons Dijon mustard
- ¼ teaspoon freshly ground black pepper
- 2 portobello mushrooms, stems discarded, caps thinly sliced
- 2 bunches kale, stems discarded, leaves torn into bite-size pieces
- ½ teaspoon sea salt
- 1 large ripe avocado, pitted and cut into small chunks

In a large skillet, heat 2 teaspoons of the olive oil over medium heat, and brown the turkey bacon until crisp, 4 to 5 minutes, then set aside on a paper towel to drain.

Pour the rendered fat into a small bowl and whisk in the vinegar, mustard, and pepper.

Clean the skillet and place it back on the stove over medium-high heat. Add the remaining 2 tablespoons olive oil. When it is shimmering, add the sliced portobellos. Cook for 5 to 6 minutes, stirring often, until the mushrooms are soft.

Meanwhile, place the kale in a large serving bowl and sprinkle it with sea salt. Using your hands, massage the kale until it begins to "wilt," about 2 minutes.

Once the mushrooms are cooked through, add them to the kale along with the dressing, and mix to incorporate. Crumble the bacon over the greens and top with the avocado.

Leftover salad can be stored in an airtight container in the refrigerator for up to 1 day.

Nutritional analysis per serving: calories 276, fat 24 g, saturated fat 18 g, cholesterol 45 mg, fiber 4 g, protein 12 g, carbohydrate 8 g, sodium 542 mg

MEDITERRANEAN STEAMED MUSSELS

10D

Mussels are one of the tastiest foods from the sea, and this salty, spicy blend of flavors only emphasizes how sweet and satisfying they are. A great source of protein, these are absolutely perfect as an appetizer or as a larger meal-size serving.

Serves: 2   Prep time: 10 minutes   Cook time: 10 minutes
- 4 large garlic cloves
- 2 tablespoons capers
- 4 anchovies
- 1 small dried red chile
- ½ teaspoon sea salt
- 1 tablespoon extra virgin olive oil
- 2 cups low-sodium chicken stock
- 3 pounds mussels, rinsed well, beards removed
- ¼ cup parsley leaves, roughly chopped
- zest of 1 lemon

Combine the garlic, capers, anchovies, red chile, and sea salt on a cutting board and chop until they become a paste. You can also use a mortar and pestle if you have one.

In a 5- or 6-quart Dutch oven, warm the olive oil over medium-high heat. Add the prepared garlic paste and cook for about 2 minutes, stirring often. Pour in the chicken stock and bring to a boil. Carefully add the mussels.

Place the lid on the pot and steam the mussels until all have opened up, 4 to 5 minutes. Divide the mussels between two bowls, then pour ¾ to 1 cup of broth over them and serve. Add the parsley and lemon zest and toss.

Nutritional analysis per serving: calories 370, fat 13 g, saturated fat 2 g, cholesterol 112 mg, fiber 0.2 g, protein 47 g, carbohydrate 14 g, sodium 1,298 mg

GRILLED SHRIMP SALAD

10D

Light and elegant, this salad is a snap once the grill is warm. It makes a wonderful appetizer for any summer meal and is super-low-carb.

Serves: 4   Prep time: 20 minutes   Cook time: 15 minutes
- ¼ cup plus 1 tablespoon extra virgin olive oil
- 1 pound large shrimp, peeled and deveined
- 2 teaspoons sea salt
- 1 large tomato, roughly chopped
- 2 tablespoons prepared horseradish
- 3 tablespoons lemon juice
- 2 tablespoons filtered water
- 2 hearts of romaine, quartered lengthwise
- 1 small red onion, thinly sliced into rings

Prepare a grill pan or an outdoor gas grill with 1 tablespoon of the olive oil. Season the shrimp with 1 teaspoon of the sea salt and place them on the hot grill. Cook the shrimp for 2 to 3 minutes per side, until fully cooked.

To make the vinaigrette, place the tomato, horse-radish, lemon juice, remaining 1 teaspoon salt, water, and remaining ¼ cup olive oil into a blender. Blend on high and puree until smooth.

To serve, place 2 quarters of the romaine on each plate. Sprinkle with the red onion and then top with 4 to 5 shrimp each. Drizzle the salad with the vinaigrette and serve.

Nutritional analysis per serving: calories 220, fat 13 g, saturated fat 2 g, cholesterol 162 mg, fiber 1 g, protein 22 g, carbohydrate 7 g, sodium 169 mg

SMOKY EGG SALAD

The chipotle adds an incredible smoky flavor to this versatile dish. It's perfect on its own, as a sandwich filling, or as a topping for crackers and vegetables. Kids love it! Feel free to adjust the spice level for them as needed.

Serves: 4   Prep time: 15 minutes   Cook time: 15 minutes (plus cooling time)
- 6 eggs
- 1 celery stalk, finely diced
- 1 large carrot, peeled and finely diced
- 1 small onion, finely diced
- 1 cup mayonnaise
- 1 tablespoon lemon juice

- 1 teaspoon paprika
- ½ teaspoon chipotle powder
- ½ teaspoon sea salt
- ¼ teaspoon freshly ground black pepper
- 6 ounces baby arugula

Place the eggs in a large saucepan and cover with filtered water by about 1 inch. Bring to a boil over high heat and cook for 1 minute. Immediately remove the pan from the heat, cover, and let stand for 5 minutes. Meanwhile, fill a large bowl with ice water.

Pour off the water in the pan, then carefully transfer the eggs to the ice water. Let stand until completely cooled, then remove the eggs and wipe them dry. Carefully crack and peel the eggs and place them in a medium bowl. Using a fork, mash the eggs, leaving them a bit chunky. Add the celery, carrot, and onion.

In a small bowl, combine the mayonnaise, lemon juice, and seasonings. Stir to combine well, then fold the mayonnaise into the egg and vegetable mixture.

To serve, divide the arugula among four plates. Top each plate of greens with a quarter of the egg salad.

The egg salad is best stored in an airtight container in the refrigerator and consumed within 3 to 4 days.

Nutritional analysis per serving: calories 339, fat 26 g, saturated fat 5 g, cholesterol 261 mg, fiber 1 g, protein 9 g, carbohydrate 18 g, sodium 527 mg

Grass-Fed Beef Chili

10D

Yum. Who doesn't love chili? This protein-rich version has a unique flavor you may not have tasted before. With garbanzo beans and a cilantro topping, it is extra-delicious. You'll definitely be making this over and over!

Serves: 4   Prep time: 20 minutes   Cook time: 1½ hours
- 2 tablespoons extra virgin olive oil
- 1 pound grass-fed ground beef
- 1 large yellow onion, finely chopped
- 2 large green bell peppers, stemmed, seeded, and finely chopped
- 3 tablespoons chili powder
- 1 tablespoon paprika
- 2 teaspoons ground cumin
- 2 teaspoons dried oregano
- 2 teaspoons dried thyme
- 1 teaspoon ground mustard
- ½ teaspoon chipotle powder
- 2 garlic cloves, finely chopped
- 1 (15-ounce) can garbanzo beans, drained and rinsed
- 1 (28-ounce) can crushed tomatoes
- 4 cups filtered water
- 2 teaspoons sea salt
- 1 cup loosely packed cilantro leaves, roughly chopped

Heat a 6-quart Dutch oven over medium-high heat. Add the olive oil, and, once it is shimmering, add the beef. Use a wooden spoon to break up the beef into small pieces, and allow it to sear and brown for about 3 minutes.

Once the beef is mostly cooked (about three-quarters of the way cooked), add the onion and peppers, stirring well. Cook until the vegetables are soft, 4 to 5 minutes, and then stir in the seasonings. Add the garbanzo beans, tomatoes, and water, and bring to a simmer.

Cover, reduce the heat to medium, and cook slowly until the chili has reduced and thickened, about 1 hour. Finish the chili by seasoning with sea salt and stirring in the cilantro.

Chili is delicious on its own but can also be served over rice or roasted cauliflower or alongside a big green salad. Small portions can be frozen for up to 3 months or stored in an airtight container in the refrigerator for 4 to 5 days.

Nutritional analysis per serving: calories 946, fat 44 g, saturated fat 14 g, cholesterol 105 mg, fiber 27 g, protein 57 g, carbohydrate 89 g, sodium 510 mg

Rainbow Salad with Healthy Fats

10D

This delicious low-carb meal is loaded with all sorts of amazing flavors, crunchy textures, and plenty of healthy fats to keep you energized and happy.

Serves: 4   Prep time: 15 minutes
- ¼ cup extra virgin olive oil
- 2 tablespoons lemon juice
- pinch of sea salt
- ¼ teaspoon freshly ground black pepper
- 8 cups mixed greens
- 2 celery stalks, trimmed and thinly sliced
- 12 cherry tomatoes, halved
- ½ cup pitted Kalamata olives, halved
- 1 large ripe avocado, peeled and diced
- 2 tablespoons pumpkin seeds

Whisk together the olive oil, lemon juice, salt, and pepper.

Divide the greens, celery, and tomatoes among four plates. Top with the olives, avocado, and pumpkin seeds.

Drizzle the vinaigrette over the salad and serve immediately.

Nutritional analysis per serving: calories 323, fat
27 g, saturated fat 5 g, cholesterol 0 mg, fiber 0.3 g,
protein 6 g, carbohydrate 21 g, sodium 75 mg

Tempeh, Quinoa, and Veggie Bowl

10D

Everyone loves the nutty flavor of quinoa and the protein punch that it packs. But the tangy sauerkraut and
olives give it a unique and delightful twist that comple-
ments the earthy taste and satisfying texture of tempeh.

*Serves: 4   Prep time: 15 minutes   Cook time: 15 minutes, plus
cooling time*
- 1 cup quinoa
- 2 cups filtered water
- 1 (8-ounce) block organic GMO-free tempeh
- 1 teaspoon sea salt
- 2 tablespoons coconut oil
- 1 cup sauerkraut
- 2 large carrots, peeled and grated
- 1 cup bean sprouts
- 12 large green olives, pitted
- 2 tablespoons extra virgin olive oil
- 1 lemon, quartered

Place the quinoa in a saucepan with the water. Cover, bring to a boil over medium-high heat, and cook for 10 to 12 minutes or just until the water is almost fully absorbed. Remove the pan from the heat and let stand, covered, for 10 minutes. Transfer the quinoa to a bowl and allow it to come to room temperature.

While the quinoa cools, cut the tempeh in half horizontally, then cut each half in half on a diagonal and sprinkle with sea salt. Heat a large skillet over medium-high heat. Add the coconut oil, and, once it is shimmering, brown the tempeh, about 2 minutes per side. Set aside.

Divide the cooked quinoa among four bowls, and add 1 slice of the tempeh to each. Top with the sauerkraut, carrots, sprouts, and olives.

Drizzle each bowl with olive oil and serve with a lemon wedge.

Nutritional analysis per serving: calories 456, fat 26 g, saturated fat 9 g, cholesterol 0 mg, fiber 6 g, protein 20 g, carbohydrate 42 g, sodium 674 mg

DINNER

BEEF CURRY

10D

Flavorful and hearty, this is comfort food at its most delicious and soul nourishing. The spices aid in digestion and are anti-inflammatory and warming. Feel free to adjust the vegetables to include what's in season or what you like. There are endless possibilities here! The curry also gets better with age, so feel free to make it a day or two ahead of time.

Serves: 4   Prep time: 15 minutes   Cook time: 2 hours
- 1 teaspoon cumin seed
- ½ teaspoon coriander seed
- ½ teaspoon whole black peppercorns
- 1 whole dried red chile
- 1-inch piece fresh ginger, peeled and minced
- 4 garlic cloves, minced
- 1 large shallot, minced
- 2 teaspoons avocado oil
- 1½ cups full-fat unsweetened coconut milk
- 1½ pounds grass-fed beef stew meat
- 2 large red bell peppers, stemmed, seeded, and cut into large chunks
- 1 cup chicken stock

- 1 head broccoli, cut into small florets
- ¼ cup fish sauce
- 1 cup basil leaves, torn into small pieces

In a small sauté pan over medium-high heat, cook the cumin, coriander, black pepper, and red chile just until the mixture begins to turn brown, 2 to 3 minutes. Remove from the heat, and, using a mortar and pestle or spice grinder, grind the mixture into a powder. Add the ginger, garlic, and shallot and blend until the mixture forms a paste. If you don't have a mortar and pestle, use a small food processor or blender to make the paste.

Heat the avocado oil in a 5-quart Dutch oven over medium-high heat until shimmering. Add the spice paste, stir well, and cook until fragrant, about 2 minutes. Pour in the coconut milk and bring to a simmer. Add the beef and red bell pepper, along with the chicken stock. Bring to a simmer and then reduce the heat to medium, partially cover, and simmer until the beef is tender, about 1½ hours.

Stir in the broccoli and fish sauce, cover again, and allow the broccoli to steam until tender, about 10 more minutes.

Divide among 4 bowls, top with the basil leaves, and serve.

The curry gets better after sitting for a day or two, so store in an airtight container in the refrigerator until ready to serve, and consume within 5 to 6 days.

Nutritional analysis per serving: calories 411, fat 15 g, saturated fat 8 g, cholesterol 152 mg, fiber 2 g, protein 55 g, carbohydrate 10 g, sodium 1,713 mg

BRAISED CHICKEN WITH FENNEL AND ENDIVE

10D

This will definitely become a favorite standby. It's delicious and incredibly easy. Fennel is great for your skin, bones, and digestion, and the endive contains lots of fiber and may help lower blood sugar levels. The flavors are simple, yet mouthwateringly perfect.

Serves: 4   Prep time: 15 minutes   Cook time: 30 minutes
- 8 bone-in, skin-on chicken drumsticks or thighs
- 1 teaspoon sea salt
- ½ teaspoon freshly ground black pepper
- 1 tablespoon avocado oil
- ½ cup white wine
- ¾ cup chicken stock
- 1 large shallot, thinly sliced
- 2 fennel bulbs, trimmed, halved, and thinly sliced (reserve fronds for garnish)
- 4 heads Belgian endive, trimmed and cut lengthwise into quarters
- 1 tablespoon lemon juice
- 2 tablespoons extra virgin olive oil
- ¼ cup parsley leaves, finely chopped

Season the chicken with the salt and pepper. In a large cast-iron pan, heat the avocado oil over medium-high heat. In 2 batches, add the chicken, skin side down, and cook until evenly browned, about 5 minutes. Turn the pieces over and cook the other side for another 3 minutes. Transfer the chicken to a plate and drain the excess oil from the pan.

Return the pan to the stovetop (still over medium-high heat), add the wine, and scrape up any brown bits left on the bottom of the pan. Boil the liquid until it is reduced by half (about 3 minutes), then add the chicken stock, followed by the reserved chicken. Top the chicken with the sliced shallot, fennel, and endive. Bring the liquid to a boil, then cover and reduce the heat to medium.

Continue to cook for 25 to 30 minutes, or until the chicken is tender and reaches an internal temperature of 165°F. Remove the lid and transfer the chicken and veggies to a serving platter. Add the lemon juice, olive oil, and parsley to the remaining liquid in the pan and stir to combine. Pour the sauce over the chicken and vegetables and serve immediately.

Store leftovers in an airtight container in the refrigerator and use within 3 to 4 days.

Nutritional analysis per serving: calories 426, fat 23 g, saturated fat 5 g, cholesterol 95 mg, fiber 20 g, protein 29 g, carbohydrate 27 g, sodium 877 mg

Piri Piri Baked Tempeh with Asparagus

10D

The flavoring of this spicy dish is amazing, and it adds a wonderful balance to the earthy tempeh and lighter asparagus. This is a perfect choice for spring, when asparagus is in season, and it's packed with tons of vitamins and fiber.

Serves: 4   Prep time: 30 minutes   Cook time: 35 minutes

- 2 tablespoons extra virgin olive oil
- 1 large red bell pepper, stemmed, seeded, and diced
- 1 small yellow onion, diced
- 2 chile peppers (such as serrano, jalapeño, or cayenne), stemmed, seeded, and finely chopped
- 2 large garlic cloves, minced
- 1 tablespoon paprika
- 2 tablespoons apple cider vinegar
- ¼ cup filtered water
- 1 teaspoon sea salt
- 2 bunches asparagus, woody ends trimmed
- 2 (8-ounce) blocks organic GMO-free tempeh, cut into 8 squares

Preheat the oven to 350°F.

Heat the olive oil in a large skillet over medium heat until shimmering. Add the bell pepper and onion, stirring occasionally, and cook until soft, 4 to 5 minutes. Stir in the chile peppers, garlic, and paprika, and continue cooking for 2 more minutes. Remove the pan from the stove and allow it to cool for 10 minutes before transferring its contents to a blender. Add the vinegar, water, and sea salt. Cover the blender and process on high until well pureed.

In a 9- x 13-inch glass baking dish, arrange the asparagus in one even layer. Layer the tempeh on top of the asparagus and then cover it all with the piri piri sauce. Place in the oven and bake for 20 minutes. Carefully remove from the oven and serve immediately.

Nutritional analysis per serving: calories 330, fat 20 g, saturated fat 4 g, cholesterol 0 mg, fiber 5 g, protein 24 g, carbohydrate 22 g, sodium 545 mg

SEARED SCALLOPS WITH CURRIED CAULIFLOWER

10D

A unique and flavorful dish that's simple to prepare and relatively hands-free while it's cooking. Scallops are almost pure protein, so this is a deceptively hearty dish.

Serves: 4   Prep time: 15 minutes   Cook time: 15 minutes

- 2 tablespoons ghee
- 1 head cauliflower, cut into small florets
- 1 tablespoon curry powder
- 8 ounces full-fat unsweetened coconut milk
- 1 teaspoon sea salt
- 1 pound large sea scallops, side muscles removed
- ¼ cup cilantro leaves, roughly chopped
- 1 lemon, quartered

Heat 1 tablespoon of the ghee in a large skillet over medium heat until shimmering. Add the cauliflower and cook, stirring occasionally, for 4 minutes. Stir in the curry powder, coconut milk, and sea salt, and simmer until the cauliflower is tender, 3 to 4 minutes.

Meanwhile, heat another large skillet over high heat with the remaining 1 tablespoon ghee. Once the ghee is hot, add the scallops and cook for 2 minutes, allowing them to sear and brown on the bottom. Carefully flip the scallops and cook for an additional minute, then transfer to a platter.

When the cauliflower is tender, divide it among four plates and top with the scallops. Sprinkle each plate with cilantro and garnish with a lemon wedge.

Nutritional analysis per serving: calories 368, fat 18 g, saturated fat 13 g, cholesterol 103 mg, fiber 3 g, protein 39 g, carbohydrate 13 g, sodium 917 mg

Skillet Tofu with Broccoli and Peppers

10D

This is a tasty and super-easy meal that can be on the table in less than 20 minutes. You can easily use 1 pound of chicken or beef in place of the tofu as well as different vegetables depending on what's available and in season.

Serves: 4   Prep time: 10 minutes   Cook time: 15 minutes
- 2 teaspoons sesame oil
- 1 large red bell pepper, stemmed, seeded, and julienned
- 2 large broccoli heads (about 1 pound total), cut into small florets
- ½-inch piece fresh ginger, peeled and minced
- 1 pound non-GMO firm tofu, drained and crumbled
- 2 tablespoons wheat-free tamari
- 1 tablespoon rice wine vinegar
- ½ cup vegetable broth or filtered water
- 1 tablespoon arrowroot
- 2 tablespoons filtered water
- 1 tablespoon white sesame seeds
- ¼ cup loosely packed cilantro leaves, roughly chopped

Heat the sesame oil in a large skillet or wok over medium-high heat until shimmering. Add the peppers and broccoli, toss to combine, and cook, stirring occasionally, until soft, 3 to 4 minutes. Stir in the ginger and cook for 1 minute. Then add the crumbled tofu and stir until the tofu is well combined.

Add the tamari, vinegar, and broth, and bring to a simmer. While the tofu cooks, combine the arrowroot with the water and pour the mixture into the pan. Stir well and simmer for another 2 to 3 minutes to allow the liquid to thicken.

Divide the tofu among four bowls and serve immediately, garnished with the sesame seeds and cilantro. This dish serves up nicely with the Coconut-Cauliflower Rice on page 473.

Nutritional analysis per serving: calories 176, fat 9 g, saturated fat 1 g, cholesterol 0 mg, fiber 4 g, protein 14 g, carbohydrate 13 g, sodium 382 mg

HERB-MARINATED CHICKEN BREASTS

10D

This is a classic comfort-food dish that the whole family will enjoy, made with ingredients you probably always have on hand. Onions are anti-inflammatory and great immune boosters. Combine that with the protein in the chicken, and you've got a solid cure-all. The fish sauce can be omitted or replaced with soy sauce.

Serves: 4   Prep time: 20 minutes, plus overnight marinating   Cook time: 20 minutes

- 1 large onion, roughly chopped
- ½ cup loosely packed parsley leaves
- ½ cup loosely packed basil leaves
- ¼ cup loosely packed mint leaves
- 2 tablespoons oregano leaves
- 4 large garlic cloves
- 2 tablespoons fish sauce
- zest of 2 lemons
- ¼ cup extra virgin olive oil
- ¼ teaspoon cayenne pepper
- 4 boneless, skin-on chicken breasts

Place the onion, herbs, garlic, fish sauce, cayenne pepper, lemon zest, and olive oil in a blender. Puree on high until well blended, about 45 seconds. Set aside ¼ cup of the marinade, and pour the rest into a bowl with the chicken breasts. Mix well until the chicken is evenly coated, cover the bowl with aluminum or plastic wrap, and transfer to the refrigerator to marinate for 6 to 8 hours or overnight.

Preheat the oven to 375°F.

Transfer the chicken, skin side down, onto a baking dish. Place the chicken in the oven and roast for 10 to 12 minutes, or until firm and fully cooked. Allow the chicken to rest for a few minutes after taking it out of the oven.

Slice the chicken against the grain, in ½-inch slices, then serve, drizzled with the reserved marinade.

Nutritional analysis per serving: calories 324, fat 20 g, saturated fat 4 g, cholesterol 82 mg, fiber 1 g, protein 30 g, carbohydrate 5 g, sodium 766 mg

GRILLED SALMON WITH PARSLEY-WALNUT BUTTER

10D

The parsley-walnut butter in this dish elevates the already delicious salmon to a whole new level and adds even more essential fatty acids to your meal. Don't be afraid of all the healthy fats here—your brain and your body need them! The butter also goes extremely well with crackers, vegetables, eggs, chicken, and other kinds of fish.

Serves: 4   Prep time: 20 minutes   Cook time: 10–15 minutes

- 4 tablespoons (½ stick) unsalted grass-fed butter, at room temperature
- ⅓ cup toasted walnuts, finely chopped
- 1 garlic clove, minced
- ¼ cup loosely packed parsley leaves, finely chopped
- 1 teaspoon sea salt
- ¼ cup extra virgin olive oil

- 4 (4- to 6-ounce) wild salmon fillets
- 1 large cucumber, thinly sliced
- 2 tablespoons red wine vinegar
- 1 tablespoon finely chopped chives

Place the butter in a small bowl and mash with a fork until smooth and spreadable. Add the walnuts, garlic, and parsley, along with ½ teaspoon of the sea salt.

Prepare a grill pan or an outdoor gas grill with 1 tablespoon of the olive oil. Season the salmon with the remaining ½ teaspoon sea salt and place on the hot grill. Cook for 3 to 4 minutes and then carefully flip the fillets and grill for an additional 3 to 4 minutes.

While the salmon cooks, combine the cucumber in a bowl with the red wine vinegar, remaining 3 tablespoons olive oil, and chives. Toss well to incorporate.

Divide the dressed cucumber among 4 plates. When the salmon is ready, plate the fillets and immediately top each with 1 tablespoon of the seasoned butter, allowing it to melt into the flesh. Serve immediately.

Nutritional analysis per serving: calories 486, fat 44 g, saturated fat 16 g, cholesterol 100 mg, fiber 1 g, protein 25 g, carbohydrate 4 g, sodium 610 mg

SIDES AND SNACKS

SOUTHWESTERN GUACAMOLE

10D

The crunch of toasted pumpkin seeds, rich cumin flavor, and tangy tomatillos make this a unique and insanely flavorful addition to any meal. Plus you get some added protein from the seeds along with the healthy fats, so it's a win-win!

Makes: 2 cups   Prep time: 20 minutes
- 2 ripe avocados
- 1 large shallot, finely minced
- 2 teaspoons hot sauce
- ½ teaspoon ground cumin seed
- ½ teaspoon sea salt
- ¼ cup loosely packed cilantro leaves, finely chopped
- 3 tomatillos, coarsely chopped
- 2 tablespoons toasted pumpkin seeds

Cut the avocados in half lengthwise, then remove and discard the pit. Make crosshatch slices in the avocado flesh with a paring knife. Scoop the flesh out with a spoon and place it in a medium bowl. Add the shallot, hot sauce, cumin, and sea salt. Use a fork to mash the avocado with the spices. Leave chunky or continue to mash until the avocado is smooth.

Gently fold in the cilantro, tomatillos, and pumpkin seeds. Serve immediately alongside sliced vegetables, on a salad, or as part of a taco meal.

Nutritional analysis per serving (2 tablespoons): calories 241, fat 22 g, saturated fat 5 g, cholesterol 0 mg, fiber 8 g, protein 3 g, carbohydrate 12 g, sodium 306 mg

COCONUT-CAULIFLOWER RICE

10D

Decadently flavorful and richly satisfying without an ounce of guilt—or grains! Made from cauliflower and flavored coconut milk with crunchy pistachios and toasted coconut to top it off, this creamy alternative to rice can be used for stir-fries or as an accompaniment for grilled vegetables, chicken, or fish.

Serves: 4   Prep time: 10 minutes   Cook time: 15 minutes
- 1 head cauliflower, cut into small florets
- 8 ounces full-fat unsweetened coconut milk
- 2 cardamom pods
- ½ teaspoon sea salt
- ¼ cup pistachios, roughly chopped
- 2 tablespoons toasted shredded coconut

Place half of the cauliflower into an 11-cup or larger food processor and pulse to chop it into smaller pieces, 11 to 12 pulses. Transfer the processed cauliflower to a 4-cup saucepan. Process the remaining cauliflower and add it to the saucepan.

Add the coconut milk, cardamom, and sea salt to the saucepan and cover. Cook the cauliflower mixture over medium heat until the milk is absorbed, 8 to 10 minutes.

Remove the lid and fold in the pistachios and coconut before serving.

Store in an airtight container in the refrigerator for 3 to 4 days.

Nutritional analysis per serving (½ cup): calories 274, fat 24 g, saturated fat 20 g, cholesterol 0 mg, fiber 7 g, protein 5 g, carbohydrate 14 g, sodium 302 mg

CHICKEN LIVER PÂTÉ

10D

Organs are amazing. Their nutritional content is off the charts, and when they're prepared correctly, their flavor is mind-blowing. This elegant pâté is delicious on crackers, vegetables, or cheese, and it's also great right off the spoon. A wonderful beginner food for little ones (adjusted to their tastes as needed)!

Makes: 2 cups   Prep time: 10 minutes   Cook time: 20 minutes

- 2 tablespoons ghee
- 1 large onion, thinly sliced
- 2 to 3 garlic cloves, thinly sliced
- 1 pound chicken livers
- ½ cup red wine
- ½ pound unsalted grass-fed butter, at room temperature
- 1 teaspoon sea salt
- 1 large sprig rosemary, stem removed, leaves finely chopped

Warm a large skillet over medium-high heat. Add 1 tablespoon of the ghee, and, once it's shimmering, add the onion. Cook until the onion slices are translucent and lightly browned, stirring often, 8 to 10 minutes. In the final 2 minutes of cooking, add the garlic and cook until fragrant, about 30 seconds. Transfer to a plate and then return the pan to the stove.

Melt the remaining 1 tablespoon ghee in the pan over medium-high heat and carefully add the livers. Cook the livers for 2 to 3 minutes, then flip and cook them another 1 to 2 minutes. I prefer to leave the livers slightly undercooked so they blend better. Transfer the livers to the plate with the onions.

Return the pan to the stove, add the red wine, and heat over medium-high heat. Use a wooden spoon to scrape up any bits left on the bottom of the pan as you reduce the wine by half. Remove from the stove and let cool.

Place the livers, onions, and reduced red wine into a food processor and blend until smooth. Use a rubber spatula to scrape down the sides. Once the mixture is smooth, run the machine and drop the butter in by the spoonful, allowing it to fully incorporate before adding more. Continue until all the butter is blended in. Add the salt and rosemary, transfer to a serving bowl, and serve with your favorite gluten-free crackers.

Store leftover pâté in a sealed glass container in the refrigerator for up to 4 days. You can fill 4-ounce mason jars with the pâté and freeze for up to 3 months.

Nutritional analysis per serving (2 tablespoons): calories 231, fat 20 g, saturated fat 12 g, cholesterol 259 mg, fiber 0.3 g, protein 10 g, carbohydrate 2 g, sodium 295 mg

Slow-Roasted Tomatoes

10D

These are perfection on a roasting pan—great alone, as a side dish, in salsas, in salads, blended into sauces, or as a topping for just about anything you can think of (pizza, pasta, soups, stir-fries). You can roast the summer's bounty up and freeze them for use in dishes throughout the year when tomatoes are no longer in season. These are delicious with roasted fish, grilled chicken, or sautéed vegetables.

Makes: 20 to 24 tomato halves   Prep time: 5 minutes   Cook time: 3 hours
- 2 pounds Roma tomatoes, halved
- 2 tablespoons extra virgin olive oil
- 1 tablespoon dried thyme
- 2 teaspoons dried oregano
- 1 teaspoon dried basil
- 1 teaspoon sea salt
- ½ teaspoon freshly ground black pepper

Preheat the oven to 325°F.

Gently toss the tomatoes in a large bowl with the remaining ingredients.

Place the tomatoes, skin side down, in a single layer on a rimmed baking sheet. Roast for 3 hours. Carefully remove them from the oven and allow them to cool completely.

Store the tomatoes in the refrigerator in a sealed container for up to 4 days.

Nutritional analysis per serving (5 tomato halves): calories 403, fat 30 g, saturated fat 4 g, cholesterol 0 mg, fiber 11 g, protein 8 g, carbohydrate 35 g, sodium 44 mg

Spinach Falafels

Everyone loves falafel. This version has even more protein than usual thanks to the chia seeds, and it is cooked in healthy saturated fats that stay stable at high temperatures, rather than the usual vegetable oil. This is also a great way to get more greens into kids' (and grown-ups') diets.

Makes: 1 dozen falafels   Prep time: 10 minutes, plus overnight soaking   Cook time: 15 minutes

- 1 cup dried chickpeas
- 4 cups filtered water
- 1 tablespoon apple cider vinegar
- 2 cups spinach, roughly chopped
- 1 small onion, minced
- 2 garlic cloves, minced
- 2 tablespoons freshly ground chia seeds
- 1 teaspoon sea salt
- 1 teaspoon baking powder
- ¼ cup ghee or coconut oil
- 1 lemon, cut into wedges

Soak the chickpeas in the water and apple cider vinegar at room temperature for 8 to 12 hours. Once they're soaked, drain and rinse them well.

Place the chickpeas in a food processor and pulse, using a rubber spatula to scrape down the sides, until they are the size of grains of rice. They should stick together when you press them between your fingers.

Add the spinach, onion, garlic, ground chia, sea salt, and baking powder to the food processor and pulse to incorporate. Once thoroughly mixed, form the mixture into 12 (1-inch) patties. Make sure they are packed tightly so they don't crumble during cooking.

Heat 2 tablespoons of the ghee in a large skillet over medium-high heat. Once the fat is shimmering, add 6 falafel patties without overcrowding the pan. Fry until golden brown on each side, 2 to 3 minutes per side. Place the cooked falafels on a paper towel to drain. Heat the remaining 2 tablespoons ghee and cook the remaining falafel patties as before.

Serve the falafels warm with a squeeze of lemon.

Store leftovers in an airtight container in the fridge for 3 to 4 days or in the freezer for up to 4 weeks.

Nutritional analysis per serving (3 falafels): calories 323, fat 17 g, saturated fat 8 g, cholesterol 33 mg, fiber 11 g, protein 16 g, carbohydrate 35 g, sodium 494 mg

SWEET POTATO DIP

Hummus is a family-friendly staple, and this version takes the classic to a whole new level. Sweet potato adds extra vitamins and minerals, including energizing vitamin B, as well as incredible flavor. It pairs perfectly with the protein-rich chickpeas. You'll always want to have this on hand. It's a treat to watch everyone you make it for go crazy over it!

Makes: 2 cups   Prep time: 5 minutes   Cook time: 15 minutes
- 1 large sweet potato, peeled and cut pieces
- 1 tablespoon extra virgin olive oil
- 1 small onion, thinly sliced
- 1 garlic clove, minced
- 1 (15-ounce) can chickpeas, rinsed and drained
- ¼ cup tahini
- 1 tablespoon lemon juice
- 2 teaspoons chili powder
- 1 teaspoon sea salt

Place the sweet potato in a saucepan and add 1 cup of filtered water. Cover and cook over high heat until the sweet potato is tender, about 10 minutes. Remove the lid, drain, and allow the sweet potato chunks to cool completely.

Meanwhile, heat a skillet over medium-high heat. Add the olive oil, and, once it's shimmering, add the onion. Cook, stirring occasionally, until the onion slices are soft and translucent, 5 to 6 minutes. Add the garlic and cook until fragrant, about 1 minute. Remove the pan from the heat and set aside to cool.

In a food processor, combine the sweet potato, onion, and chickpeas. Pulse the mixture until it begins to puree, 6 to 7 pulses. Scrape down the sides with a rubber spatula, then add the remaining ingredients.

Run the machine until the dip becomes smooth

and creamy, about 1 minute. Serve immediately or transfer the dip to an airtight container and refrigerate for up to 4 days.

Nutritional analysis per serving (2 tablespoons): calories 278, fat 9 g, saturated fat 1 g, cholesterol 0 mg, fiber 11 g, protein 12 g, carbohydrate 39 g, sodium 30 mg

HERB-ROASTED MUSHROOMS

10D

We often think of roasted mushrooms as heavy and stuffed with cheese. These are much lighter, although they're still a hearty side or topping for any meal. Plus, they're packed with flavor and nutrition. Good luck not eating them all before they even hit the plates!

Serves: 4   Prep time: 10 minutes   Cook time: 30 minutes
- 1 pound cremini or white button mushrooms
- 3 tablespoons extra virgin olive oil
- 2 large garlic cloves, minced
- 1 large sprig rosemary, stem removed, leaves roughly chopped
- ¼ cup packed parsley leaves, roughly chopped
- 2 sprigs thyme, stems removed, leaves roughly chopped

- 2 teaspoons sea salt
- ½ teaspoon freshly ground black pepper

Preheat the oven to 350°F.

Use a towel to wipe any dirt from the mushrooms, then place them in a large bowl. Add the remaining ingredients and toss well to incorporate.

Spread the mushrooms out on a rimmed baking sheet and place it in the oven. Roast the mushrooms until they are soft and slightly golden, 25 to 30 minutes. Carefully remove them from the oven and serve immediately. Any extra mushrooms can be stored in an airtight container in the fridge for up to 3 days.

Nutritional analysis per serving (1 cup of cooked mushrooms): calories 61, fat 5 g, saturated fat 1 g, cholesterol 0 mg, fiber 0.6 g, protein 2 g, carbohydrate 3 g, sodium 4 mg

DESSERTS

Warm Spiced Apple Slices

Decadent *and* healthy? This incredible dessert achieves the seemingly impossible. It makes for a beautiful presentation, and you can swap out the apple for other fruits depending on what's in season.

Serves: 4   Prep time: 5 minutes   Cook time: 12 minutes
- 2 large, crisp apples (preferably Fuji)
- 2 tablespoons ghee or coconut oil
- ¼ teaspoon ground cinnamon
- scant pinch of ground clove
- optional: 1 tablespoon maple syrup
- 2 tablespoons coconut cream
- 3 tablespoons hazelnuts, roughly chopped
- 1 tablespoon toasted coconut flakes

Peel each apple, cut it in half, remove the core, and slice it into ⅛-inch slices. Melt the ghee in a large skillet over medium heat. Add the apples and cook for 3 to 4 minutes, stirring occasionally to prevent them from burning.

Stir in the cinnamon and clove, and cook for 1 minute. Then add the maple syrup (if using) and coconut cream. Allow the liquid to simmer and thicken, 2 to 3 minutes. Stir in the hazelnuts and coconut flakes and serve immediately.

Nutritional analysis per serving (with maple syrup): calories 171, fat 11 g, saturated fat 6 g, cholesterol 16 mg, fiber 3 g, protein 1 g, carbohydrate 20 g, sodium 3 mg, sugars 15 g

BLUEBERRY SOFT SERVE

Who doesn't love ice cream? This creamy treat is packed full of antioxidants, and the coconut oil provides incredible fuel and nutrition while helping lower cholesterol levels. It's the perfect dessert for grown-ups and kids alike.

Serves: 4   Prep time: 5 minutes, plus chilling time

- 4 cups frozen blueberries
- ½ cup full-fat coconut milk
- ¼ cup coconut oil
- 2 tablespoons basil leaves, minced
- optional: 1 tablespoon honey
- zest of 1 lime
- ½ teaspoon alcohol-free, gluten-free pure vanilla extract
- 4 tablespoons bee pollen, for garnish

It's best to make this recipe in two batches. Combine half of the blueberries, coconut milk, oil, basil, honey (if using), lime zest, and vanilla in a blender, and blend on high, using the tamper to push the berries down toward the blade. Process until the mixture is smooth, thick, and creamy, about 1 minute. Transfer the mixture to a large bowl and place the bowl in the freezer. Repeat with the other half of the ingredients (except the bee pollen) and add to the first batch. Keep the first batch in the freezer only while you're making the second batch.

Scoop the ice cream into 4 bowls. Sprinkle each portion with 1 tablespoon bee pollen. Serve immediately. It's best to eat this ice cream right away. Freezing it for too long will make it icy.

Nutritional analysis per serving: calories 260, fat 16 g, saturated fat 13 g, cholesterol 0 mg, fiber 6 g, protein 3 g, carbohydrate 30 g, sodium 2 mg, sugars 21 g

ALMOND BUTTER TRUFFLES

Once you've tasted these, you'll always want to have them on hand. You can experiment by adding crushed nuts or cacao nibs. Cacao has four times the antioxidants of regular dark chocolate and tons of other nutrients, making these guilt-free treats.

Makes: 24 cookies   Prep time: 15 minutes, plus chilling time
- 3 soft Medjool dates, pitted
- 3 tablespoons unsalted grass-fed butter
- ½ cup smooth unsalted almond butter
- 3 tablespoons coconut oil

- ¾ cup shredded coconut
- 2 tablespoons cacao powder
- ½ teaspoon alcohol-free, gluten-free pure vanilla extract
- ⅛ teaspoon sea salt

Place the dates in a food processor and pulse 8 to 10 times to coarsely chop. Add the butter, almond butter, and coconut oil, then process the mixture until it is smooth and creamy. Add the shredded coconut, cacao powder, vanilla, and salt and pulse until well combined.

Line a baking sheet with parchment paper.

Drop ½-tablespoon portions onto the baking sheet. Place the sheet in the refrigerator or freezer for 20 minutes so the truffles can harden.

Store any remaining truffles in an airtight container in the fridge for 3–4 days or the freezer for up to 1 month.

Nutritional analysis per serving (1 truffle): calories 482, fat 43 g, saturated fat 22 g, cholesterol 23 mg, fiber 9 g, protein 9 g, carbohydrate 27 g, sodium 62 mg, sugars 15 g

Fudgy Carob Brownies

A chocolate-, refined-sugar-, and gluten-free treat that we promise you'll go crazy over! You won't even miss the sugar and chocolate in these brownies. Carob helps digestion and maple syrup provides necessary minerals while boosting immune and heart health.

Makes: 8 brownies   Prep time: 10 minutes   Cook time: 30 to 35 minutes, plus cooling

- ½ cup plus 2 tablespoons unsalted grass-fed butter
- ½ cup coconut flour
- ½ cup carob powder
- 3 eggs, at room temperature
- ¼ cup maple syrup
- 1 teaspoon alcohol-free, gluten-free pure vanilla extract

Preheat the oven to 325°F. Grease a 9 × 10 glass baking dish with 2 tablespoons of the butter.

In a medium bowl, combine the coconut flour and carob powder. Add the remaining ½ cup butter and the eggs, maple syrup, and vanilla, and mix to combine.

Pour the mixture into the baking dish and bake in the oven for 30 to 35 minutes or until a toothpick inserted into the center comes out clean.

Cool for 30 minutes before cutting the brownies or removing them from the pan.

These store well in an airtight container at room temperature or in the refrigerator for up to 7 days.

Nutritional analysis per serving (1 brownie): calories 360, fat 27 g, saturated fat 16 g, cholesterol 184 mg, fiber 2 g, protein 5 g, carbohydrate 25 g, sodium 215 mg, sugars 18 g

RASPBERRY-LEMON ICE POPS

Gelatin powder adds a sneaky protein kick to these sweet frozen treats. They're perfect as post-workout recovery fuel, and an easy and delicious way to get important nutrients into busy kiddos. You'll need ice pop molds for these.

Makes: 4 to 6 pops   Prep time: 15 minutes, plus freezer time
- 2¼ cups full-fat coconut milk
- 2½ teaspoons unflavored gelatin powder
- ¼ cup maple syrup
- zest of 1 lemon
- ½ teaspoon ground cardamom
- 1 teaspoon alcohol-free, gluten-free pure vanilla extract
- ⅛ teaspoon sea salt
- ½ cup fresh or frozen raspberries

Place ¼ cup of the coconut milk in a medium heat-proof bowl. Sprinkle the gelatin over it and set it aside to bloom for 5 minutes.

Heat the remaining 2 cups coconut milk with the maple syrup, lemon zest, cardamom, vanilla, and sea salt in a saucepan over medium-high heat for 5 minutes. Whisk the softened gelatin into the saucepan and continue whisking until all of it is dissolved.

Allow the mixture to chill for 15 to 20 minutes. Place 3 to 4 raspberries in each ice pop mold, then fill with the liquid. Place the pops in the freezer to set for a minimum of 4 hours.

Nutritional analysis per serving (1 ice pop):
calories 130, fat 6 g, saturated fat 6 g, cholesterol 0 mg, fiber 1 g, protein 3 g, carbohydrate 16 g, sodium 69 mg, sugars 12 g

FLOURLESS CASHEW BUTTER COOKIES

Now you'll never have to wonder what to make when you need something gluten-free to please a crowd. These cookies have a fantastic texture, and the protein from the nut butter makes them incredibly satiating; a perfect snack any time of the day.

Makes: 12 cookies   Prep time: 10 minutes   Cook time: 8 to 10 minutes

- 1 cup cashew or almond butter
- 2 tablespoons coconut palm sugar or maple syrup
- 1 large egg
- 1 teaspoon alcohol-free, gluten-free pure vanilla extract
- 1 teaspoon baking soda
- 1 teaspoon ground cinnamon
- ½ teaspoon ground ginger
- ½ teaspoon ground nutmeg
- ½ teaspoon sea salt

Preheat the oven to 350°F. Line a baking sheet with parchment paper.

In a mixing bowl, combine the cashew butter and coconut palm sugar. Beat in the egg and vanilla and mix well. In a separate bowl, combine the baking soda, cinnamon, ginger, nutmeg, and salt. Add the baking soda mixture to the almond butter mixture, and combine until well incorporated.

Form the dough into 12 evenly sized balls and place them on the baking sheet. Using the back of a fork, partially flatten each ball, making crosshatch marks.

Place the baking sheet in the oven and bake for 8 to 10 minutes. Remove the sheet from the oven and carefully transfer the cookies to a cooling rack.

Once fully cooled, the cookies can be stored in an airtight container for 3 to 4 days.

Nutritional analysis per serving (1 cookie): calories 296, fat 22 g, saturated fat 5 g, cholesterol 47 mg, fiber 1 g, protein 9 g, carbohydrate 19 g, sodium 513 mg, sugars 8 g

CHOCOLATE CHIP COOKIE DOUGH SPREAD

This may be an icing, but that doesn't mean it has to go on a cake. It's a perfect spread on apple slices or frozen into little bites...or eaten right off the spoon. Healthy saturated fat from the butter keeps your body and brain well satiated and fueled for anything.

Makes: 8 portions   Prep time: 5 minutes
- 1 stick unsalted grass-fed butter, at room temperature
- 2 tablespoons cacao nibs
- ½ teaspoon ground cinnamon
- 1 teaspoon alcohol-free, gluten-free pure vanilla extract
- optional: 1 tablespoon maple sugar

Place the butter in a medium-size bowl and, using the back of a spoon or a rubber spatula, mash it until it's soft and spreadable. Add the remaining ingredients and mix to incorporate.

Enjoy by spreading 1 tablespoon onto ripe pear or apple slices, or freeze 1-tablespoon dollops until firm for a frozen treat.

Nutritional analysis per serving (1 tablespoon): calories 208, fat 24 g, saturated fat 16 g, cholesterol 60 mg, fiber 0 g, protein 0 g, carbohydrate 2 g, sodium 0 mg, sugars 2 g

Acknowledgments

This book was grown in the rich soil of experience and collaboration, from the work of the scientists and clinicians who laid the groundwork for our modern understanding of the way our bodies interact with the food we eat. But it could not have been written without the help and support of so many people who have inspired, guided, and helped me along the way.

First, I must thank my patients, who are my greatest teachers. Only with their trust and goodwill have I been able to learn so much about using food as medicine.

My views are not based solely on the academic science of nutrition, but also on my observations of real people over decades as they've changed their diets. And of course, on the tireless, often tedious, careful work of scientists and researchers who have pointed me in the right direction.

And then there are all those who have taught and inspired me, including Jeffrey Bland, David Ludwig, Robert Lustig, Michael Pollan, Mark Bittman, Michael Moss, Andrew Weil, Chris Kresser, Marc David, and so many others.

My teams at The UltraWellness Center and at Cleveland Clinic Center for Functional Medicine work hard every day to deliver innovative healing to our patients and communities using food as the primary medicine. You all are key actors in the transformation of health care, and I couldn't do what I do without all of you. Thank you. A special thanks to Liz Boham, Todd LePine, and Kathie Swift for two decades of work together and mutual support. And, Kathie, thank you for introducing me to the world of functional medicine and a new way of thinking about nutrition.

I cannot express enough gratitude to Toby Cosgrove, the CEO of Cleveland Clinic, for what he has done to advance the progress of functional medicine by building a functional medicine program at Cleveland Clinic. This program is now led by Tawny Jones, Patrick Hanaway, Michele Beidelschies, Elizabeth Bradley, and Mary Curran. You are all amazing. And I am deeply grateful to all the health care providers and caregivers there doing the work to make functional medicine the standard of care.

There are so many others without whom this book would never have happened. Bill Tonelli helped me translate my vision into a reality. Anahad O'Connor gathered and helped me translate the science behind *Food*. Kaya Purohit, as always, delivered amazing insights about the links between food, the environment, and our health. Dhru Purohit is the glue that holds it all together and makes things happen. Grateful beyond words. Chef Frank Giglio translates my vision of healthy eating into astoundingly delicious recipes. Audria Brumberg was super great helping with the cover design.

Of course there is no way I could do the work I do to communicate the message of healing without my publishing team at Little, Brown—especially Tracy Behar, who believed in me way back almost 20 years ago. And Richard Pine, my agent, who has guided and supported my work also for almost 20 years. Without him I wouldn't have been able to realize my dreams. Thank you, Ian Straus, for helping with the manuscript.

Without Anne McLaughlin, who always says yes, I would not have been able to keep all the pieces of my life together. You are the best, ever. There are so many to thank, but a few need special mention for stepping up: Denise Curtin, Tammy Boyd, and Dianna Galia.

The support of my family allows me to do my work and be fully expressed. Thank you. And, Mia, my extraordinary wife, thank you for always believing in me and for being the solid ground on which I stand.

Notes

Part I

1. Ravnskov U, DiNicolantonio JJ, Harcombe Z, Kummerow FA, Okuyama H, Worm N. The questionable benefits of exchanging saturated fat with polyunsaturated fat. *Mayo Clin Proc.* 2014 Apr;89(4):451–53.
2. Lesser LI, Ebbeling CB, Goozner M, Wypij D, Ludwig DS. Relationship between funding source and conclusion among nutrition-related scientific articles. *PLoS Med.* 2007 Jan;4(1):e5.
3. Executive summary. *Dietary Guidelines for Americans, 2015–2020*, 8th ed. Office of Disease Prevention and Health Promotion. https://health.gov/dietaryguidelines/2015/guidelines/execut ive-summary/.
4. Chronic diseases: the leading cause of death and disability in the United States. Centers for Disease Control and Prevention. https://www.cdc.gov/chronicdisease/overview/. Updated June 28, 2017.
5. Office of the Assistant Secretary for Planning and Evaluation. US Department of Health and Human Services. Effects of health care spending on the U.S. economy. https://aspe.hhs.gov/ basic-report/effects-health-care-spending-us-economy. February 22, 2005.
6. Basch CE. Healthier students are better learners: a missing link in school reforms to close the achievement gap. *J Sch Health.* 2011 Oct;81(10):593–98.

7. Too fat to fight. Council for a Strong America. https://www .strongnation.org/articles/23-too-fat-to-fight. April 10, 2010.

8. Hidden cost of industrial agriculture. Union of Concerned Scientists. http://www.ucsusa.org/food_and_agriculture/our -failing-food-system/industrial-agriculture/hidden-costs-of -industrial.html#.WSIrTDOZNPM.

9. Gilbert N. One third of our greenhouse gas emissions come from agriculture. *Nature.* http://www.nature.com/news/one -third-of-our-greenhouse-gas-emissions-come-from-agri culture-1.11708. October 2012.

10. Lawrence F. Omega-3, junk food and the link between violence and what we eat. *Guardian.* October 17, 2006. https:// www.theguardian.com/politics/2006/oct/17/prisonsandpro bation.ukcrime.

11. Nestle M. Food marketing and childhood obesity—a matter of policy. *N Engl J Med.* 2006 Jun 15;354(24):2527–29.

12. Kessler DA. Toward more comprehensive food labeling. *N Engl J Med.* 2014 Jul 17;371(3):193–95.

13. Siegel KR, McKeever Bullard K, Imperatore G, et al. Association of higher consumption of foods derived from subsidized commodities with adverse cardiometabolic risk among US adults. *JAMA Intern Med.* 2016;176(8):1124–32.

14. Siegel KR, McKeever Bullard K, Imperatore G, et al. Association of higher consumption of foods derived from subsidized commodities with adverse cardiometabolic risk among US adults. *JAMA Intern Med.* 2016;176(8):1124–32.

15. Brownell KD, Ludwig DS. The Supplemental Nutrition Assistance Program, soda, and USDA policy: who benefits? *JAMA.* 2011;306(12):1370–71.

16. Teicholz Nina. The scientific report guiding the US dietary guidelines: is it scientific? *BMJ.* 2015;351:h4962.

17. Finkelstein EA, Zhen C, Nonnemaker J, Todd JE. Impact of

targeted beverage taxes on higher- and lower-income households. *Arch Intern Med.* 2010;170(22):2028–34.

18. Nestle M. New study: Big Food's ties to registered dietitians. *Food Politics.* http://www.foodpolitics.com/2013/01/new-study -big-foods-ties-to-registered-dietitians/. January 22, 2013.

19. The Daniel Plan. http://www.danielplan.com/.

20. Rapaport L. Antibiotics in animal feed may endanger kids, doctors warn. *Scientific American.* https://www.scientificam erican.com/article/antibiotics-in-animal-feed-may-endanger -kids-doctors-warn/. November 16, 2015.

21. Schillinger D, Jacobson MF. Science and public health on trial: warning notices on advertisements for sugary drinks. *JAMA.* 2016;316(15):1545–46.

22. Gilbert N. One-third of our greenhouse gas emissions come from agriculture. *Nature.* https://www.nature.com/news/one-third-of -our-greenhouse-gas-emissions-come-from-agriculture-1.11708. October 31, 2012.

23. Ludwig DS, Majzoub JA, Al-Zahrani A, Dallal GE, Blanco I, Roberts SB. High glycemic index foods, overeating, and obesity. *Pediatrics.* 1999 Mar;103(3):E26.

24. Millen BE, Abrams S, Adams-Campbell L, et al. The 2015 Dietary Guidelines Advisory Committee Scientific Report: development and major conclusions. *Adv Nutr.* 2016 May 16;7(3):438–44.

25. Tobias DK, Chen M, Manson JE, Ludwig DS, Willett W, Hu FB. Effect of low-fat diet interventions versus other diet interventions on long-term weight change in adults: a systematic review and meta-analysis. *Lancet Diabetes Endocrinol.* 2015 Dec;3(12):968–79.

26. Ebbeling CB, Swain JF, Feldman HA, et al. Effects of dietary composition on energy expenditure during weight-loss maintenance. *JAMA.* 2012 Jun 27;307(24):2627–34.

27. Ludwig DS, Willett WC. Three daily servings of reduced-fat milk: an evidence-based recommendation? *JAMA Pediatr.* 2013 Sep;167(9):788–89.

28. Chowdhury R, Warnakula S, Kunutsor S, et al. Association of dietary, circulating, and supplement fatty acids with coronary risk: a systematic review and meta-analysis. *Ann Intern Med.* 2014 Mar 18;160(6):398–406. doi: 10.7326/M13-1788. Review.

29. Ramsden CE, Zamora D, Leelarthaepin B, et al. Use of dietary linoleic acid for secondary prevention of coronary heart disease and death: evaluation of recovered data from the Sydney Diet Heart Study and updated meta-analysis. *BMJ.* 2013 Feb 4;346:e8707.

Part II

Meat

1. Chowdhury R, Warnakula S, Kunutsor S, et al. Association of dietary, circulating, and supplement fatty acids with coronary risk: a systematic review and meta-analysis. *Ann Intern Med.* 2014 Mar 18;160(6):398–406.

2. van Vliet S, Burd NA, van Loon LJ. The skeletal muscle anabolic response to plant- versus animal-based protein consumption. *J Nutr.* 2015 Sep;145(9):1981–91.

3. Whalen KA, Judd S, McCullough ML, Flanders WD, Hartman TJ, Bostick RM. Paleolithic and Mediterranean diet pattern scores are inversely associated with all-cause and cause-specific mortality in adults. *J Nutr.* 2017 Feb 8.

4. Scheu A, Powell A, Bollongino R, et al. The genetic prehistory of domesticated cattle from their origin to the spread across Europe. *BMC Genet.* 2015 May 28;16:54.

5. Cordain L, Eaton SB, Miller JB, et al. The paradoxical nature

of hunter-gatherer diets: meat-based, yet non-atherogenic. *Eur J Clin Nutr.* 2002 Mar;56 Suppl 1:S42–S52.

6. Newport F. In U.S., 5 percent consider themselves vegetarians. Gallup. July 26, 2012.

7. Leu, C.. Know your meat—and bugs: introducing the periodic table of protein. *Wired.* https://www.wired.com/2016/07/sustainable-proteins/#slide-1. July 2016.

8. Nelson GC. *Genetically Modified Organisms in Agriculture: Economics and Politics.* 1st ed. San Diego, CA: Academic Press; 2001.

9. Hayes KC. Saturated fats and blood lipids: new slant on an old story. *Can J Cardiol.* 1995 Oct;11 Suppl G:39G–48G.

10. Dreon DM, Fernstrom HA, Campos H, et al. Change in dietary saturated fat intake is correlated with change in mass of large low-density-lipoprotein particles in men. *Am J Clin Nutr.* 1998 May;67(5):828–36.

11. Siri PW, Krauss RM. Influence of dietary carbohydrate and fat on LDL and HDL particle distributions. *Curr Atheroscler Rep.* 2005 Nov;7(6):455–59.

12. Yerushalmy J, Hilleboe HE. Fat in the diet and mortality from heart disease; a methodologic note. *NY State J Med.* 1957 Jul 15;57(14):2343–54.

13. US Department of Health and Human Services; US Department of Agriculture. *2015–2020 Dietary Guidelines for Americans.* 8th ed. December 2015.

14. McAdams M. How much saturated fat should you have per day? *SFGate.* http://healthyeating.sfgate.com/much-saturated-fats-should-per-day-5488.html. February 15, 2017.

15. American Heart Association. Saturated fats. https://www.heart.org/HEARTORG/HealthyLiving/HealthyEating/Nutrition/Saturated-Fats_UCM_301110_Article.jsp. February 14, 2017.

16. Sachdeva A, Cannon CP, Deedwania PC, et al. Lipid levels in patients hospitalized with coronary artery disease: an analysis of 136,905 hospitalizations in Get with the Guidelines. *Am Heart J.* 2009 Jan;157(1):111–17.

17. Pencina MJ, D'Agostino RB, Larson MG, et al. Predicting the 30-year risk of cardiovascular disease. The Framingham Heart Study. *Circulation.* 2009;119:3078-84. Wilson PWF, Anderson KM. HDL cholesterol and triglycerides as risk factors for CHD. *Atherosclerosis and Cardiovascular Disease.* 1990:609–15.

18. Astrup A, Dyerberg J, Elwood P, et al. The role of reducing intakes of saturated fat in the prevention of cardiovascular disease: where does the evidence stand in 2010? *Am J Clin Nutr.* 2011 Apr;93(4):684–88.

19. Ramsden CE, Zamora D, Majchrzak-Hong S, et al. Re-evaluation of the traditional diet-heart hypothesis: analysis of recovered data from Minnesota Coronary Experiment (1968–73). *BMJ.* 2016 Apr 12;353:i1246.

20. Chowdhury R, Warnakula S, Kunutsor S, et al. Association of dietary, circulating, and supplement fatty acids with coronary risk: a systematic review and meta-analysis. *Ann Intern Med.* 2014 Mar 18;160(6):398–406.

21. Grasgruber P, Sebera M, Hrazdira E, et al. Food consumption and the actual statistics of cardiovascular diseases: an epidemiological comparison of 42 European countries. *Food Nutr Res.* 2016 Sep 27;60:31694.

22. Johnston L. Potatoes and cereals are health risk, while dairy is good for you, says new study. *Express.* October 16, 2016.

23. Nissen SE. U.S. dietary guidelines: an evidence-free zone. *Ann Intern Med.* 2016 Apr 19;164(8):555–59.

24. Salim Y. Nutrition and CVD: data from 17 countries on 150,000 people. *Cardiology Update 2017.* Davos, Switzerland. February 12, 2017.

25. Campbell WW, Barton ML Jr, Cyr-Campbell D, et al. Effects of an omnivorous diet compared with a lactoovovegetarian diet on resistance-training-induced changes in body composition and skeletal muscle in older men. *Am J Clin Nutr.* 1999 Dec;70(6):1032–39.

26. Pannemans DL, Wagenmakers AJ, Westerterp KR, et al. Effect of protein source and quantity on protein metabolism in elderly women. *Am J Clin Nutr.* 1998 Dec;68(6): 1228–35.

27. Bouvard V, Loomis D, Guyton KZ, et al. Carcinogenicity of consumption of red and processed meat. *Lancet Oncol.* 2015 Dec;16(16):1599–1600.

28. Alexander DD, Cushing CA. Red meat and colorectal cancer: a critical summary of prospective epidemiologic studies. *Obes Rev.* 2011 May;12(5):e472–e493.

29. Lin J, Zhang SM, Cook NR, et al. Dietary fat and fatty acids and risk of colorectal cancer in women. *Am J Epidemiol.* 2004 Nov 15;160(10):1011–22.

30. National Research Council (US) Committee on Drug Use in Food Animals. *The Use of Drugs in Food Animals: Benefits and Risks.* Washington, DC: National Academies Press; 1999.

31. Sapkota AR, Lefferts LY, McKenzie S, et al. What do we feed to food-production animals? A review of animal feed ingredients and their potential impacts on human health. *Environ Health Perspect.* 2007 May;115(5):663–70.

32. Brady H. Red Skittles spilling onto Wisconsin highway were headed for cattle. *National Geographic.* January 23, 2017.

33. Schultz R. Feeding candy to cows is sweet for their digestion. *Wisconsin State Journal.* January 29, 2017.

34. Mackinnon E. Candy not corn for cows in drought. *Live Science.* August 23, 2012.

35. Ibid.

36. Nagaraja TG, Chengappa MM. Liver abscesses in feedlot cattle: a review. *J Anim Sci.* 1998 Jan;76(1):287–98.

37. Uwituze S, Parsons GL, Shelor MK, et al. Evaluation of dried distillers grains and roughage source in steam-flaked corn finishing diets. *J Anim Sci.* 2010 Jan;88(1):258–74.

38. Rock A. How safe is your ground beef? *Consumer Reports.* December 21, 2015.

39. Ibid.

40. Daley CA, Abbott A, Doyle PS, et al. A review of fatty acid profiles and antioxidant content in grass-fed and grain-fed beef. *Nutr J.* 2010 Mar 10;9:10.

41. Ibid.

42. Leheska JM, Thompson LD, Howe JC, et al. Effects of conventional and grass-feeding systems on the nutrient composition of beef. *J Anim Sci.* 2008 Dec;86(12):3575–85.

43. Hall N, Schonfeldt HC, Pretorius B. Fatty acids in beef from grain- and grass-fed cattle: the unique South African scenario. *South Afr J Clin Nutr.* 2016;29(2).

44. Leheska JM, Thompson LD, Howe JC, et al. Effects of conventional and grass-feeding systems on the nutrient composition of beef. *J Anim Sci.* 2008 Dec;86(12):3575–85.

45. Castro-Webb N, Ruiz-Narvaez EA, Campos H. Cross-sectional study of conjugated linoleic acid in adipose tissue and risk of diabetes. *Am J Clin Nutr.* 2012 Jul;96(1):175–81.

46. Ochoa JJ, Farquharson AJ, Grant I, et al. Conjugated linoleic acids (CLAs) decrease prostate cancer cell proliferation: different molecular mechanisms for cis-9, trans-11 and trans-10, cis-12 isomers. *Carcinogenesis.* 2004 Jul;25(7):1185–91.

47. Dilzer A, Park Y. Implication of conjugated linoleic acid (CLA) in human health. *Crit Rev Food Sci Nutr.* 2012;52(6): 488–513.

48. Why grass-fed beef costs more. *Consumer Reports*. August 24, 2015.

49. Rock A. How safe is your ground beef? *Consumer Reports*. December 21, 2015.

50. US Department of Agriculture. National Nutrient Database for Standard Reference. Beef, liver, raw. https://ndb.nal.usda.gov/ndb/foods/show/3787. February 18, 2017. Kresser C. Liver: nature's most potent superfood. Chris Kresser. https://chriskresser.com/natures-most-potent-superfood/. April 11, 2008.

51. Phillips DH. Polycyclic aromatic hydrocarbons in the diet. *Mutat Res*. 1999 Jul 15;443(1–2).

52. Key TJ, Thorogood M, Appleby PN, Burr ML. Dietary habits and mortality in 11,000 vegetarians and health conscious people: results of a 17 year follow up. *BMJ*. 1996;313(7060): 775–79.

53. Mihrshahi S, Ding D, Gale J, Allman-Farinelli M, Banks E, Bauman AE. Vegetarian diet and all-cause mortality: evidence from a large population-based Australian cohort—the 45 and Up Study. *Prev Med*. 2017 Apr;97:1–7.

54. Goodland R, Anhang J. Livestock and climate change: what if the key actors in climate change are . . . cows, pigs and chickens? *World Watch Magazine*. 2009 November–December; 22(6).

55. Mekonnen MM, Hoekstra AY. *The Green, Blue and Grey Water Footprint of Farm Animals and Animal Products*. Value of Water Research Report Series No. 48. Delft, Netherlands: UNESCO-IHE Institute for Water Education; December 2010.

56. Puangsombat K, Smith JS. Inhibition of heterocyclic amine formation in beef patties by ethanolic extracts of rosemary. *J Food Sci*. 2010 Mar;75(2):T40–T47.

57. Smith JS, Ameri F, Gadgil P. Effect of marinades on the

formation of heterocyclic amines in grilled beef steaks. *J Food Sci*. 2008 Aug;73(6):T100–T105.

Poultry and Eggs

1. Shin JY, Xun P, Nakamura Y, He K. Egg consumption in relation to risk of cardiovascular disease and diabetes: a systematic review and meta-analysis. *Am J Clin Nutr*. 2013 Jul;98(1):146–59. doi: 10.3945/ajcn.112.051318. Review.
2. National Chicken Council. *Per Capita Consumption of Poultry and Livestock, 1965 to Estimated 2016, in Pounds*. September 21, 2016.
3. Ponte PI, Prates JA, Crespo JP, et al. Restricting the intake of a cereal-based feed in free-range-pastured poultry: effects on performance and meat quality. *Poult Sci*. 2008 Oct;87(10): 2032–42. Ponte PI, Alves SP, Bessa RJ, et al. Influence of pasture intake on the fatty acid composition, and cholesterol, tocopherols, and tocotrienols content in meat from free-range broilers. *Poult Sci*. 2008 Jan;87(1):80–88.
4. Mateo-Gallego R, Perez-Calahorra S, Cenarro A, et al. Effect of lean red meat from lamb v. lean white meat from chicken on the serum lipid profile: a randomized, cross-over study in women. *Br J Nutr*. 2012 May;107(10):1403–7.
5. Hu FB, Stampfer MJ, Rimm EB, et al. A prospective study of egg consumption and risk of cardiovascular disease in men and women. *JAMA*. 1999 Apr 21;281(15):1387–94.
6. Fuller NR, Caterson ID, Sainsbury A, et al. The effect of a high-egg diet on cardiovascular risk factors in people with type 2 diabetes: the Diabetes and Egg (DIABEGG) Study—a 3-mo randomized controlled trial. *Am J Clin Nutr*. 2015 Apr;101(4):705–13.
7. Rong Y, Chen L, Zhu T, et al. Egg consumption and risk of

coronary heart disease and stroke: dose-response meta-analysis of prospective cohort studies. *BMJ.* 2013 Jan 7;346:e8539.

8. US Department of Health and Human Services; US Department of Agriculture. *Scientific Report of the 2015 Dietary Guidelines Advisory Committee.* Washington, DC; February 2015.

9. O'Connor A. Nutrition panel calls for less sugar and eases cholesterol and fat restrictions. *New York Times.* February 19, 2015.

10. Povoledo E. Raw eggs and no husband since '38 keep her young at 115. *New York Times.* February 14, 2015.

11. Koeth RA, Wang Z, Levison BS, et al. Intestinal microbiota metabolism of L-carnitine, a nutrient in red meat, promotes atherosclerosis. *Nat Med.* 2013 May;19(5):576–85.

12. Wang Z, Klipfell E, Bennett BJ, et al. Gut flora metabolism of phosphatidylcholine promotes cardiovascular disease. *Nature.* 2011 Apr 7;472(7341):57–63.

13. Cho CE, Taesuwan S, Malysheva OV, et al. Trimethylamine-N-oxide (TMAO) response to animal source foods varies among healthy young men and is influenced by their gut microbiota composition: a randomized controlled trial. *Mol Nutr Food Res.* 2017 Jan;61(1).

14. Ufnal M, Zadlo A, Ostaszewski R. TMAO: a small molecule of great expectations. *Nutrition.* 2015 Nov–Dec;31(11–12): 1317–23.

15. Chan JM, Wang F, Holly EA. Pancreatic cancer, animal protein and dietary fat in a population-based study, San Francisco Bay Area, California. *Cancer Causes Control.* 2007 Dec;18(10):1153–67.

16. Kolahdooz F, van der Pols JC, Bain JC, et al. Meat, fish, and ovarian cancer risk: results from 2 Australian case-control studies, a systematic review, and meta-analysis. *Am J Clin Nutr.* 2010 Jun;91(6):1752–63.

17. Daniel CR, Cross AJ, Graubard BI, et al. Prospective investigation of poultry and fish intake in relation to cancer risk. *Cancer Prev Res (Phila)*. 2011 Nov;4(11):1903–11.

18. US Department of Agriculture Food Safety and Inspection Service. Meat and poultry labeling terms. https://www.fsis.usda.gov/wps/portal/fsis/topics/food-safety-education/get-answers/food-safety-fact-sheets/food-labeling/meat-and-poultry-labeling-terms. Retrieved March 5, 2017. Updated August 10, 2015.

19. Curry L. Ground-breaking animal welfare organic rules moving forward. *Civil Eats*. January 12, 2017.

20. Grossman E. Absent federal policy, states take lead on animal welfare. *Civil Eats*. February 15, 2017.

21. Centers for Disease Control and Prevention. Salmonella and chicken: what you should know and what you can do. https://www.cdc.gov/features/SalmonellaChicken/index.html. Updated September 11, 2017.

22. Food and Drug Administration. Department of Health and Human Services. *2012 Summary Report on Antimicrobials Sold or Distributed for Use in Food-Producing Animals*. https://www.fda.gov/downloads/ForIndustry/UserFees/AnimalDrugUserFeeActADUFA/UCM416983.pdf. September 2014.

23. Consumer Reports. Dangerous contaminated chicken. http://www.consumerreports.org/cro/magazine/2014/02/the-high-cost-of-cheap-chicken/index.htm. Updated January 2014.

24. Klein S, Witmer J, Tian A, DeWaal CS. *The Ten Riskiest Foods Regulated by the U.S. Food and Drug Administration*. Center for Science in the Public Interest. October 7, 2009.

25. Ibid.

26. National Center for Biotechnology Information. PubChem Compound Database: CID=24455, Sodium tripolyphosphate. https://pubchem.ncbi.nlm.nih.gov/compound/24455. August 8, 2005.

27. Eagle H, Doak GO. The biological activity of arsenosoben-zenes in relation to their structure. *Pharmacol Rev.* 1951 Jun;3(2):107–43.

28. IARC. *Monographs on the Evaluation of Carcinogenic Risks to Humans: Drinking Water Disinfectants and Contaminants, including Arsenic.* Lyon: International Agency for Research on Cancer; 2007.

29. Schmidt CW. Arsenical association: inorganic arsenic may accumulate in the meat of treated chickens. *Environ Health Perspect.* 2013 Jul;121(7):A226.

30. Environment America. *America's Next Top Polluter: Corporate Agribusiness: Company Profile, Tyson Foods, Inc.* http://environ mentnewyork.org/sites/environment/files/reports/Env_Am _Tyson_v4_1.pdf.

31. Kristof N. Abusing chickens we eat. *New York Times.* December 3, 2014.

Milk and Dairy

1. Ludwig DS, Willett WC. Three daily servings of reduced-fat milk: an evidence-based recommendation? *JAMA Pediatr.* 2013 Sep;167(9):788–89.

2. Bischoff-Ferrari HA, Dawson-Hughes B, Baron JA, et al. Milk intake and risk of hip fracture in men and women: a meta-analysis of prospective cohort studies. *J Bone Miner Res.* 2011;26(4):833–39.

3. Pimpin L, Wu JH, Haskelberg H, Del Gobbo L, Mozaffarian D. Is butter back? A systematic review and meta-analysis of butter consumption and risk of cardiovascular disease, diabetes, and total mortality. *PLoS One.* 2016 Jun 29;11(6).

4. Danby FW. Acne, dairy and cancer: the 5alpha-P link. *Dermatoendocrinol.* 2009 Jan;1(1):12–16.

5. Chowdhury R, Warnakula S, Kunutsor S, et al. Association of dietary, circulating, and supplement fatty acids with coronary risk: a systematic review and meta-analysis. *Ann Intern Med.* 2014 Mar 18;160(6):398–406.

6. Heyman MB. Lactose intolerance in infants, children and adolescents. *Pediatrics.* 2006 Sep;118(3):1279–86.

7. Aune D, Navarro Rosenblatt DA, Chan DS, et al. Dairy products, calcium, and prostate cancer risk: a systematic review and meta-analysis of cohort studies. *Am J Clin Nutr.* 2015 Jan;101(1):87–117.

8. Carroccio A, Brusca I, Mansueto P, et al. Fecal assays detect hypersensitivity to cow's milk protein and gluten in adults with irritable bowel syndrome. *Clin Gastroenterol Hepatol.* 2011 Nov;9(11):965–71.

9. Gerbault P, Liebert A, Itan Y, et al. Evolution of lactase persistence: an example of human niche construction. *Philos Trans R Soc London B Biol Sci.* 2011 Mar 27;366(1566):863–77.

10. Howchwallner H, Schulmeister U, Swoboda I, et al. Cow's milk allergy: from allergens to new forms of diagnosis, therapy and prevention. *Methods.* 2014 Mar;66(1):22–33.

11. Hochwallner H, Schulmeister U, Swoboda I, et al. Microarray and allergenic activity assessment of milk allergens. *Clin Exp Allergy.* 2010 Dec;40(12):1809–18.

12. Katta R, Schlichte M. Diet and dermatitis: food triggers. *J Clin Aesthet Dermatol.* 2014 Mar;7(3):30–36.

13. Juntti H, Tikkanen S, Kokkonen J, et al. Cow's milk allergy is associated with recurrent otitis media during childhood. *Acta Otolaryngol.* 1999;119(8):867–73.

14. Lill C, Loader B, Seemann R, et al. Milk allergy is frequent in patients with chronic sinusitis and nasal polyposis. *Am J Rhinol Allergy.* 2011 Nov–Dec;25(6):e221–e224.

15. United States Department of Agriculture: Choose MyPlate.

10 tips: got your dairy today? https://www.choosemyplate.gov/ten-tips-got-your-dairy-today. Updated August 4, 2017.

16. IBISWorld. Dairy farms in the US: market research report. https://www.ibisworld.com/industry/default.aspx?indid=49. June 2017.

17. Center for Responsive Politics. Dairy: long-term contribution trends. https://www.opensecrets.org/industries/totals.php. December 22, 2016.

18. Dietitians for Professional Integrity. How industry lobbying shapes the dietary guidelines. http://integritydietitians.org/2015/11/18/how-industry-lobbying-shapes-the-dietary-guidelines/. November 18, 2015.

19. Lesser LI, Ebbeling CB, Goozner M, et al. Relationship between funding source and conclusion among nutrition-related scientific articles. *PLoS Med.* 2007 Jan;4(1):e5.

20. Lanou AJ. Should dairy be recommended as part of a healthy vegetarian diet? Counterpoint. *Am J Clin Nutr.* 2009 May; 89(5):1638S–1642S.

21. Bischoff-Ferrari HA, Dawson-Hughes B, Baron JA, et al. Milk intake and risk of hip fracture in men and women: a meta-analysis of prospective cohort studies. *J Bone Miner Res.* 2011 Apr;26(4):833–39.

22. Bischoff-Ferrari HA, Dawson-Hughes B, Baron JA, et al. Calcium intake and hip fracture risk in men and women: a meta-analysis of prospective cohort studies and randomized controlled trials. *Am J Clin Nutr.* 2007 Dec;86(6):1780–90.

23. Feskanich D, Willett WC, Stampfer MJ, et al. Milk, dietary calcium, and bone fractures in women: a 12-year prospective study. *Am J Public Health.* 1997;87:992–97.

24. Michaelsson K, Melhus H, Bellocco R, et al. Dietary calcium and vitamin D in relation to osteoporotic fracture risk. *Bone.* 2003;32:694–703.

25. Winzenberg T, Shaw K, Fryer J, et al. Effects of calcium supplementation on bone density in healthy children: meta-analysis of randomized controlled trials. *BMJ.* 2006 Oct 14;333(7572):775.

26. Lanou AJ, Berkow SE, Barnard ND. Calcium, dairy products, and bone health in children and young adults: a reevaluation of the evidence. *Pediatrics.* 2005 Mar;115(3):736–43.

27. Lloyd T, Chinchilli VM, Johnson-Rollings N, et al. Adult female hip bone density reflects teenage sports-exercise patterns but not teenage calcium intake. *Pediatrics.* 2000 Jul; 106(1 Pt 1):40–44.

28. Heaney RP. The bone remodeling transient: interpreting interventions involving bone-related nutrients. *Nutr Rev.* 2001;59(10):327–34.

29. World's Healthiest Foods. Calcium. http://www.whfoods .com/genpage.php?tname=nutrient&dbid=45.

30. Feskanich D, Willett WC, Colditz GA. Calcium, vitamin D, milk consumption, and hip fractures: a prospective study among postmenopausal women. *Am J Clin Nutr.* 2003 Feb; 77(2):504–11.

31. Ludwig DS, Willett WC. Three daily servings of reduced-fat milk: an evidence-based recommendation? *JAMA Pediatr.* 2013;167(9):788–89.

32. Teppala S, Shankar A, Sabanayagam C. Association between IGF-1 and chronic kidney disease among US adults. *Clin Exp Nephrol.* 2010 Oct;14(5):440–44.

33. Friedrich N, Thuesen B, Jorgensen T, et al. The association between IGF-1 and insulin resistance: a general population study in Danish adults. *Diabetes Care.* 2012 Apr;35(4):768–73.

34. Andreassen M, Raymond I, Kistorp C, et al. IGF1 as predictor of all cause mortality and cardiovascular disease in an elderly population. *Eur J Endocrinol.* 2009 Jan;160(1):25–31.

35. Heaney RP, McCarron DA, Dawson-Hughes B, et al. Dietary changes favorably affect bone remodeling in older adults. *J Am Diet Assoc.* 1999;99:1228–33.

36. Ahn J, Albanes D, Peters U, et al. Dairy products, calcium intake and risk of prostate cancer in the prostate, lung, colorectal and ovarian cancer screening trial. *Cancer Epidemiol Biomarkers Prev.* 2007 Dec;16(12):2623–30.

37. Song Y, Chavarro JE, Cao Y, et al. Whole milk intake is associated with prostate cancer–specific mortality among U.S. male physicians. *J Nutr.* 2013 Feb;143(2):189–96.

38. Chowdhury R, Wamakula S, Kunutsor S, et al. Association of dietary, circulating and supplement fatty acids with coronary risk: a systematic review and meta-analysis. *Ann Intern Med.* 2014 Mar 18;160(6):398–406.

39. Yakoob MY, Shi P, Willett WC, et al. Circulating biomarkers of dairy fat and risk of incident diabetes mellitus among men and women in the United States in two large prospective cohorts. *Circulation.* 2016 Apr 26;133(17):1645–54.

40. Berkey CS, Rockett HR, Willett WC, et al. Milk, dairy fat, dietary calcium and weight gain: a longitudinal study of adolescents. *Arch Pediatr Adolesc Med.* 2005 Jun;159(6):543–50. Mozaffarian D, Hao T, Rimm EB, et al. Changes in diet and lifestyle and long-term weight gain in women and men. *N Engl J Med.* 2011;364(25):2392–2404.

41. The Dairy Practices Council. *Guideline for Vitamin A & D Fortification of Fluid Milk.* http://phpa.dhmh.maryland.gov/OEHFP/OFPCHS/Milk/Shared%20Documents/DPC053_Vitamin_AD_Fortification_Fluid_Milk.pdf. July 2001.

42. Pimpin L, Wu JH, Haskelberg H, et al. Is butter back? A systematic review and meta-analysis of butter consumption and risk of cardiovascular disease, diabetes and total mortality. *PLoS One.* 2016 Jun 29;11(6).

43. Robinson J. Super natural milk. Eatwild.com. http://www
    .eatwild.com/articles/superhealthy.html.

44. Botta A, Ghosh S. Exploring the impact of n-6 PUFA-rich oil-
    seed production on commercial butter compositions world-
    wide. *J Agric Food Chem*. 2016;64(42):8026–34.

45. Jianqin S, Leiming X, Lu X, Yelland GW, Ni J, Clarke AJ.
    Effects of milk containing only A2 beta casein versus milk con-
    taining both A1 and A2 beta casein proteins on gastrointestinal
    physiology, symptoms of discomfort, and cognitive behavior of
    people with self-reported intolerance to traditional cows' milk.
    Nutrition Journal. 2016;15:35.

46. Deth R, Clarke A, Ni J, Trivedi M. Clinical evaluation of glu-
    tathione concentrations after consumption of milk contain-
    ing different subtypes of β-casein: results from a randomized,
    cross-over clinical trial. *Nutr J*. 2016 Sep 29;15(1):82.

47. Elliott RB, Harris DP, Hill JP, Bibby NJ, Wasmuth HE. Type
    I (insulin-dependent) diabetes mellitus and cow milk: casein
    variant consumption. *Diabetologia*. 1999 Mar;42(3):292–96.

48. Raw milk laws state by state as of April 19, 2016. http://milk
    .procon.org/view.resource.php?resourceID=005192#sales
    -prohibited.

49. Mungai EA, Behravesh CB, Gould LH. Increased outbreaks
    associated with nonpasteurized milk, United States, 2007–
    2012. *Emerg Infect Dis*. 2015 Jan;21(1):119–22.

50. Kresser C. Raw milk reality: benefits of raw milk. Chris Kresser.
    https://chriskresser.com/raw-milk-reality-benefits-of-raw-milk/.
    May 18, 2012.

51. Hoekstra AY. The hidden water resource use behind meat and
    dairy. *Animal Frontiers*. 2012;2(2):3–8.

52. Good K. Milk life? How about milk destruction: the shocking
    truth about the dairy industry and the environment. One

Green Planet. http://www.onegreenplanet.org/animalsandna
ture/the-dairy-industry-and-the-environment/. April 22, 2016.

Fish and Seafood

1. Harvest of fears: farm-raised fish may not be free of mercury and other pollutants. *Scientific American.* https://www.scientificam erican.com/article/farm-raised-fish-not-free-mercury -pcb-dioxin/.
2. Braun DR, Harris JW, Levin NE, et al. Early hominin diet included diverse terrestrial and aquatic animals 1.95 Ma in East Turkana, Kenya. *Proc Natl Acad Sci U S A.* 2010 Jun 1;107(22):10002–7.
3. Innis SM. Dietary omega 3 fatty acids and the developing brain. *Brain Res.* 2008 Oct 27;1237:35–43.
4. Mozaffarian D, Wu JH. Omega-3 fatty acids and cardiovascular disease: effects on risk factors, molecular pathways, and clinical events. *J Am Coll Cardiol.* 2011 Nov 8;58(20): 2047–67.
5. Nkondjock A, Receveur O. Fish-seafood consumption, obesity, and type 2 diabetes: an ecological study. *Diabetes Metab.* 2003 Dec;29(6):635–42.
6. Simopoulos AP. Omega-3 fatty acids in inflammation and autoimmune diseases. *J Am Coll Nutr.* 2002;21(6):495–505.
7. Li F, Liu X, Zhang D. Fish consumption and risk of depression: a meta-analysis. *J Epidemiol Community Health.* 2016; 70:299–304.
8. Johns Hopkins Bloomberg School of Public Health. Global shift in farmed fish feed may impact nutritional benefits ascribed to consuming seafood. http://www.jhsph.edu/research/ centers-and-institutes/johns-hopkins-center-for-a

   -livable-future/news-room/News-Releases/2016/global-shift
   -in-farmed-fish-feed-may-impact-nutritional-benefits
   -ascribed-to-consuming-seafood.html. March 14, 2016.

9. Done HY, Halden RU. Reconnaissance of 47 antibiotics and
   associated microbial risks in seafood sold in the United States.
   J Hazard Mater. 2015 Jan 23;282:10–17.

10. Fry JP, Love DC, MacDonald GK, et al. Environmental
    health impacts of feeding crops to farmed fish. *Environ Int.*
    2016 May;91:201–14.

11. Mozaffarian D, Rimm EB. Fish intake, contaminants, and
    human health: evaluating the risks and the benefits. *JAMA.*
    2006;296(15):1885–99. Del Gobbo LC, Imamura F, Aslibekyan
    S, et al. ω-3 Polyunsaturated fatty acid biomarkers and coronary
    heart disease: pooling project of 19 cohort studies. *JAMA Intern
    Med.* 2016 Aug 1;176(8):1155–66.

12. Miles EA, Calder PC. Influence of marine n-3 polyunsatu-
    rated fatty acids on immune function and a systematic review
    of their effects on clinical outcomes in rheumatoid arthritis.
    Br J Nutr. 2012 Jun;107 Suppl 2:S171–S184.

13. GISSI-Prevenzione Investigators. Dietary supplementation with
    n-3 polyunsaturated fatty acids and vitamin E after myocardial
    infarction: results of the GISSI-Prevenzione trial. *Lancet.* 1999
    Aug 7;354(9177):447–55.

14. Yokoyama M, Origasa H, Matsuzaki M, et al. Effects of eicos-
    apentaenoic acid on major coronary events in hypercholester-
    olaemic patients (JELIS): a randomized open-label, blinded
    endpoint analysis. *Lancet.* 2007 Mar 31;369(9567):1090–98.

15. Simopoulos AP. Omega-3 fatty acids in health and disease
    and in growth and development. *Am J Clin Nutr.* 1991
    Sep;54(3):438–63.

16. Simopoulos AP. The importance of the ratio of omega-6/

omega-3 essential fatty acids. *Biomed Pharmacother.* 2002 Oct;56(8):365–79. Review.

17. US Department of Agriculture; US Department of Health and Human Services. *Dietary Guidelines for Americans 2015–2020.* 8th ed. https://health.gov/dietaryguidelines/2015/guide lines/chapter-1/a-closer-look-inside-healthy-eating-patterns/. January 2016.

18. US Department of Agriculture. High omega-3 fish analysis. https://health.gov/DietaryGuidelines/dga2005/report/HTML/table_g2_adda2.htm. January 8, 2017.

19. Tanskanen A, Hibbeln JR, Hintikka J. Fish consumption, depression, and suicidality in a general population. *Arch Gen Psychiatry.* 2001;58(5):512–13.

20. Bloch MH, Qawasmi A. Omega-3 fatty acid supplementation for the treatment of children with attention-deficit/hyperactivity disorder symptomatology: systematic review and meta-analysis. *J Am Acad Child Adolesc Psychiatry.* 2011 Oct;50(10): 991–1000.

21. Zaalberg A, Nijman H, Bulten E, et al. Effects of nutritional supplements on aggression, rule-breaking, and psychopathology among young adult prisoners. *Aggress Behav.* 2010 Mar –Apr;36(2):117–26.

22. Lewis MD, Hibbeln JR, Johnson JE, et al. Suicide deaths of active-duty US military and omega-3 fatty-acid status: a case-control comparison. *J Clin Psychiatry.* 2011 Dec;72(12): 1585–90.

23. National Institutes of Health. Study links low DHA levels to suicide risk among U.S. military personnel. https://www.nih.gov/news-events/news-releases/study-links-low-dha-levels-suicide-risk-among-us-military-personnel. August 23, 2011.

24. Hibbeln JR, Gow RV. Omega-3 fatty acid and nutrient

deficits in adverse neurodevelopment and childhood behaviors. *Child Adolesc Psychiatr Clin N Am.* 2014 Jul;23(3):555–90.

25. Draft Updated Advice by FDA and EPA. Fish: what pregnant women and parents should know. http://www.fda.gov/Food/FoodborneIllnessContaminants/Metals/ucm393070.htm. June 2014.

26. Oken E, Radesky JS, Wright RO, et al. Maternal fish intake during pregnancy, blood mercury levels, and child cognition at age 3 years in a US cohort. *Am J Epidemiol.* 2008 May 15;167(10):1171–81.

27. Food and Drug Administration. FDA and EPA issue draft updated advice for fish consumption. http://www.fda.gov/news events/newsroom/pressannouncements/ucm397929.htm. June 10, 2014.

28. Colombo J, Carlson SE, Cheatham CL, et al. Long-term effects of LCPUFA supplementation on childhood cognitive outcomes. *Am J Clin Nutr.* 2013 Aug;98(2):403–12.

29. Oceana. Deceptive dishes: seafood swaps found worldwide. September 2016.

30. National Oceanic and Atmospheric Administration. Grand jury indicts Santa Monica restaurant and sushi chefs on federal charges related to sale of protected whale meat. http://www.nmfs.noaa.gov/ole/newsroom/stories/13/grand_jury_indicts_santa_monica_restaurant.html. 2013.

31. Weintraub K. AskWell: canned vs. fresh fish. *New York Times.* October 7, 2015.

32. Environmental Working Group. Consumer guide to seafood. http://www.ewg.org/research/ewg-s-consumer-guide-seafood/why-eat-seafood-and-how-much. September 2014.

33. Weaver KL, Ivester P, Chilton JA, et al. The content of favorable and unfavorable polyunsaturated fatty acids found in

commonly eaten fish. *J Am Diet Assoc.* 2008 Jul;108(7): 1178–85.

34. Hites RA, Foran JA, Schwager SJ, et al. Global assessment of polybrominated diphenyl ethers in farmed and wild salmon. *Environ Sci Technol.* 2004 Oct 1;38(19):4945–49.

35. Hamilton MC, Hites RA, Schwager SJ, et al. Lipid composition and contaminants in farmed and wild salmon. *Environ Sci Technol.* 2005 Nov 15;39(22):8622–29.

36. Guallar E, Sanz-Gallardo MI, van't Veer P, et al. Mercury, fish oils, and the risk of myocardial infarction. *N Engl J Med.* 2002 Nov 28;347(22):1747–54.

37. Food and Drug Administration. Mercury levels in commercial fish and shellfish (1990–2010). http://www.fda.gov/food/foodborneillnesscontaminants/metals/ucm115644.htm. October 8, 2014.

38. Crinnion WJ. The role of persistent organic pollutants in the worldwide epidemic of type 2 diabetes mellitus and the possible connection to farmed Atlantic salmon (*Salmo salar*). *Altern Med Rev.* 2011 Dec;16(4):301–13. Review.

39. Bayen S, Barlow P, Lee HK, et al. Effect of cooking on the loss of persistent organic pollutants from salmon. *J Toxicol Environ Health.* 2005 Feb 27;68(4):253–65.

40. Hori T, Nakagawa R, Tobiishi K, et al. Effects of cooking on concentrations of polychlorinated dibenzo-p-dioxins and related compounds in fish and meat. *J Agric Food Chem.* 2005 Nov 2;53(22):8820–28.

41. Lewis MD, Bailes J. Neuroprotection for the warrior: dietary supplementation with omega-3 fatty acids. *Mil Med.* 2011 Oct;176(10):1120–27. Review.

42. Yurko-Mauro K, Kralovec J, Bailey-Hall E, et al. Similar eicosapentaenoic acid and docosahexaenoic acid plasma levels

achieved with fish oil or krill oil in a randomized double-blind four-week bioavailability study. *Lipids Health Dis.* 2015 Sep 2;14:99.

43. Lane K, Derbyshire E, Li W, et al. Bioavailability and potential uses of vegetarian sources of omega-3 fatty acids: a review of the literature. *Crit Rev Food Sci Nutr.* 2014;54(5):572–79.

Vegetables

1. Worthington V. Nutritional quality of organic versus conventional fruits, vegetables, and grains. *J Altern Complement Med.* 2001 Apr;7(2):161–73.
2. Craig WJ. Health effects of vegan diets. *Am J Clin Nutr.* 2009 May;89(5):1627S–33S.
3. Kaczmarczyk MM, Miller MJ, Freund GG. The health benefits of dietary fiber: beyond the usual suspects of type 2 diabetes mellitus, cardiovascular disease and colon cancer. *Metabolism.* 2012 Aug;61(8):1058–66.
4. King DE, Mainous AG 3rd, Lamburne CA. Trends in dietary fiber intake in the United States, 1999–2008. *J Acad Nutr Diet.* 2012 May;112(5):642–48.
5. Pandey KB, Rizvi SI. Planty polyphenols as dietary antioxidants in human health and disease. *Oxid Med Cell Longev.* 2009 Nov–Dec;2(5):270–78.
6. Robinson J. Breeding the nutrition out of food. *New York Times.* http://www.nytimes.com/2013/05/26/opinion/sunday/breeding-the-nutrition-out-of-our-food.html. May 25, 2013.
7. Zhang L, Hou D, Chen X, et al. Exogenous plant MIR168a specifically targets mammalian LDLRAP1: evidence of cross-kingdom regulation by microRNA. *Cell Research.* 2012;22:107–26.
8. Mascio PD, Kaiser S, Sies H. Lycopene as the most efficient

biological carotenoid singlet oxygen quencher. *Biochemistry and Biophysics.* 1989 Nov;274(2):532–38.

9. Alavanja MCR. Pesticide use and exposure extensive worldwide. *Rev Environ Health.* 2009 Oct–Dec;24(4):303–9.

10. Priyadarshi A, Khuder SA, Schaub EA, et al. A meta-analysis of Parkinson's disease and exposure to pesticides. *Neurotoxicology.* 2000 Aug;21(4):435–40.

11. Bassil KL, Vakil C, Sanborn M, et al. Cancer health effects of pesticides: systematic review. *Can Fam Physician.* 2007 Oct;53 (10):1704–11.

12. Beard JD, Umbach DM, Hoppin JA, et al. Pesticide exposure and depression among male private pesticide applicators in the agricultural health study. *Environ Health Perspect.* 2014 Sept;122(9):984–91.

13. Curl CL, Beresford SAA, Fenske RA, et al. Estimating pesticide exposure from dietary intake and organic food choices: the multi-ethnic study of atherosclerosis (MESA). *Environ Health Perspect.* 2015 May;123(5):475–83.

14. Environmental Working Group. All 48 fruits and vegetables with pesticide residue data. https://www.ewg.org/foodnews/list.php. January 11, 2017.

15. Cavagnaro PF, Camargo A, Galmarini CR, Simon PW. Effect of cooking on garlic (*Allium sativum L.*) antiplatelet activity and thiosulfinates content. *J Agric Food Chem.* 2007 Feb 21;55(4):1280–88.

16. Vermeulen M, Klöpping-Ketelaars IW, van den Berg R, Vaes WH. Bioavailability and kinetics of sulforaphane in humans after consumption of cooked versus raw broccoli. *J Agric Food Chem.* 2008 Nov 26;56(22):10505–9.

17. Rabin RC. Are frozen fruits and vegetables as nutritious as fresh? *New York Times.* November 18, 2016.

18. Oyebode O, Gordon-Dseagu V, Walker A, et al. Fruit and

vegetable consumption and all-cause, cancer and CVD mortality: analysis of health survey for England data. *J Epidemiol Community Health.* 2014 Sep;68(9):856–62.

19. Childers NF, Margoles MS. An apparent relation of night-shades (*Solanaceae*) to arthritis. *J Neurol Orthop Med Surg.* 1993;12:227–31. Childers NF. *Arthritis: Childers' Diet That Stops It! Nightshades, Aging, and Ill Health,* 4th ed. Florida: Horticultural Publications; 1993:19–21.

20. Krishnaiah D, Rosalam S, Prasad DMR, et al. Mineral content of some seaweeds from Sabah's South China Sea. *Asian J Scientific Res.* 2008;1:166–70.

21. McGovern PE, Zhang J, Tang J, et al. Fermented beverages of pre- and proto-historic China. *Proc Natl Acad Sci U S A.* 2004 Dec 21;101(51):17593–98.

22. Pathak DR, He JP, Charzewska J. Joint association of high cabbage/sauerkraut intake at 12–13 years of age and adulthood with reduced breast cancer risk in Polish migrant women: results from the US component of the Polish Women's Health Study (PWHS). AACR Fourth Annual Conference on Frontiers in Cancer Prevention Research, Baltimore; 2005.

23. Martinez-Villaluenga C, Penas E, Frias J, et al. Influence of fermentation conditions on glucosinolates, ascorbigen, and ascorbic acid content in white cabbage cultivated in different seasons. *J Food Sci.* 2009 Jan–Feb;74(1):C62–67.

24. Breidt F, McFeeters RF, Perez-Diaz I, et al. Fermented vegetables. *Food Microbiology: Fundamentals and Frontiers.* 4th ed. Washington, DC: ASM Press; 2013.

25. Foster-Powell K, Holt SHA, Brand-Miller JC. International table of glycemic index and glycemic load values: 2002. *Am J Clin Nutr.* 2002;76:5–56. http://ajcn.nutrition.org/content/76/1/5.full.pdf+html.

26. Heiman ML, Greenway FL. A healthy gastrointestinal microbiome is dependent on dietary diversity. *Mol Metab*. 2016 Mar 5;5(5):317–20.

Fruit

1. Centers for Disease Control and Prevention. Obesity and overweight. https://www.cdc.gov/nchs/fastats/obesity-overweight .htm. January 20, 2017.
2. Centers for Disease Control and Prevention. Diabetes latest. https://www.cdc.gov/Features/DiabetesFactSheet/. January 20, 2017.
3. Lampe JW. Health effects of vegetables and fruit: assessing mechanisms of action in human experimental studies. *Am J Clin Nutr*. 1999 Sep;70(3):475–90.
4. Coe SA, Clegg M, Armengol M, et al. The polyphenol-rich baobab fruit (*Adansonia digitata L.*) reduces starch digestion and glycemic response in humans. *Nutr Res*. 2013 Nov;33(11):888–96.
5. Wang X, Ouyang Y, Liu J, et al. Fruit and vegetable consumption and mortality from all causes, cardiovascular disease, and cancer: systematic review and dose-response meta-analysis of prospective cohort studies. *BMJ*. 2014 Jul 29;349:g4490. Muraki I, Imamura F, Manson JE, et al. Fruit consumption and risk of type 2 diabetes: results from three prospective longitudinal cohort studies. *BMJ*. 2013;347:f5001. Joshipura KJ, Hu FB, Manson JE, et al. The effect of fruit and vegetable intake on risk for coronary heart disease. *Ann Intern Med*. 2001 Jun 19;134(12):1106–14.
6. Produce for Better Health Foundation. *State of the Plate: 2015 Study on America's Consumption of Fruit & Vegetables*. http:// pbhfoundation.org/pdfs/about/res/pbh_res/State_of_the _Plate_2015_WEB_Bookmarked.pdf. February 2015.

7. Imamura F, O'Connor L, Ye Z, et al. Consumption of sugar sweetened beverages, artificially sweetened beverages, and fruit juice and incidence of type 2 diabetes: systematic review, meta-analysis, and estimation of population attributable fraction. *BMJ.* 2015 Jul 21;351:h3576. doi: 10.1136/bmj.h3576. Review.

8. Cohen JC, Schall R. Reassessing the effects of simple carbohydrates on the serum triglyceride responses to fat meals. *Am J Clin Nutr.* 1988;48:1031–34.

9. Maersk M, Belza A, Stodkilde-Jorgensen H, et al. Sucrose-sweetened beverages increase fat storage in the liver, muscle, and visceral fat depot: a 6-mo randomized intervention study. *Am J Clin Nutr.* 2012;95:283–89.

10. Stanhope KL, Havel PJ. Fructose consumption: considerations for future research on its effects on adipose distribution, lipid metabolism, and insulin sensitivity in humans. *J Nutr.* 2009;139:1236S–1241S.

11. Te Morenga L, Mallard S, Mann J. Dietary sugars and body weight: systematic review and meta-analyses of randomized controlled trials and cohort studies. *BMJ.* 2012 Jan 15;346: e7492.

12. Ludwig DS. Examining the health effects of fructose. *JAMA.* 2013;310(1):33–34.

13. Meyer BJ, de Bruin EJ, Du Plessis DG, et al. Some biochemical effects of a mainly fruit diet in man. *S Afr Med J.* 1971;45(10):253–61.

14. He FJ, Nowson CA, Lucas M, et al. Increased consumption of fruit and vegetables is related to a reduced risk of coronary heart disease: meta-analysis of cohort studies. *J Hum Hypertens.* 2007 Sep;21(9):717–28.

15. Nooyens AC, Bueno-de-Mesquita HB, van Boxtel MP, et al. Fruit and vegetable intake and cognitive decline in middle-

aged men and women: the Doetinchem Cohort Study. *Br J Nutr.* 2011 Sep;106(5):752–61.

16. He FJ, Nowson CA, MacGregor GA. Fruit and vegetable consumption and stroke: meta-analysis of cohort studies. *Lancet.* 2006 Jan 28;367(9507):320–26.

17. Aune D, Chan DS, Vieira AR, et al. Fruits, vegetables and breast cancer risk: a systematic review and meta-analysis of prospective studies. *Breast Cancer Res Treat.* 2012 Jul;134(2): 479–93.

18. Jenkins DJA, Srichaikul K, Kendall CWC, et al. The relation of low glycemic index fruit consumption to glycemic control and risk factors for coronary heart disease in type 2 diabetes. *Diabetologia.* 2011 Feb;54(2):271–79.

19. Foster-Powell K, Holt SHA, Brand-Miller JC. International table of glycemic index and glycemic load values: 2002. *Am J Clin Nutr.* 2002;76:5–56.

20. The Antioxidant Food Table. http://www.orac-info-portal.de/download/ORAC_R2.pdf.

21. Environmental Working Group. 2017 shopper's guide to pesticides in produce. https://www.ewg.org/foodnews/summary.php.

22. US Department of Agriculture. *2014 Pesticide Data Program Annual Summary.* January 11, 2016.

23. Walker B, Lunder S. "Pesticides + poison gases = cheap, year-round strawberries." Environmental Working Group. https://www.ewg.org/foodnews/strawberries.php.

24. Gilliam C. Alarming levels of glyphosate found in popular American foods. *EcoWatch.* November 14, 2016.

25. Bouzari A, Holstege D, Barrett DM. Vitamin retention in eight fruits and vegetables: a comparison of refrigerated and frozen storage. *J Agric Food Chem.* 2015 Jan 28;63(3):957–62.

26. Rodriguez-Mateos A, Cifuentes-Gomez T, George TW, et al.

Impact of cooking, proving, and baking on the (poly)phenol content of wild blueberry. *J Agric Food Chem*. 2014 May 7;62(18):3979–86.

27. Rodriguez-Mateos A, Rendeiro C, Bergillos-Meca T, et al. Intake and time dependence of blueberry flavonoid-induced improvements in vascular function: a randomized, controlled, double-blind, crossover intervention study with mechanistic insights into biological activity. *Am J Clin Nutr*. 2013 Nov;98(5): 1179–91.

28. de Graaf C. Why liquid energy results in overconsumption. *Proc Nutr Soc*. 2011 May;70(2):162–70.

29. US Department of Agriculture Economic Research Service. Agricultural trade. https://www.ers.usda.gov/data-products/ag-and-food-statistics-charting-the-essentials/agricultural-trade/. Retrieved February 6, 2017. Updated May 5, 2017.

30. Weber CL, Matthews HS. Food-miles and the relative climate impacts of food choices in the United States. *Environ Sci Technol*. 2008 May 15;42(10):3508–13.

31. Siddique, H. Rising avocado prices fueling illegal deforestation in Mexico. *Guardian*. August 10, 2016.

32. Guasch-Ferre M, Babio N, Martinez-Gonzalez MA, et al. Dietary fat intake and risk of cardiovascular disease and all-cause mortality in a population at high risk of cardiovascular disease. *Am J Clin Nutr*. 2015 Dec;102(6):1563–73.

33. Dulloo AG, Fathi M, Mensi N, et al. Twenty-four-hour energy expenditure and urinary catecholamines of humans consuming low-to-moderate amounts of medium-chain triglycerides: a dose-response study in a human respiratory chamber. *Eur J Clin Nutr*. 1996 Mar;50(3):152–58.

34. Guasch-Ferre M, Hu FB, Martinez-Gonzalez MA, et al. Olive oil intake and risk of cardiovascular disease and mortality in the PREDIMED Study. *BMC Med*. 2014;12:78.

Fats and Oils

1. Hyman M. *Eat Fat, Get Thin.* Chapter 6. Boston: Little, Brown; 2016.
2. Tobias, Deirdre K, et al. Effect of low-fat diet interventions versus other diet interventions on long term weight change in adults: a systematic review and meta-analysis, *Lancet Diabetes & Endocrinology,* 3(12):968–79.
3. Ebbeling CB, Swain JF, Feldman HA, et al. Effects of dietary composition on energy expenditure during weight-loss maintenance. *JAMA.* 2012 Jun 27;307(24):2627–34.
4. Mason M. A dangerous fat and its risky alternatives. *New York Times.* October 10, 2006.
5. Ebbeling CB, Swain JF, Feldman HA, et al. Effects of dietary composition on energy expenditure during weight-loss maintenance. *JAMA.* 2012 Jun 27;307(24):2627–34.
6. Bazzano LA, Hu T, Reynolds K, et al. Effects of low-carbohydrate and low-fat diets: a randomized trial. *Ann Intern Med.* 2014 Sep 2;161(5):309–18.
7. Thomas DE, Elliot EJ, Baur L. Low glycemic index or low glycemic load diets for overweight and obesity. *Cochrane Database Syst Rev.* 2007 Jul 18;3.
8. Tobias DK, Chen M, Manson JE, et al. Effect of low-fat diet interventions versus other diet interventions on long-term weight change in adults: a systematic review and meta-analysis. *Lancet Diabetes Endocrinol.* 2015 Dec;3(12):968–79.
9. Ludwig DS. The forty-year low-fat folly. *Medium.* December 3, 2015.
10. Flegal KM, Carroll MD, Kit BK, et al. Prevalence of obesity and trends in the distribution of body mass index among US adults, 1999–2010. *JAMA.* 2012 Feb 1;307(5):491–97.
11. Fryar CD, Carroll MD, Ogden CL. Prevalence of overweight and obesity among children and adolescents: United States,

1963–1965 through 2011–2012. Atlanta, GA: National Center for Health Statistics; 2014.

12. Mozaffarian D, Ludwig DS. Lifting the ban on total dietary fat. *JAMA*. 2015;313(24):2421–22.

13. Gillingham LG, Harris-Janz S, Jones PJ. Dietary monounsaturated fatty acids are protective against metabolic syndrome and cardiovascular disease risk factors. *Lipids*. 2011 Mar;46(3):209–28. Appel LJ, Sacks FM, Carey VJ, et al. Effects of protein, monounsaturated fat, and carbohydrate intake on blood pressure and serum lipids: results of the OmniHeart randomized trial. *JAMA*. 2005 Nov 16;294(19):2455–64.

14. Parlesak A, Eckoldt J, Winkler K, et al. Intercorrelations of lipoprotein subfractions and their covariation with lifestyle factors in healthy men. *J Clin Biochem Nutr*. 2014 May;54(3): 174–80.

15. Sanchez-Muniz FJ. Oils and fats: changes due to culinary and industrial processes. *Int J Vitam Nutr Res*. 2006 Jul;76(4): 230–37.

16. Lorente-Cebrian S, Costa AG, Navas-Carretero S, et al. Role of omega-3 fatty acids in obesity, metabolic syndrome, and cardiovascular diseases: a review of the evidence. *J Physiol Biochem*. 2013 Sep;69(3):633–51. Carrie L, Abellan Van Kan G, Rolland Y, et al. PUFA for prevention and treatment of dementia? *Curr Pharm Des*. 2009;15(36):4173–85.

17. Loef M, Walach H. The omega-6/omega-3 ratio and dementia or cognitive decline: a systematic review on human studies and biological evidence. *J Nutr Gerontol Geriatr*. 2013;32(1):1–23. Hibbeln JR. Depression, suicide and deficiencies of omega-3 essential fatty acids in modern diets. *World Rev Nutr Diet*. 2009;99:17–30.

18. Simopoulos AP. The importance of the ratio of omega-6/

omega-3 essential fatty acids. *Biomed Pharmacother.* 2002 Oct;56(8):365–79.

19. De Lorgeril M, Salen P, Martin JL, et al. Mediterranean dietary pattern in a randomized trial: prolonged survival and possible reduced cancer rate. *Arch Intern Med.* 1998 Jun;158 (11):1181–87.

20. Hiza HAB, Bente L. *Nutrient Content of the U.S. Food Supply, 1909–2004: A Summary Report.* USDA Center for Nutrition Policy and Promotion. February 2007.

21. Kris-Etherton PM, Taylor DS, Yu-Poth S, et al. Polyunsaturated fatty acids in the food chain in the United States. *Am J Clin Nutr.* 2000 Jan;71(1 Suppl):179S–188S. Review.

22. Ramsden CE, Zamora D, Leelarthaepin B, et al. Use of dietary linoleic acid for secondary prevention of coronary heart disease and death: evaluation of recovered data from the Sydney Diet Heart Study and updated meta-analysis. *BMJ.* 2013 Feb 4;346:e8707.

23. A full list of dietary saturated fats can be found at https://en.wikipedia.org/wiki/List_of_saturated_fatty_acids.

24. Siri-Tarino PW, Sun Q, Hu FB, et al. Saturated fat, carbohydrate, and cardiovascular disease. *Am J Clin Nutr.* 2010;91(3): 502–9.

25. Volk BM, Kunces LJ, Freidenreich DJ, et al. Effects of stepwise increases in dietary carbohydrate on circulating saturated fatty acids and palmitoleic acid in adults with metabolic syndrome. *PLoS One.* 2014 Nov 21;9(11):e113605.

26. Chowdhury R, Warnakula S, Kunutsor S, et al. Association of dietary, circulating, and supplement fatty acids with coronary risk: a systematic review and meta-analysis. *Ann Intern Med.* 2014 Mar 18;160(6):398–406.

27. Aarsland A, Wolfe RR. Hepatic secretion of VLDL fatty acids

during stimulated lipogenesis in men. *J Lipid Res.* 1998;39(6): 1280–86.

28. Sacks FM, et al.; American Heart Association. Dietary Fats and Cardiovascular Disease: A Presidential Advisory from the American Heart Association. Circulation. 2017 Jul 18;136(3): e1-e23.

29. Ramsden CE, et al. Re-evaluation of the traditional diet-heart hypothesis: analysis of recovered data from Minnesota Coronary Experiment (1968–73). *BMJ.* 2016 Apr 12;353:i1246.

30. Dehghan M, Mente A, Zhang X, et al. Associations of fats and carbohydrate intake with cardiovascular disease and mortality in 18 countries from five continents (PURE): a prospective cohort study. *Lancet.* 2017 Aug 29.

31. Masterjohn C. Saturated fat does a body good. Weston A. Price Foundation. May 6, 2016.

32. National Institutes of Health. Cooking with healthier fats and oils. https://www.nhlbi.nih.gov/health/educational/wecan/down loads/tip-fats-and-oils.pdf. Retrieved March 9, 2017.

33. Ramsden CE, Zamora D, Leelarthaepin B, et al. Use of dietary linoleic acid for secondary prevention of coronary heart disease and death: evaluation of recovered data from the Sydney Diet Heart Study and updated meta-analysis. *BMJ.* 2013 Feb 4;346:e8707.

34. Good J. Smoke point of oils for healthy cooking. Baseline of Health Foundation. https://jonbarron.org/diet-and-nutrition/ healthiest-cooking-oil-chart-smoke-points. April 17, 2012.

35. De Souza RJ, Mente A, Maroleanu A, et al. Intake of saturated and trans unsaturated fatty acids and risk of all cause mortality, cardiovascular disease, and type 2 diabetes: systematic review and meta-analysis of observational studies. *BMJ.* 2015 Aug 11;351:h3978.

36. Potera C. Food companies have three years to eliminate trans fats. *Am J Nurs.* 2015;115(9):14.

37. Vallverdú-Queralt A, Regueiro J, Rinaldi de Alvarenga JF, et al. Home cooking and phenolics: effect of thermal treatment and addition of extra virgin olive oil on the phenolic profile of tomato sauces. *J Agric Food Chem.* 2014 Mar 27.

38. Perez-Jimenez F, Ruano J, Perez-Martinez P, et al. The influence of olive oil on human health: not a question of fat alone. *Mol Nutr Food Res.* 2007 Oct;51(10):1199–1208.

39. Achitoff-Gray N. Cooking fats 101: what's a smoke point and why does it matter? *Serious Eats.* May 16, 2014.

40. Mueller T. Slippery business: the trade in adulterated olive oil. *The New Yorker.* August 13, 2007.

41. Smith M. Italy arrests 33 accused of olive oil fraud. *Olive Oil Times.* February 16, 2017.

42. Frankel EN, Mailer RJ, Shoemaker CF, et al. *Tests Indicate that Imported "Extra Virgin" Olive Oil Often Fails International and USDA Standards.* UC Davis Olive Center. July 2010.

43. Prior IA, Davidson F, Salmond CE, Czochanska Z. Cholesterol, coconuts, and diet on Polynesian atolls: a natural experiment: the Pukapuka and Tokelau island studies. *Am J Clin Nutr.* 1981 Aug;34(8):1552–61.

44. St-Onge MP, Jones PJ. Greater rise in fat oxidation with medium-chain triglyceride consumption relative to long-chain triglyceride is associated with lower initial body weight and greater loss of subcutaneous adipose tissue. *Int J Obes Relat Metab Disord.* 2003 Dec;27(12):1565–71. Assunção ML, Ferreira HS, dos Santos AF, et al. Effects of dietary coconut oil on the biochemical and anthropometric profiles of women presenting abdominal obesity. *Lipids.* 2009 Jul;44(7):593–601.

45. Brandhorst S, Choi IY, Wei M, et al. A periodic diet that mimics fasting promotes multi-system regeneration, enhanced cognitive performance, and healthspan. *Cell Metab*. 2015 Jul 7;22(1):86–99.

46. Roberts MN, et al. A ketogenic diet extends longevity and healthspan in adult mice. *Cell Metab*. 2017 Sep5;26(3):539–546:e5.

47. Liu YM, Wang HS. Medium-chain triglyceride ketogenic diet, an effective treatment for drug-resistant epilepsy and a comparison with other ketogenic diets. *Biomed J*. 2013 Jan–Feb; 36(1):9–15.

48. Sevier L. Drizzle with care. *The Ecologist*. August 7, 2008.

Beans

1. Miller V, Mente A, Dehghan M, et al. Fruit, vegetable, and legume intake, and cardiovascular disease and deaths in 18 countries (PURE): a prospective cohort study. *Lancet*. 2017 Aug 29.

2. Frauenknecht V, Thiel S, Storm L, et al. Plasma levels of manna-binding lectin (MBL)-associated serine proteases (MASPs) and MBL-associated protein in cardio- and cerebrovascular diseases. *Clin Exp Immunolo*. 2013 Jul;173(1):112–20.

3. Greer F, Pusztai A. Toxicity of kidney bean (Phaseolus vulgaris) in rats: changes in intestinal permeability. *Digestion*. 1985;32(1):42–46.

4. Freed DLJ. Do dietary lectins cause disease? *BMJ*. 1999 Apr 17;318(7190):1023–24.

5. Fujita S, Volpi E. Amino acids and muscle loss with aging. *J Nutr*. 2006 Jan;136(1 Suppl):277S–80S.

6. Krebs JD, Parry Strong A, Cresswell P, et al. A randomized trial of the feasibility of a low carbohydrate diet vs standard

carbohydrate counting in adults with type 1 diabetes taking body weight into account. *Asia Pac J Clin Nutr.* 2016;25(1): 78–84.

7. Rodriguez NR. Introduction to Protein Summit 2.0: continued exploration of the impact of high-quality protein on optimal health. *Am J Clin Nutr.* 2015 Apr 29.

8. Gebhardt SE, Thomas RG. *Nutritive Values of Foods.* Beltsville, MD: US Department of Agriculture, Agricultural Research Service, Nutrient Data Laboratory; 2002. https://www.ars.usda .gov/is/np/NutritiveValueofFoods/NutritiveValueofFoods.pdf.

9. Birt DF, Boylston T, Hendrich S, et al. Resistant starch: promise for improving human health. *Adv Nutr.* 2013 Nov 6;4(6):587–601.

10. Cummings JH, Macfarlane GT, Englyst HN. Prebiotic digestion and fermentation. *Am J Clin Nutr.* 2001 Feb;73(2 Suppl):415S–420S.

11. Jenkins DJ, Kendall CW, Augustin LS, et al. Effect of legumes as part of a low glycemic index diet on glycemic control and cardiovascular risk factors in type 2 diabetes mellitus: a randomized controlled trial. *Arch Intern Med.* 2012:1–8.

12. Yadav BS, Sharma A, Yadav RB. Studies on effect of multiple heating/cooling cycles on the resistant starch formation in cereals, legumes and tubers. *Int J Food Sci Nutr.* 2009;60 Suppl 4:258–72.

13. Winham DM, Hutchins AM. Perceptions of flatulence from bean consumption among adults in 3 feeding studies. *Nutr J.* 2011;10:128.

14. Ford AC, Moayyedi P, Lacy BE, et al. American College of Gastroenterology monograph on the management of irritable bowel syndrome and chronic idiopathic constipation. *Am J Gastroenterol.* 2014 Aug;109 Suppl 1:S2–S26.

15. Dent J, El-Serag HB, Wallander M-A, et al. Epidemiology of

gastro-oesophageal reflux disease: a systematic review. *Gut.* 2005 May;54(5):710–17.

16. Elyassi AR, Rowshan HH. Perioperative management of the glucose-6-phosphate dehydrogenase deficient patient: a review of literature. *Anesth Prog.* 2009 Fall;56(3):86–91.

17. Provvisiero DP, Pivonello C, Muscogiuri G, et al. Influence of bisphenol A on type 2 diabetes mellitus. *Int J Environ Res Public Health.* 2016 Oct 6;13(10). pii:E989. Review.

18. Bae S, Hong YC. Exposure to bisphenol A from drinking canned beverages increases blood pressure: randomized crossover trial. *Hypertension.* 2015 Feb;65(2):313–19.

19. Yang CZ, Yaniger SI, Jordan VC, et al. Most plastic products release estrogenic chemicals: a potential health problem that can be solved. *Environ Health Perspect.* 2011 Jul;119(7):989–96. Liao C, Kannan K. Concentrations and profiles of bisphenol A and other bisphenol analogues in foodstuffs from the United States and their implications for human exposure. *J Agric Food Chem.* 2013 May 15;61(19):4655–62.

20. US Department of Agriculture. Adoption of genetically engineered crops in the U.S. https://www.ers.usda.gov/data-products/adoption-of-genetically-engineered-crops-in-the-us/. October 19, 2016.

21. Patterson E, Wall R, Fitzgerald GF, et al. Health implications of high dietary omega-6 polyunsaturated fatty acids. *J Nutr Metab.* 2012;2012:539426. Maingrette F, Renier G. Linoleic acid increases lectin-like oxidized LDL receptor-1 (LOX-1) expression in human aortic endothelial cells. *Diabetes.* 2005 May;54(5):1506–13. Barsch H, Nair J, Owen RW. Dietary polyunsaturated fatty acids and cancers of the breast and colorectum: emerging evidence for their role as risk modifiers. *Carcinogenesis.* 1999 Dec;20(12):2209–18. Hibbeln JR, Gow RV. The potential for military diets to reduce depression, suicide, and

impulsive aggression: a review of current evidence for omega-3 and omega-6 fatty acids. *Mil Med.* 2014 Nov;179(11 Suppl): 117–28.

22. Henrgy AG, Brooks AS, Piperno DR. Microfossils in calculus demonstrate consumption of plants and cooked foods in Neanderthal diets (Shanidar III, Iraq; Spy I and II, Belgium). *Proc Natl Acad Sci U S A.* 2011 Jan 11;108(2):486–91.

Grains

1. Fasano A, Sapone A, Zevallos V, Schuppan D. Nonceliac gluten sensitivity. *Gastroenterology.* 2015 May;148(6):1195–1204.

2. Dietary Guidelines Advisory Committee. *Report of the Dietary Guidelines Advisory Committee on the Dietary Guidelines for Americans, 2010.* Washington, DC: US Department of Agriculture Research Service; 2011.

3. Schwingshackl L, Hoffmann G. Long-term effects of low glycemic index/load vs. high glycemic index/load diets on parameters of obesity and obesity-associated risks: a systematic review and meta-analysis. *Nutr Metab Cardiovasc Dis.* 2013 Aug;23(8):699–706. doi: 10.1016/j.numecd.2013.04.008. Epub 2013 Jun 17. Review.

4. Mirrahimi A, de Souza RJ, Chiavaroli L, et al. Associations of glycemic index and load with coronary heart disease events: a systematic review and meta-analysis of prospective cohorts. *J Am Heart Assoc.* 2012 Oct;1(5).

5. Seetharaman S, Andel R, McEvoy C, Dahl Aslan AK, Finkel D, Pedersen NL. Blood glucose, diet-based glycemic load and cognitive aging among dementia-free older adults. *J Gerontol A Biol Sci Med Sci.* 2015 Apr;70(4):471–79.

6. Dong JY, Qin LQ. Dietary glycemic index, glycemic load, and risk of breast cancer: meta-analysis of prospective cohort

studies. *Breast Cancer Res Treat.* 2011 Apr;126(2):287–94. doi: 10.1007/s10549-011-1343-3. Epub 2011 Jan 11. Review.

7. Braconnier, D. Farming to blame for our shrinking size and brains. Phys.org. https://phys.org/news/2011-06-farming-blame -size-brains.html. June 15, 2011.

8. Ripsin CM, Keenan JM, Jacobs DR Jr, et al. Oat products and lipid lowering. A meta-analysis. *JAMA.* 1992 Jun 24;267(24): 3317–25.

9. Keenan JM, Pins JJ, Frazel C, et al. Oat ingestion reduces systolic and diastolic blood pressure in patients with mild or borderline hypertension: a pilot trial. *J Fam Pract.* 2002 Apr;51(4):369.

10. Pereira MA, O'Reilly E, Augustsson K, et al. Dietary fiber and risk of coronary heart disease: a pooled analysis of cohort studies. *Arch Intern Med.* 2004 Feb 23;164(4):370–76.

11. Klement RJ, Kammerer U. Is there a role for carbohydrate restriction in the treatment and prevention of cancer? *Nutr Metab (Lond).* 2011;8:75.

12. Peet M. International variations in the outcome of schizo-phrenia and the prevalence of depression in relation to national dietary practices: an ecological analysis. *Br J Psychia-try.* 2004 May;184:404–8.

13. de Munter JS, Hu FB, Spiegelman D, et al. Whole grain, bran, and germ intake and risk of type 2 diabetes: a prospec-tive cohort study and systematic review. *PLoS Med.* 2007 Aug;4(8):e261.

14. Quealy K, Sanger-Katz M. Is sushi "healthy"? What about granola? Where Americans and nutritionists disagree. *New York Times.* July 5, 2016.

15. Atkinson FS, Foster-Powell K, Brand-Miller JC. International tables of glycemic index and glycemic load values: 2008. *Dia-betes Care.* 31:2281–83.

16. Farrell RJ, Kelly CP. Celiac sprue. *N Engl J Med.* 2002 Jan 17;346(3):180–88. Review.

17. Uhde M, Ajamian M, Caio G, et al. Intestinal cell damage and systemic immune activation in individuals reporting sensitivity to wheat in the absence of coeliac disease. *Gut.* 2016;65:1930–37.

18. Sturgeon C, Fasano A. Zonulin, a regulator of epithelial and endothelial barrier functions, and its involvement in chronic inflammatory diseases. *Tissue Barriers.* 2016 Oct 21;4(4): e1251384.

19. Rubio-Tapia A, Kyle RA, Kaplan EL, et al. Increased prevalence and mortality in undiagnosed celiac disease. *Gastroenterology.* 2009 Jul;137(1):88–93.

20. Byrnes SE, Miller JC, Denyer GS. Amylopectin starch promotes the development of insulin resistance in rats. *J Nutr.* 1995 Jun;125(6):1430–37.

21. Samsel A, Seneff S. Glyphosate, pathways to modern diseases II: celiac sprue and gluten intolerance. *Interdisciplinary Toxicology.* 2013;6(4):159–84. Samsel A, Seneff S. Glyphosate's suppression of cytochrome P450 enzymes and amino acid biosynthesis by the gut microbiome: pathways to modern diseases. *Entropy.* 2013;15:1416–63.

22. Environmental Working Group. Sugar in children's cereals: healthy breakfast tips. December 12, 2011.

23. Thies F, Masson LF, Boffetta P, et al. Oats and CVD risk markers: a systematic literature review. *Br J Nutr.* 2014 Oct;112 Suppl 2:S19–S30.

24. Ravnskov U, Diamond DM, Hama R, et al. Lack of an association or an inverse association between low-density-lipoprotein cholesterol and mortality in the elderly: a systematic review. *BMJ Open.* 2016 Jun 12;6(6):e010401.

25. Ebbeling CB, Swain JF, Feldman HA, et al. Effects of dietary composition on energy expenditure during weight-loss maintenance. *JAMA*. 2012 Jun 27;307(24):2627–34.

26. Abdel-Aal el-SM, Akhtar H, Zaheer K, et al. Dietary sources of lutein and zeaxanthin carotenoids and their role in eye health. *Nutrients*. 2013 Apr 9;5(4):1169–85.

27. US Department of Agriculture. Adoption of genetically engineered crops in the U.S.: recent trends in GE adoption. November 3, 2016.

28. Hayes TB, Khoury V, Narayan A, et al. Atrazine induces complete feminization and chemical castration in male African clawed frogs (Xenopus laevis). *Proc Natl Acad Sci U S A*. 2010 Mar 9;107(10):4612–17. Sass JB, Colangelo A. European Union bans atrazine, while the United States negotiates continued use. *Int J Occup Environ Health*. 2006 Jul–Sep; 12(3):260–67.

29. Agopian AJ, Lupo PJ, Canfield MA, et al. Case-control study of maternal residential atrazine exposure and male genital malformations. *Am J Med Genet A*. 2013 May;161A(5):977–82.

30. Sun Q, Spiegelman D, van Dam RM, et al. White rice, brown rice, and risk of type 2 diabetes in US men and women. *Arch Intern Med*. 2010 June 14;170(11):961–69.

31. Deng GF, Xu XR, Zhang Y, et al. Phenolic compounds and bioactivities of pigmented rice. *Crit Rev Food Sci Nutr*. 2013;53(3):296–306.

32. Consumer Reports. Arsenic in your food. http://www.consumerreports.org/cro/magazine/2012/11/arsenic-in-your-food/index.htm. November 2012. Consumer Reports. How much arsenic is in your rice? http://www.consumerreports.org/cro/magazine/2015/01/how-much-arsenic-is-in-your-rice/index.htm. January 2015.

33. US Food and Drug Administration. US Department of

Health and Human Services. Guidance for industry and FDA staff. Whole grain label statements. February 2006.

34. US Department of Agriculture. Pesticide data program. https:// www.ams.usda.gov/datasets/pdp. Retrieved March 8, 2017.

35. Woodcock BA, Isaac NJ, Bullock JM, et al. Impacts of neonicotinoid use on long-term population changes in wild bees in England. *Nat Commun.* 2016 Aug 16;7:12459.

Nuts and Seeds

1. Su X, Tamimi RM, Collins LC, et al. Intake of fiber and nuts during adolescence and incidence of proliferative benign breast disease. *Cancer Causes Control.* 2010 Jul;21(7):1033–46.

2. Savoie K. Food pyramid perils. *Health Perspectives.* February 2003.

3. Sabate J. Nut consumption and body weight. *Am J Clin Nutr.* 2003 Sep;78(3 Suppl):647S–650S.

4. Babio N, Toledo E, Estruch R, et al., PREDIMED Study Investigators. Mediterranean diets and metabolic syndrome status in the PREDIMED randomized trial. *CMAJ.* 2014 Nov 18;186(17):E649–E657.

5. Storniolo CE, Casillas R, Bullo M, et al. A Mediterranean diet supplemented with extra virgin olive oil or nuts improves endothelial markers involved in blood pressure control in hypertensive women. *Eur J Nutr.* 2017 Feb;56(1):89–97.

6. Estruch R, Sierra C. Commentary: frequent nut consumption protects against cardiovascular and cancer mortality, but the effects may be even greater if nuts are included in a healthy diet. *Int J Epidemiol.* 2015 Jun;44(3):1049–50.

7. Asghari G, Ghorbani Z, Mirmiran P, Azizi F. Nut consumption is associated with lower incidence of type 2 diabetes: the Tehran Lipid and Glucose Study. *Diabetes Metab.* 2017 Feb;43(1):18–24.

8. Gopinath B, Flood VM, Burlutsky G, et al. Consumption of nuts and risk of total and cause-specific mortality over 15 years. *Nutr Metab Cardiovasc Dis.* 2015 Dec;25(12):1125–31.

9. Estruch R, Ros E, Salas-Salvadó J, et al. Primary prevention of cardiovascular disease with a Mediterranean diet. *NEJM.* 2013 Apr 4;368(14):1279–90.

10. Ibarrola-Jurado N, Bullo M, Guasch-Ferre M, et al. Cross-sectional assessment of nut consumption and obesity, metabolic syndrome and cardiometabolic risk factors: the PREDIMED study. *PLoS One.* 2013;8(2):e57367.

11. Storniolo CE, Casillas R, Bullo M, et al. A Mediterranean diet supplemented with extra virgin olive oil or nuts improves endothelial markers involved in blood pressure control in hypertensive women. *Eur J Nutr.* 2017 Feb;56(1):89–97.

12. Casas R, Sacanella E, Urpi-Sarda M, et al. The effects of the Mediterranean diet on biomarkers of vascular wall inflammation and plaque vulnerability in subjects with high risk for cardiovascular disease. A randomized trial. *PLoS One.* 2014 Jun 12;9(6):2100084.

13. Jenkins DJ, Wong JM, Kendall CW, et al. Effect of a 6-month vegan low-carbohydrate ("Eco-Atkins") diet on cardiovascular risk factors and body weight in hyperlipidaemic adults: a randomized controlled trial. *BMJ Open.* 2014 Feb 5;4(2):e003505.

14. Aune D, Keum N, Giovannucci E, et al. Nut consumption and risk of cardiovascular disease, total cancer, all-cause and cause-specific mortality: a systematic review and dose-response meta-analysis of prospective studies. *BMC Medicine.* 2016 December;14:207.

15. Ros E. Health benefits of nut consumption. *Nutrients.* 2010 Jul;2(7):652–82.

16. Bes-Rastrollo M, Sabaté J, Gómez-Gracia E, et al. Nut

consumption and weight gain in a Mediterranean cohort: the SUN study. *Obesity (Silver Spring)*. 2007 Jan;15(1):107–16.

17. Smith JD, Hou T, Ludwig DS, et al. Changes in intake of protein foods, carbohydrate amount and quality, and long-term weight change: results from 3 prospective cohorts. *Am J Clin Nutr*. 2015 Jun;101(6):1216–24.

18. US Department of Agriculture, Agricultural Research Service. 2010. Oxygen radical absorbance capacity (ORAC) of selected foods, release 2. Nutrient Data Laboratory Home Page: https://www.ars.usda.gov/northeast-area/beltsville-md/beltsville -human-nutrition-research-center/nutrient-data-laboratory/docs/ oxygen-radical-absorbance-capacity-orac-of-selected-foods -release-2-2010/. Updated August 13, 2016.

19. Cortés B, Núñez I, Cofán M, et al. Acute effects of high-fat meals enriched with walnuts or olive oil on postprandial endo-thelial function. *J Am Coll Cardiol*. 2006 Oct 17;48(8): 1666–71.

20. Yang J, Liu RH, Halim L. Antioxidant and antiproliferative activities of common edible nut seeds. *LWT-Food Science and Technology*. 2009;42(1):1–8.

21. Rajaram S, Burke K, Connell B, Myint T, Sabaté J. A mono-unsaturated fatty acid–rich pecan-enriched diet favorably alters the serum lipid profile of healthy men and women. *J Nutr*. 2001 Sep;131(9):2275–79.

22. Knekt P, Heliovaara M, Aho K, et al. Serum selenium, serum alpha-tocopherol, and the risk of rheumatoid arthritis. *Epide-miology*. 2000 Jul;11(4):402–5.

23. Cominetti C, de Bortoli MC, Garrido AB Jr, et al. Brazilian nut consumption improves selenium status and glutathione peroxidase activity and reduces atherogenic risk in obese women. *Nutr Res*. 2012 Jun;32(6):403–7.

24. Orem A, Yucesan FB, Orem C, et al. Hazelnut-enriched diet improves cardiovascular risk biomarkers beyond a lipid-lowering effect in hypercholesterolemic subjects. *J Clin Lipidol.* 2013 Mar–Apr;7(2):123–31.

25. Aldemir M, Okulu E, Neşelioğlu S, Erel O, Kayıgil O. Pistachio diet improves erectile function parameters and serum lipid profiles in patients with erectile dysfunction. *Int J Impot Res.* 2011 Jan–Feb;23(1):32–38.

26. Griel AE, Cao Y, Bagshaw DD, et al. A macadamia nut–rich diet reduces total and LDL-cholesterol in mildly hypercholesterolemic men and women. *J Nutr.* 2008 Apr;138(4):761–67.

27. Calani L, Dall'Asta M, Derlindati E, et al. Colonic metabolism of polyphenols from coffee, green tea, and hazelnut skins. *J Clin Gastroenterol.* 2012 Oct;46 Suppl:S95–S99.

28. Demark-Wahnefried W, Polascik TJ, George SL, et al. Flaxseed supplementation (not dietary fat restriction) reduces prostate cancer proliferation rates in men pre-surgery. *Cancer Epidemiol Biomarkers Prev.* 2008 Dec;17(12):3577–87. Flower G, Fritz H, Balneaves LG, et al. Flax and breast cancer: a systematic review. *Integr Cancer Ther.* 2014 May;13(3):181–92.

29. Singh KK, Mridula D, Rehal J, et al. Flaxseed: a potential source of food, feed and fiber. *Crit Rev Food Sci Nutr.* 2011 Mar;51(3):210–22. Kajla P, Sharma A, Sood DR. Flaxseed-a potential functional food source. *J Food Sci Technol.* 2015.

30. Nachbar MS, Oppenheim JD. Lectins in the United States diet: a survey of lectins in commonly consumed foods and a review of the literature. *Am J Clin Nutr.* 1980 Nov;33(11):2338–45.

31. Sisson M. The lowdown on lectins. Mark's Daily Apple. June 4, 2010.

32. Macfarlane BJ, Bezwoda WR, Bothwell TH, et al. Inhibitory effect of nuts on iron absorption. *Am J Clin Nutr.* 1988 Feb;47(2):270–74.

33. Pierson D. California farms lead the way in almond production. *Los Angeles Times.* January 12, 2014.
34. Bland A. California drought has wild salmon competing with almonds for water. NPR. August 21, 2014.

Sugar and Sweeteners

1. Softic S, Cohen DE, Kahn CR. Role of dietary fructose and hepatic de novo lipogenesis in fatty liver disease. *Dig Dis Sci.* 2016 May;61(5):1282–93. doi: 10.1007/s10620-016-4054-0. Epub 2016 Feb 8. Review.
2. Yang Q, Zhang Z, Gregg EW, Flanders WD, Merritt R, Hu FB. Added sugar intake and cardiovascular diseases mortality among US adults. *JAMA Intern Med.* 2014;174(4):516–24.
3. Chowdhury R, Warnakula S, Kunutsor S, et al. Association of dietary, circulating, and supplement fatty acids with coronary risk: a systematic review and meta-analysis. *Ann Intern Med.* 2014;160:398–406.
4. Lenoir M, Serre F, Cantin L, Ahmed SH. Intense sweetness surpasses cocaine reward. *PLoS One* 2007 Aug 1;2(8):e698.
5. Lenoir M, Serre F, Cantin L, Ahmed SH. Intense sweetness surpasses cocaine reward. *PLoS One.* 2007 Aug 1;2(8):e698.
6. Suez J, Korem T, Zeevi D, et al. Artificial sweeteners induce glucose intolerance by altering the gut microbiota. *Nature.* 2014 Oct 9;514(7521):181–86.
7. Ruanpeng D, Thongprayoon C, Cheungpasitporn W, Harindhanavudhi T. Sugar and artificially-sweetened beverages linked to obesity: a systematic review and meta-analysis. *QJM.* 2017 Apr 11.
8. Popkin BM, Hawkes C. Sweetening of the global diet, particularly beverages: patterns, trends and policy responses. *Lancet Diabetes Endocrinol.* 2016 Feb;4(2):174–86.

9. Yang Q, Zhang Z, Gregg EW, et al. Added sugar intake and cardiovascular diseases mortality among US adults. *JAMA Intern Med.* 2014 Apr;174(4):516–24.

10. Westover AN, Marangell LB. A cross-national relationship between sugar consumption and major depression? *Depress Anxiety.* 2002;16(3):118–20.

11. 2015 Dietary Guidelines Advisory Committee. *Scientific Report of the 2015 Dietary Guidelines Advisory Committee.* Office of Disease Prevention and Health Promotion. http:// www.health.gov/dietaryguidelines/2015-scientific-report/. December 2016.

12. US Department of Agriculture, Economic Research Service. Per capita wheat flour consumption declines along with other starches. https://www.ers.usda.gov/data-products/chart-gallery/ gallery/chart-detail/?chartId=81227. Updated November 28, 2016.

13. Ferdman RA. Where people around the world eat the most sugar and fat. *Washington Post.* https://www.washingtonpost .com/news/wonk/wp/2015/02/05/where-people-around-the -world-eat-the-most-sugar-and-fat/. February 5, 2015.

14. Te Morenga L, Mallard S, Mann J. Dietary sugars and body weight: systematic review and meta-analyses of randomized controlled trials and cohort studies. *BMJ.* 2013;346:e7492.

15. Singh GM, Micha R, Khatibzadeh S, et al. Estimated global, regional, and national disease burdens related to sugar-sweetened beverage consumption in 2010. *Circulation.* 2015 Aug 25;132 (8):639–66.

16. World Health Organization. Sugars intake for adults and children. http://www.who.int/nutrition/publications/guidelines/ sugars_intake/en/. March 2015.

17. American Heart Association. Kids and added sugars: how

much is too much? http://news.heart.org/kids-and-added-sugars -how-much-is-too-much/. August 2016.

18. Kuhnle GG, Tasevska N, Lenties MA, et al. Association between sucrose intake and risk of overweight and obesity in a prospective sub-cohort of the European prospective investigation into cancer in Norfolk (EPIC-Norfolk). *Public Health Nutr.* 2015 Oct;18(15):2815–24.

19. Drewnowski A, Rehm CD. Consumption of added sugars among US children and adults by food purchase location and food source. *Am J Clin Nutr.* 2014 Sep;100(3):901–7.

20. World Health Organization, *Global Report on Diabetes.* Geneva, Switzerland: WHO Press; 2016. http://apps.who.int/iris/bitstr eam/10665/204871/1/9789241565257_eng.pdf.

21. Te Morenga LA, Howatson AJ, Jones RM, et al. Dietary sugars and cardiometabolic risk: systematic review and meta-analyses of randomized controlled trials of the effects on blood pressure and lipids. *Am J Clin Nutr.* 2014 Jul;100(1):65–79. Ruff RR. Sugar-sweetened beverage consumption is linked to global adult morbidity and mortality through diabetes mellitus, cardiovascular disease and adiposity-related cancers. *Evid Based Med.* 2015 Dec;20(6):223–24.

22. Krone CA, Ely JT. Controlling hyperglycemia as an adjunct to cancer therapy. *Integr Cancer Ther.* 2005 Mar;4(1):25–31. Meyerhardt JA, Sato K, Niedzwiecki D, et al. Dietary glycemic load and cancer recurrence and survival in patients with stage III colon cancer: findings from CALGB 89803. *J Natl Cancer Inst.* 2012 Nov 21;104(22):1702–11.

23. Mastrocola R, Nigro D, Cento AS, et al. High-fructose intake as risk factor for neurodegeneration: key role for carboxy methyllysine accumulation in mice hippocampal neurons. *Neurobiol Dis.* 2016 May;89:65–75.

24. Stephan BC, Wells JC, Brayne C, et al. Increased fructose intake as a risk factor for dementia. *J Gerontol A Biol Sci Med Sci.* 2010 Aug;65(8):809–14.

25. Felix DR, Costenaro F, Gottschall CB, et al. Non-alcoholic fatty liver disease (Nafld) in obese children—effect of refined carbohydrates in diet. *BMC Pediatr.* 2016 Nov 15;16(1):187. Kavanagh K, Wylie AT, Tucker KL, et al. Dietary fructose induces endotoxemia and hepatic injury in calorically controlled primates. *Am J Clin Nutr.* 2013 Aug;98(2):349–57.

26. Yang Q. Gain weight by "going diet"? Artificial sweeteners and the neurobiology of sugar cravings: Neuroscience 2010. *Yale Journal of Biology and Medicine.* 2010;83(2):101–8.

27. Banting W. Letter on corpulence, addressed to the public. *Obes Res.* 1993 Mar;1(2):153–63.

28. US Department of Agriculture; US Department of Health and Human Services. Nutrition and your health: dietary guidelines for Americans. *Home and Garden Bulletin.* 1980 Feb;232. https://health.gov/dietaryguidelines/1980thin.pdf?_ga=2.1803 72961.77605286.1503837658-755408361.1503663254.

29. Malik VS. Sugar sweetened beverages and cardiometabolic health. *Curr Opin Cardiol.* 2017 Sep;32(5):572–79.

30. Teicholz N. *The Big Fat Surprise.* New York: Scribner; 2014.

31. Yerushalmy J, Hilleboe HE. Fat in the diet and mortality from heart disease; a methodologic note. *NY State J Med.* 1957 Jul 15;57(14):2343–54.

32. Szanto S, Yudkin J. The effect of dietary sucrose on blood lipids, serum insulin, platelet adhesiveness and body weight in human volunteers. *Postgrad Med J.* 1969 Sep;45(527):602–7.

33. Yudkin J. Dietary factors in arteriosclerosis: sucrose. *Lipids.* 1978 May;13(5):370–72.

34. Yudkin J, Lustig RH. *Pure, White, and Deadly: How Sugar Is*

Killing Us and What We Can Do to Stop It. New York: Penguin Books; 2013.

35. Kearns CE, Schmidt LA, Glantz SA. Sugar industry and coronary heart disease research: a historical analysis of internal industry documents. *JAMA Intern Med.* 2016;176(11):1680–85.

36. O'Connor A. Coca-Cola funds scientists who shift blame for obesity away from bad diets. *New York Times.* August 9, 2015.

37. Choi C. How candy makers shape nutrition science. Associated Press. June 2, 2016.

38. Erickson J, Sadeghirad B, Lytvyn L, et al. The scientific basis of guideline recommendations on sugar intake: a systematic review. *Ann Intern Med.* 2016 Dec 20. [Epub ahead of print.]

39. Lennerz BS, Alsop DC, Holsen LM, et al. Effects of dietary glycemic index on brain regions related to reward and craving in men. *Am J Clin Nutr.* 2013 Sep;98(3):641–47.

40. Avena NM, Rada P, Hoebel BG. Evidence for sugar addiction: behavioral and neurochemical effects of intermittent, excessive sugar intake. *Neurosci Biobehav Rev.* 2008;32(1):20–39.

41. Lustig RH, Mulligan K, Noworolski SM, et al. Isocaloric fructose restriction and metabolic improvement in children with obesity and metabolic syndrome. *Obesity (Silver Spring).* 2016 Feb;24(2):453–60.

42. Gugliucci A, Lustig RH, Caccavello R, et al. Short-term isocaloric fructose restriction lowers apoC-III levels and yields less atherogenic lipoprotein profiles in children with obesity and metabolic syndrome. *Atherosclerosis.* 2016 Oct;253:171–77.

43. Vos MB, Lavine JE. Dietary fructose in nonalcoholic fatty liver disease. *Hepatology.* 2013 Jun;57(6):2525–31.

44. Rapin JR, Wiernsperger N. Possible links between intestinal permeability and food processing: a potential therapeutic niche for glutamine. *Clinics (Sao Paulo).* 2010 Jun;65(6):635–43.

45. Bray GA, Nielsen SJ, Popkin BM. Consumption of high-fructose corn syrup in beverages may play a role in the epidemic of obesity. *Am J Clin Nutr.* 2004 Apr;79(4):537–43.

46. Nettleton JA, Lutsey PL, Wang Y, et al. Diet soda intake and risk of incident metabolic syndrome and type 2 diabetes in the Multi-Ethnic Study of Atherosclerosis (MESA). *Diabetes Care.* 2009;32(4):688–94.

47. Soffritti M, Belpoggi F, Manservigi M, et al. Aspartame administered in feed, beginning prenatally through life span, induces cancers of the liver and lung in male Swiss mice. *Am J Ind Med.* 2010 Dec;53(12):1197–1206.

48. Suez J, Korem T, Zeevi D, et al. Artificial sweeteners induce glucose intolerance by altering the gut microbiota. *Nature.* 2014;514(7521):181–86.

49. Maher TJ, Wurtman RJ. Possible neurologic effects of aspartame, a widely used food additive. *Environ Health Perspect.* 1987 Nov;75:53–57.

50. Wang QP, Lin YQ, Zhang L, et al. Sucralose promotes food intake through NPY and a neuronal fasting response. *Cell Metab.* 2016 Jul 12;24(1):75–90. Swithers SE, Davidson TL. A role for sweet taste: calorie predictive relations in energy regulation by rats. *Behav Neurosci.* 2008 Feb;122(1):161–73.

51. Feijó Fde M, Ballard CR, Foletto KC, et al. Saccharin and aspartame, compared with sucrose, induce greater weight gain in adult Wistar rats, at similar total caloric intake levels. *Appetite.* 2013 Jan;60(1):203–7.

52. Borges MC, Louzada ML, de Sa TH, et al. Artificially sweetened beverages and the response to the global obesity crisis. *PLoS Med.* 2017 Jan 3;14(1):e1002195.

53. Hootman KC, Trezzi JP, Kraemer L, et al. Erythritol is a pentose-phosphate pathway metabolite and associated with adiposity gain in young adults. *Proc Natl Acad Sci U S A.*

2017 May 23;114(21):E4233–E4240. doi: 10.1073/pnas.16200 79114.

54. Phillips KM, Carlsen MH, Blomhoff R. Total antioxidant content of alternatives to refined sugar. *J Am Diet Assoc.* 2009 Jan;109(1):64–71.

55. Clay J. *World Agriculture and the Environment: A Commodity-By-Commodity Guide to Impacts and Practices.* Washington, DC: Island Press; March 1, 2004.

56. Elizabeth K. UNCW professors study Splenda in Cape Fear River. *Star News Online.* March 10, 2013.

57. Wu-Smart J, Spivak M. Sub-lethal effects of dietary neonicotinoid insecticide exposure on honey bee queen fecundity and colony development. *Sci Rep.* 2016 Aug 26;6:32108.

58. Tey SL, Salleh NB, Henry J, Forde CG. Effects of aspartame-, monk fruit-, stevia- and sucrose-sweetened beverages on postprandial glucose, insulin and energy intake. *Int J Obes (Lond).* 2017 Mar;41(3):450–57.

Beverages

1. Ibarra-Reynoso LDR, López-Lemus HL, Garay-Sevilla ME, Malacara JM. Effect of restriction of foods with high fructose corn syrup content on metabolic indices and fatty liver in obese children. *Obes Facts.* 2017 Aug 5;10(4):332–40.

2. Smith-Warner SA, Spiegelman D, Yaun SS, et al. Alcohol and breast cancer in women: a pooled analysis of cohort studies. *JAMA.* 1998 Feb 18;279(7):535–40.

3. Hyman M. *Eat Fat, Get Thin.* New York: Little, Brown; 2016.

4. Singh GM, Micha R, Khatibzadeh S, et al. Estimated global, regional and national disease burdens related to sugar-sweetened beverage consumption in 2010. *Circulation.* 2015 Aug 25;132 (8):639–66.

5. Ruanpeng D, Thongprayoon C, Cheungpasitporn W, Harind-hanavudhi T. Sugar and artificially-sweetened beverages linked to obesity: a systematic review and meta-analysis. *QJM*. 2017 Apr 11.

6. Greenwood DC, Threapleton DE, Evans CE, et al. Association between sugar-sweetened and artificially sweetened soft drinks and type 2 diabetes: systematic review and dose-response meta-analysis of prospective studies. *Br J Nutr*. 2014 Sep 14;112(5):725–34.

7. Wijarnpreecha K, Thongprayoon C, Edmonds PJ, Cheung-pasitporn W. Associations of sugar- and artificially sweetened soda with nonalcoholic fatty liver disease: a systematic review and meta-analysis. *QJM*. 2016 Jul;109(7):461–66.

8. Cheungpasitporn W, Thongprayoon C, O'Corragain OA, Edmonds PJ, Kittanamongkolchai W, Erickson SB. Associations of sugar-sweetened and artificially sweetened soda with chronic kidney disease: a systematic review and meta-analysis. *Nephrology (Carlton)*. 2014 Dec;19(12):791–97.

9. Cheungpasitporn W, Thongprayoon C, Edmonds PJ, et al. Sugar and artificially sweetened soda consumption linked to hypertension: a systematic review and meta-analysis. *Clin Exp Hypertens*. 2015;37(7):587–93.

10. Malik VS. Sugar sweetened beverages and cardiometabolic health. *Curr Opin Cardiol*. 2017 Sep;32(5):572–79.

11. Victor D. I don't drink coffee. Should I start? *New York Times*. http://well.blogs.nytimes.com/2016/02/24/i-dont-drink-coffee-should-i-start/. February 24, 2016.

12. Ding M, Satija A, Bhupathiraju SN, et al. Association of coffee consumption with total and cause-specific mortality in 3 large prospective cohorts. *Circulation*. 2015 November;132: 2305–15. Kennedy OJ, Roderick P, Buchanan R, Fallowfield JA, Hayes PC, Parkes J. Systematic review with meta-analysis:

coffee consumption and the risk of cirrhosis. *Aliment Pharmacol Ther.* 2016 Mar;43(5):562–74. O'Keefe JH, Bhatti SK, Patil HR, et al. Effects of habitual coffee consumption on cardiometabolic disease, cardiovascular health, and all-cause mortality. *J Am Coll Cardiol.* 2013 Sep 17;62(12):1043–51. Wu L, Sun D, He Y. Coffee intake and the incident risk of cognitive disorders: a dose-response meta-analysis of nine prospective cohort studies. *Clin Nutr.* 2016 May 30. S0261 — 5614(16)30111-X.

13. Yashin A, Yashin Y, Wang JY, et al. Antioxidant and antiradical activity of coffee. *Antioxidants.* 2013 Dec;2(4):230–45.

14. Bjarnadottir A. Science: coffee is the world's biggest source of antioxidants. https://authoritynutrition.com/coffee-worlds-biggest-source-of-antioxidants/. Retrieved December 27, 2016.

15. Svilaas A, Sakhi AK, Anderson LF, et al. Intakes of antioxidants in coffee, wine, and vegetables are correlated with plasma carotenoids in humans. *J Nutr.* 2004 Mar;134(3):562–67.

16. Van Dam RM, Pasman WJ, Verhoef P. Effects of coffee consumption on fasting blood glucose and insulin concentrations: randomized controlled trials in healthy volunteers. *Diabetes Care.* 2004 Dec;27(12):2990–92.

17. Lovallo WR, Al'Absi M, Blick K, et al. Stress-like adrenocorticotropin responses to caffeine in young healthy men. *Pharmacol Biochem Behav.* 1996 Nov;55(3):365–69.

18. Environmental Working Group. Erin Brockovich carcinogen in tap water of more than 200 million Americans. http://www.ewg.org/research/chromium-six-found-in-us-tap-water. September 20, 2016.

19. Natural Resources Defense Council. The truth about tap. https://www.nrdc.org/stories/truth-about-tap.

20. Tobacman JK. Review of harmful gastrointestinal effects of carrageenan in animal experiments. *Environ Health Perspect.* 2001 Oct;109(10):983–94.

21. Kresser C. Harmful or harmless: carrageenan. Chris Kresser. https://chriskresser.com/harmful-or-harmless-carrageenan/. November 15, 2013.

22. St-Onge MP, Jones PJ. Physiological effects of medium-chain triglycerides: potential agents in the prevention of obesity. *J Nutr.* 2002 Mar;132(3):329–32.

23. Kasai M, Nosaka N, Maki H, et al. Effect of dietary medium- and long-chain triacylglycerols (MLCT) on accumulation of body fat in healthy humans. *Asia Pac J Clin Nutr.* 2003; 12(2):151–60.

24. Di Castelnuovo A, Costanzo S, Bagnardi V, et al. Alcohol dosing and total mortality in men and women: an updated meta-analysis of 34 prospective studies. *Arch Intern Med.* 2006 Dec 11–25;166(22):2437–45.

25. Costanzo S, Di Castelnuovo A, Donati MB, et al. Alcohol consumption and mortality in patients with cardiovascular disease: a meta-analysis. *J Am Coll Cardiol.* 2010 Mar 30;55 (13):1339–47.

26. Jin M, Cai S, Guo J, et al. Alcohol drinking and all cancer mortality: a meta-analysis. *Ann Oncol.* 2013 Mar;24(3):807–16.

27. Gepner Y, Golan R, Harman-Boehm I, et al. Effects of initiating moderate alcohol intake on cardiometabolic risk in adults with type 2 diabetes: a 2-year randomized, controlled trial. *Ann Intern Med.* 2015 Oct 20;163(8):569–79.

28. Saleem TSM, Basha SD. Red wine: a drink to your heart. *J Cardiovasc Dis Res.* 2010 Oct–Dec;1(4):171–76.

29. Siler SQ, Neese RA, Hellerstein MK. De novo lipogenesis, lipid kinetics, and whole-body lipid balances in humans after acute alcohol consumption. *Am J Clin Nutr.* 1999 November;70(5):928–36.

30. Tanner GJ, Colgrave ML, Blundell MJ, et al. Measuring

hordein (gluten) in beer—a comparison of ELISA and mass spectrometry. *PLoS One.* 2013;8(2).

31. Wolk BJ, Ganetsky M, Babu KM. Toxicity of energy drinks. *Curr Opin Pediatr.* 2012 Apr;24(2):243–51.

32. Carlsen MH, Halvorsen BL, Holte K, et al. The total antioxidant content of more than 3100 foods, beverages, spices, herbs and supplements used worldwide. *Nutr J.* 2010 Jan 22;9:3.

33. Mukhtar H, Ahmad N. Tea polyphenols: prevention of cancer and optimizing health. *Am J Clin Nutr.* 2000 Jun;71(6 Suppl):1698S–1702S.

34. Nagao T, Komine Y, Soga S, et al. Ingestion of a tea rich in catechins leads to a reduction in body fat and malondialdehyde-modified LDL in men. *Am J Clin Nutr.* 2005 Jan;81(1): 122–29.

35. National Cancer Institute. Tea and cancer prevention. https://www.cancer.gov/about-cancer/causes-prevention/risk/diet/tea-fact-sheet. Retrieved December 29, 2016.

36. Nastu P. Carbon footprint of Tropicana orange juice: 1.7 kg. *Environmental Leader.* January 23, 2009.

37. Levitt T. Coca-Cola just part of India's "free-for-all." *Ecologist.* December 4, 2009.

Part III

1. American Nutrition Association. Review of: Excitotoxins: The taste that kills. *Nutrition Digest.* 38(2)1995. http://americannutritionassociation.org/newsletter/review-excitotoxins-taste-kills.

2. Roach J. Gulf of Mexico "dead zone" is size of New Jersey. National Geographic News. http://news.nationalgeographic.com/news/2005/05/0525_050525_deadzone.html. May 25, 2005.

3. Food and Drug Administration. Food additive status list. http://www.fda.gov/Food/IngredientsPackagingLabeling/ FoodAdditivesIngredients/ucm091048.htm.

4. Environmental Working Group. EWG's Dirty Dozen guide to food additives: generally recognized as safe—but is it? http:// www.ewg.org/research/ewg-s-dirty-dozen-guide-food-addi tives/generally-recognized-as-safe-but-is-it. November 12, 2014.

5. Center for Science in the Public Interest. Chemical cuisine. https://cspinet.org/eating-healthy/chemical-cuisine#myco protein.

6. Frye RE, Rose S, Chacko J, et al. Modulation of mitochondrial function by the microbiome metabolite propionic acid in autism and control cell lines. *Transl Psychiatry.* 2016 Oct 25;6(10):e927. Macfabe DF. Short-chain fatty acid fermentation products of the gut microbiome: implications in autism spectrum disorders. *Microb Ecol Health Dis.* 2012 Aug 24;23.

7. Hakim D. Doubts about the promised bounty of genetically modified crops. *New York Times.* October 29, 2016.

8. Chang Q, Wang W, Regev-Yochay G, et al. Antibiotics in agriculture and the risk to human health: how worried should we be? *Evolutionary Applications.* 2015;8(3):240–47.

9. Key TJ. Diet, insulin-like growth factor-1 and cancer risk. *Proc Nutr Soc.* 2011 May 3:1–4.

10. Reed CE, Fenton SE. Exposure to diethylstilbestrol during sensitive life stages: a legacy of heritable health effects. *Birth Defects Res C Embryo Today: Reviews.* 2013;99(2):10.

11. Jiang HY, Wang F, Chen HM, Yan XJ. κ-carrageenan induces the disruption of intestinal epithelial Caco-2 monolayers by promoting the interaction between intestinal epithelial cells and immune cells. *Mol Med Rep.* 2013 Dec;8(6):1635–42.

12. Lerner A, Matthias T. Changes in intestinal tight junction permeability associated with industrial food additives explain

the rising incidence of autoimmune disease. *Autoimmun Rev.* 2015 Jun;14(6):479–89.

13. Food and Drug Administration. Questions & answers on bisphenol A (BPA) use in food contact applications. http:// www.fda.gov/Food/IngredientsPackagingLabeling/FoodAddi tivesIngredients/ucm355155.htm.

14. Provvisiero DP, Pivonello C, Muscogiuri G, et al. Influence of bisphenol A on type 2 diabetes mellitus. *Int J Environ Res Public Health.* 2016 Oct 6;13(10). pii:E989. Review.

15. Kay VR, Chambers C, Foster WG. Reproductive and developmental effects of phthalate diesters in females. *Critical Reviews in Toxicology.* 2013;43(3):200–219. http://doi.org/10 .3109/10408444.2013.766149.

16. Kobrosly RW, Evans S, Miodovnik A, et al. Prenatal phthalate exposures and neurobehavioral development scores in boys and girls at 6–10 years of age. *Environ Health Perspect.* 2014;122(5):521–28. http://doi.org/10.1289/ehp.1307063.

17. Food and Drug Administration. The FDA takes step to remove artificial trans fats in processed foods. http://www .fda.gov/NewsEvents/Newsroom/PressAnnouncements/ ucm451237.htm. June 16, 2015.

18. Doukky R, Avery E, Mangla A, et al. Impact of dietary sodium restriction on heart failure outcomes. *JACC Heart Fail.* 2016 Jan;4(1):24–35.

19. Environmental Working Group. How much is too much? Appendix B: vitamin and mineral deficiencies in the U.S. http://www.ewg.org/research/how-much-is-too-much/appen dix-b-vitamin-and-mineral-deficiencies-us. June 19, 2014.

20. Heaney RP. Long-latency deficiency disease: insights from calcium and vitamin D. *Am J Clin Nutr.* 2003 Nov;78(5):912– 19. Review.

Part IV

1. Saslow LR, et al. An online intervention comparing a very low-carbohydrate ketogenic diet and lifestyle recommendations versus a plate method diet in overweight individuals with type 2 diabetes: a randomized controlled trial. *J Med Internet Res.* 2017 Feb 13;19(2):e36.

2. Fasano A, Sapone A, Zevallos V, Schuppan D. Nonceliac gluten sensitivity. *Gastroenterology.* 2015 May;148(6):1195–1204.

3. Freed DLJ. Do dietary lectins cause disease? The evidence is suggestive—and raises interesting possibilities for treatment. *BMJ: British Medical Journal.* 1999;318(7190):1023–24.

About the Author

Mark Hyman, MD, believes that we all deserve a life of vitality—and that we have the potential to create it for ourselves. That's why he is dedicated to tackling the root causes of chronic disease by harnessing the power of functional medicine to transform health care. Dr. Hyman and his team work every day to empower people, organizations, and communities to heal their bodies and minds and to improve our social and economic resilience.

Dr. Hyman is a practicing family physician, a ten-time #1 *New York Times* bestselling author, and an internationally recognized leader, speaker, educator, and advocate in his field. He is the director of the Cleveland Clinic Center for Functional Medicine. He is also the founder and medical director of The Ultra-Wellness Center, chairman of the board of the Institute for Functional Medicine, and a medical editor of *The Huffington Post* and was a regular medical contributor on many television shows and networks, including *CBS This Morning, Today, Good Morning America*, CNN, *The View, Katie,* and *The Dr. Oz Show.*

Dr. Hyman works with individuals and organizations, as well as policy makers and influencers. He has testified before both the White House Commission on Complementary and Alternative Medicine and the Senate Working Group on Health Care Reform on Functional Medicine. He has consulted with the surgeon general on diabetes prevention and participated in the 2009 White House Forum on Prevention and Wellness. Senator Tom Harkin of Iowa nominated Dr. Hyman for the President's Advisory Group on Prevention, Health Promotion, and Integrative and Public Health. In addition, Dr. Hyman has worked with President Bill Clinton, presenting at the Clinton Foundation's Health Matters, Achieving Wellness in Every Generation conference, and the Clinton Global Initiative, as well as with the World Economic Forum on global health issues. He is the winner of the Linus Pauling Award, the Nantucket Project Award, and the Christian Book of the Year Award for *The Daniel Plan* and was inducted in the Books for Better Life Hall of Fame.

Dr. Hyman also works with fellow leaders in his field to help people and communities thrive—with Rick Warren, Dr. Mehmet Oz, and Dr. Daniel Amen, he created the Daniel Plan, a faith-based initiative that helped the Saddleback Church collectively lose 250,000 pounds. He is an adviser and guest co-host on *The Dr. Oz Show* and is on the board of Dr. Oz's HealthCorps, which tackles the obesity epidemic by educating

American students about nutrition. With Dr. Dean Ornish and Dr. Michael Roizen, Dr. Hyman crafted and helped introduce the Take Back Your Health Act of 2009 to the United States Senate to provide for reimbursement of lifestyle treatment of chronic disease. And with Tim Ryan in 2015, he helped introduce the ENRICH Act into Congress to fund nutrition in medical education. Dr. Hyman plays a substantial role in a major film produced by Laurie David and Katie Couric, released in 2014, called *Fed Up*, which addresses childhood obesity. Please join him in helping us all take back our health at www.drhyman.com, or follow him on Twitter, Facebook, and Instagram.